The Essential Guide to Practice Success for Acupuncturists

POINTS for PROFIT

Honora Wolfe

with

Marilyn Allen

Fifth, Fully-Revised Edition!

Published by:
BLUE POPPY PRESS
A Division of Blue Poppy Enterprises, Inc.
1990 N. 57th Ct. Unit A
BOULDER, CO 80301

First Edition, February 2004
Second Edition, August 2005
Third Edition, June 2007
Fourth Edition, July 2009
Fifth, fully-revised New Edition, September 2013

Original ISBN 978-1-891845-25-X
New Edition ISBN 1-891845-64-0
(13 Digit)1-978-891845-64-2

LCCN #2013946988

**COPYRIGHT © BLUE POPPY PRESS, 2004, 2013.
All Rights Reserved.**

No part of this book may be reproduced, stored in a retrieval system, transcribed in any form or by any means, electronic, mechanical, photocopy, recording, or any other means, or translated into any language without the prior written permission of the publisher.

DISCLAIMER: The information in this book is given in good faith. However, the author and the publishers cannot be held responsible for any error or omission. The publishers will not accept liabilities for any injuries or damages caused to the reader that may result from the reader's acting upon or using the content contained in this book. The publishers make this information available to English language readers for research and scholarly purposes only.

The publishers do not advocate nor endorse self-medication by laypersons. Chinese medicine is a professional medicine. Laypersons interested in availing themselves of the treatments described in this book should seek out a qualified professional practitioner of Chinese medicine.

10 9 8 7 6 (6th Printing, New Edition)

Printed at Edwards Brothers Malloy, Ann Arbor, MI
on acid free paper with soy inks.

With Appreciation...

There were many people involved with the creation of this book. A heartfelt thank you to everyone who helped:

Bruce Staff for his willingness to give me all the time needed to complete this project well.

Bob Flaws for his research, creative suggestions, and editing of the final draft.

Misha Cohen, Bob Damone, Cara Frank, Michael Gaeta, Lisa Hanfileti, Cynthia Neipris, Stuart Watts, and Ron Zaidman for being advance copy readers of various editions.

Joan Podgorski for a great book design.

Eric Brearton for design support and facilitation not to mention his unfailing good humor.

Everyone who contributed their stories, information, and quotations:

- Ryan Altman
- Jonathan B. Ammen
- Don Beans
- Nancy Bilello
- Michael Buyze
- Evelyn Kade Byram
- Larry Caldwell
- Judy Chaleff
- Steven F. Otsuka Dardis
- Valerie DeLaune
- Dagmar Ehling
- William Feather
- Laura Freeman
- John Frostad
- Bertram Furman
- Carol Green
- Lori Gritz
- Christian Hanson
- Elizabeth Healy
- George Herbert
- Valerie Hobbs
- Geoffrey Hudson
- Fred Jennes
- Steve Kauffman
- Gary Klepper
- Peter Lichtenstein
- Elizabeth Liddell
- Andrew Lininger
- Lisa Lowe
- Rande Lucas
- Maria MacKnight
- Karen Marks
- Brian Mears
- Eric Meyer-Reed
- Neal Stuart Miller
- Anna Nazos
- Michael Nolan
- Jeannette Painovich
- Mary Ann Radmacher
- Jean Jacques Rousseau
- Ihara Sai Ka Ku
- Susan Schiff
- Michael Schroeder
- Daniel Schulman
- John Scott
- Beverly Sills
- Greg Sperber
- C. Karen Stopford
- Aman Tandias
- Frank Yurasek

Contents

With Appreciation iii
Contents v

SECTION ONE: GETTING UP AND RUNNING

Chapter 1   Welcome & Introduction 1
Chapter 2   First Things First: Setting Goals 4
Chapter 3   What Could You Be Doing While You're Still in School? 15
Chapter 4   Dealing with Your Student Loan Debt 32
Chapter 5   Legal Stuff You Need to Know and Do. 37
Chapter 6   The Best Business Model for Your Practice 49
Chapter 7   Working with Others 59
Chapter 8   Getting a Job in Another Practitioner's Clinic. 70
Chapter 9   Working in Hospitals or Integrated Clinics. 80
Chapter 10   Your Community Acupuncture Clinic 93
Chapter 11   Going Where Your Skills Are Needed. 98
Chapter 12   Think About Specialization 100

SECTION TWO: WORKING ON YOUR OWN

Chapter 1   Business Basics 105
Chapter 2   Setting Your Fees and Managing Your Budget. 124
Chapter 3   How Much $$ Do You Need to Get Started? 135
Chapter 4   Finding Space and Negotiating a Lease. 148
Chapter 5   Creating a Business Plan for Your Clinic Can Be Fun . . 155
Chapter 6   Consider the Look and Feel of Your Clinic. 162
Chapter 7   Outside the Doc-in-a-Box 172
Chapter 8   Files and Recordkeeping. 184
Chapter 9   The Wonderful World of HIPAA Compliance 192
Chapter 10   Hiring and Keeping Good Employees 199
Chapter 11   The Tax Man Cometh: Here's How to Be Ready . . 211

CONTENTS

Chapter 12   Managing a Successful Herbal Dispensary 218
Chapter 13   Patient Management, or How Do You Keep Them
             Coming Back Happy?. 224
Chapter 14   Using the Services of Other Professionals 238

SECTION THREE: GETTING PAID
Chapter 1   Attitudes About Money 251
Chapter 2   Methods of Payment for Your Patients 257
Chapter 3   The Ins and Outs of Billing Insurance 275
Chapter 4   Personal Injury (PI) Patients: Yes or No?. 302
Chapter 5   Working with Workers' Compensation 315
Chapter 6   Selling Products from Your Clinic. 322
Chapter 7   Buying or Selling an Acupuncture Practice 330

SECTION FOUR: MARKETING YOUR PRACTICE
Chapter 1   Marketing From Day One: First Things First 341
Chapter 2   Marketing Inside Out. 350
Chapter 3   Community Team Builders and Marketing. 364
Chapter 4   Building & Using a Mailing List. 376
Chapter 5   Creating Your Presentation Folder 382
Chapter 6   Using Press Releases 396
Chapter 7   Marketing Your Practice on the Internet 402
Chapter 8   Marketing Odds and Ends 419
Chapter 9   Growing Your Life . . . Avoiding Burnout. 422
Chapter 10   Conclusion. 428
Resources for Going Further (books, classes, websites). 429
Appendix A–Getting a National Provider (NPI) Number 435
Appendix B–Creating Hospital Work Agreements 436
Index. 439

SECTION ONE

Getting Up and Running

Welcome & Introduction

Welcome to the new, revised edition of this book, which was first written in 2003. Back in the early days of teaching classes on practice management around the U.S. (1999-2000), Marilyn Allen and I were asked scores of times, "Do you have a book on this subject?" We didn't. That was inevitably followed by, "Can you recommend anyone else's book?" We couldn't. From the inspiration of those inquiries and with the help of a third author, Eric Strand, the first edition of this book was created. At the time, it filled an empty niche for our profession... the need for a thorough, easy-to-use book on the business of acupuncture and East Asian medicine.

At the time of this rewrite (2013), several other books on the business of acupuncture are available (see the resources section) and much has changed in our profession: Student loan amounts have skyrocketed. More research on acupuncture has moved us a few steps closer to mainstream practice in "integrated" settings. The Community Acupuncture movement has become a major force for bringing our skills to an expanded demographic. Electronic Medical Recordkeeping (EMR) is careening toward our profession at the speed of light. Still, as we talk to practitioners all around the country, the chatter about business and money problems has not changed much. People in our profession continue to struggle with these issues.

In the years since the first edition of this book, we've continued to teach and write on business, marketing, clinic management, ethics, and other subjects to help improve our chances, as a profession, for long-term success. It is still our belief that, by following even a part of the advice we give in this book, students and practitioners will be able to create more successful businesses and, hopefully, happier lives, whatever one's definitions of those things might be.

A book such as this one, which includes many legal and regulatory references, must be updated with each reprinting. This fully-revised edition includes several new chapters. In addition to chapters about working in integrated settings and on community acupuncture, there is a chapter on dealing with student loan debt and working in Western medical settings. There is also ever-expanding information about internet marketing, and basics about electronic medical records and Obamacare. All other chapters have been rewritten at least to some extent, and some completely.

▶ Tips on how to use this book and website

1. **The ⬤ Icon.** As you go through this book, you will find this icon repeated regularly. Every time you see this, it means you can find additional material on the companion website pertaining to the subject being discussed in the book. The website contains sample forms, letters, and contracts (all downloadable), a complete business plan outline, lots of web links, and a variety of other useful resources that were not very useful on paper but may be valuable if made available to you in a form that you could personalize. To access the website, go to **http://pointsforprofit.bluepoppy.com**.

2. **Practitioner Pointers.** Throughout the book we have included, wherever possible, quotes and stories from practitioners all around the country. Newer ones that I [HW] gathered for this edition are, in some cases, longer "interviews" with successful practitioners, and the boxes in those cases are larger. These boxes are titled Thoughts from Successful Practitioners. We hope you find them inspiring.

3. **Power Points.** These are specific bits of information that we want to draw special attention to. They are presented in

boxed formats, separate from the main body of the text throughout the book.

4. **Points to Ponder.** At the end of each chapter, we have listed the most important points covered in that chapter. Not sure if you want or need to read the whole chapter? Read the Points to Ponder at the end of the chapter to see what's there and why you might want to read the whole thing.

5. **Points for Teachers.** If you are using this book as a text for a practice management class, contact Blue Poppy for a teacher's guide to using this book. This companion information gives you ideas for student assignments and grading criteria. There is no charge for this guide when an order for the books is placed by your school.

6. **Related Products.** The publisher of this book has many other products to help you grow your practice, including distance-learning seminars on specific subjects related to the business of Chinese medicine as well as brochures, intake forms, and books about Chinese medicine written specifically for selling to the lay public.

7. **Business and Marketing Blog.** I have been writing blogs on subjects related to business for years. The blog is archived, so visit whenever you like. Go to www.bluepoppy.com, look for the links on the right side home page for Blue Poppy blogs and then for my Marketing Your Practice blog specifically.

Finally, I [HW] want to thank you for purchasing this book. I know there are a bazillion other books on business that you could have purchased instead of this one, but I truly believe that something here will help you be a happier and more successful practitioner in your chosen profession. Marilyn and I wish you the best of luck with your practice, but we encourage you to remember that, most of the time, luck is at least 90% perspiration and only 10% inspiration.

First Things First: Setting Goals | 2

The Buddha said, "Action follows thought as a cart follows an ox." Napoleon Hill said, "Think and grow rich." These statements are ways of saying that the mental activity of planning and goal-setting, when used effectively, helps us immeasurably to manage our behavior, prioritize our actions, motivate ourselves over the long haul, and set the bar high enough to help us excel. Thus this book begins with a chapter on goal-setting because this is where any business starts... as an idea, a thought, a dream. We believe it is important to get this part right, right from the start. So please don't skip this chapter; it can make a huge difference in your life.

Goal-setting as a daily practice has always had a powerful place in the business world and is especially important for anyone starting a new small business such as yours. You may also find, after reading this chapter, that setting goals can have a substantial benefit to your personal life. Active goal-setting is really a combination of two things. First, it is a roadmap that you create as you travel it. Second, each small goal reached as you go along is a "prize" you give yourself as you build a life in your chosen profession.

➤ Why do we need goals?

If suddenly tomorrow you woke up in the middle of the ocean in a small boat (think *Life of Pi*), your only supplies being a compass, a box of matches, and a bag of potato chips, would you sit and wait for a rescue to come along? Would you set the sails on fire hoping someone would see the smoke? Or would you use the compass to point yourself in one direction and sail, row, or both(!!) until you found land?

CHAPTER 2 | First Things First: Setting Goals

Few among us would see any sense in floating around without direction with only a bag of chips to eat! And anyone who thinks that waiting for rescue is the best idea should probably not be a small-business owner. Depending upon your situation, there may be no search and rescue team out there except yourself when you are the boss! No, the best bet as a castaway or a business owner is to pick a direction and move forward as if your life depended on it. And it is the positive action of setting goals that is your compass and your map.

The power of a goal is tremendous. Just the articulation and writing down of a goal focuses your mind, intention, and qi. Good goals give you a feeling of control over your world and your destiny. You are sending a message out to the universe that you have a set of specific plans and desires and you are going after them. Similar to placing an acupuncture needle in a specific location on the patient's body, the focusing of your energy is doing work, only this work is for your life and your success as a businessperson.

> "If there is no wind, row."
> —Anonymous

A goal successfully met increases your self-esteem. Few things make you feel as good as when you achieve a dream, and a goal is nothing other than a dream with a deadline. It is through goals that you stretch your potential, force yourself to reach just a little bit higher, take a bigger bite out of the universe of possibilities, throw more paint on the canvas of your life.

▶ Why we don't set goals

Setting a goal in and of itself is not a difficult task. Indeed, figuring out what you want and setting your sights upon achieving your dreams can be a fairly simple activity. So why don't more people set goals?

First of all, most people are unaware of the power of active goal-setting. Another reason may be that it is, consciously or unconsciously, scary to do this. It requires some courage to honestly look at where we are, acknowledge what we want, and commit *out loud,* at least to ourselves never mind to others, to the work of achieving our dreams.

Finally and possibly the most common, if least acknowledged, reason that people do not set goals is that you may set a goal and not meet it. You may fall short in patient visits, income level, personal achievement within the profession, or your larger life aspirations. This is something many people find difficult to face. However, it is by stating our dreams and desires for the future that we continue to grow, learn, and set a course of achievement for our lives.

> "Persistence and determination alone are omnipotent. The slogan 'press on' has solved and always will solve the problems of the human race."
> —*Calvin Coolidge*

▶ Dream into your goals

What is a goal, really? It can be very simple, such as a to-do list completed by a certain date, or it can be quite profound, such as what you believe is worthwhile in life, a vision of who you wish to become and what you wish to share with the world. So when you sit down to write a list of goals, start with some basics. What do you value in life? What do you believe is important: free time, family, money, philanthropy, travel, enlightenment? When we have clearly defined our values and dreams, it is easier to articulate the goals that might help us live them. Do you want to be a great parent and spouse, a trusted friend, a well-respected practitioner, or an international volunteer, or do you have more tangible desires such as a new house or car, a college fund for your children, or an early and comfortable retirement? Clarity about these aspirations can help us put a real, workable plan in motion.

▶ Wise goals are S*M*A*R*T

Knowing why we should set goals is a start. Knowing how to set a good goal is the next step. Making goals, good ones that push us to our best without defeating or discouraging us, is a learned skill. However, by following the advice of David Sandler, well-known author and founder of the Sandler Sales Institute, the task of setting good goals is easier. Sandler says that goals need to be S*M*A*R*T—**S**pecific, **M**easurable, **A**ttainable, **R**ealistic, and **T**ime-bound.

Make your goals *specific.* State exactly what it is you want to accomplish. For example, "I will make $100,000 net before taxes in the year 20XX," or, "I will see 30 patients per week by the end of June this year." The more specific your goal, the more you will be able to focus your energy on its achievement.

Make your goals *measurable.* At the end of the time period you specify, you are able to check your progress. Be it dollars, patients, classes you want to take, or places you wish to visit, you will be able to ascertain the difference between what you stated you would do and what you have actually done.

Make your goals *attainable.* They need to be possible. "I will see 100 new patients next week" is probably not attainable if you are only seeing 10 this week. So don't set pie in the sky goals; set goals that are attainable. Otherwise you will defeat yourself and become discouraged before you even start.

Make your goals *realistic.* Attainable and realistic go hand in hand, although there is a difference. While you may be able to see 100 new patients in a month (this could be accomplished in a week if you are working in a community acupuncture clinic), even if you had people lined up outside the door of your clinic and around the corner, it may be physically impossible to make the leap from 10 to 100 patients in a week and do it well. In other words, don't set a goal to be the first acupuncturist in space if you aren't a colonel in the NASA space program. Your goal must be within the realm of possibility.

Make your goals *time-bound.* Set a deadline: this week, the end of this month, February 2, every Wednesday, by December 31 of this year, etc. If a goal has no deadline, there is no way to be able to measure progress. We should be able to ascertain if we did what we set out to do.

▶ More than just an idea

Goals don't count unless you write them down. Putting your goals on paper does two things. First, it sets your intention in motion. By writing down your goals, you are making them real for yourself. Second, they are less likely to be forgotten. You are less likely to sweep them aside when another idea pops into your head. It is, of course, perfectly okay to add more goals to the ones you have written. In fact, Mark Victor Hansen, author of *The One Minute Millionaire* and *Chicken Soup for the Soul,* says that we should write down up to 100 goals every day, so that they stay clearly present in our consciousness. I must admit that I've never written down that many goals at one sitting!

There is more power in written goals than in spoken ones. Write them all down, both personal and professional. We suggest that you pick your most ambitious business goal, write it on a business card and laminate it. Then wrap the card in a one-hundred dollar bill and place it in your wallet. Keep it in your wallet until you meet your goal. You may spend the money in an emergency, but it has to be replaced within 24 hours. Carrying that Benjamin around can give you a different feeling about yourself and what's possible for you, and it can affect the way you carry yourself and operate in the world.

Personalize your goals. Create "I" or "we" statements. Making your goal a personal aspiration will increase your actual inclination to do something to realize it. If the goal is just a fuzzy hope for the future, it is unlikely that your mind (even in partnership with universal mind) will be able to make it manifest.

When writing goals, avoid words like "try," "should," "would," or "maybe." Goals should be positive and clear, not wishy-washy. "I will," "we are going to," or "I will create" are all statements of intention. Don't be afraid to state what you will accomplish and by when it will be so.

> "You may be disappointed if you fail, but you are doomed if you don't try."
> —Beverly Sills

Keep it simple. Goals can be complex, but at first keep them simple. Break larger goals into small steps. Instead of setting a goal to reach a clinic income of $75,000 within X months, set smaller, short-term goals as stepping stones to that end. Patient visits per week, new patients per month, outbound calls per week, marketing activities per week, etc. are all small stepping-stone goals that lead naturally to larger ones. When you achieve the small ones, it gives your conscious and unconscious mind the support and belief that you can achieve the greater ones as well.

Have fun with it! Goal-setting need not be somber nor should it make you miserable or fearful! It's about improving your life and realizing your dreams. You do want to challenge yourself to do better and grow into all those dreams that will improve the quality of your clinic and your life, but don't make it into some kind of gladiatorial event! Also remember that it's okay and even likely that you'll change your goals as you go. What you think is important is very likely to evolve with your life. Only you can decide upon your goals and what the path to realizing them should look like.

▸ Time lines

I personally believe that it's useful to have short-term, long-term, and lifetime goals. Just remember to articulate a time line/deadline for each one of them!

Short-term goals

These are no longer than six months, and three months is better. These will usually be smaller, stepping-stone goals. They are the action-steps which, when pieced together, will allow you to achieve a long-term goal. You should write down these goals every day and add to them with flexibility as you go.

Long-term goals

Goals with a deadline from 6–12 months are considered long-term. These goals should be larger in scope or level of achievement and may be the result of completing your smaller, short-term goals. These are the goals we set for serious financial change or personal improvement in our lives.

Lifetime goals

These goals are larger aspirations that you wish to accomplish at some point in your life, or they will relate to the sum total of what you create or achieve. Establishing lifetime goals can be fuzzy, and achieving them will be difficult if you don't have short- and long-term goals established in order to get there. Don't worry too much if these are difficult or if they change with time. I'm still working on mine, too!

▸ Seven areas for setting your goals

Goals are not just for your business. Although setting goals will surely help you make your business a success, there are more things in life than work. In fact, there are at least seven areas of life in which we can set goals. Perhaps you can think of even more.

Family goals can be as simple as "I'll spend an hour every evening this week reading to my kids" or as complicated as "I'll re-establish a relationship with my estranged sibling." Who among us could not do better in this area of life?

Financial goals are about financial stability and your relationship to the mysterious world of money. These goals include things like paying off your student loans, funding a retirement account or a college fund for your children, or creating enough patients to buy your clinic building.

Spiritual goals reflect your internal life. Religious observance, meditation practice, creating time for thought and reflection, or just being in nature, this is anything that nourishes your spirit and gives you strength. For example, "I will take a quiet walk in nature twice a week during the month of May."

Work goals could include a variety of things, but the area of clinical success may be the easiest place to begin setting goals. "I am going to see five new patients per week, every week, by the second week in September," for example, is a specific, measurable, attainable, realistic, and time-bound short-term goal. Other work-related goals may include improving your clinical or diagnostic skills through continuing education, perfecting a new clinical technique, reviewing one herbal formula per week, or reading a new clinical text each month.

Business goals are an easy set of goals to create and write down. How many patients are you seeing per day, per week, per month? It may surprise you how much the act of focusing mental energy on your patient numbers can help you grow your practice. Start with the number of new patients you see on average at present. Let's say you are seeing an average of three new patients a week. Come up with a time line to increase that number to five—by the end of the month, for example!

Social goals sound easy (unless you are really shy), but they, too, take thought and energy. "I will join the Susan B. Komen breast cancer walk-a-thon," "I will create an acupuncturist team for the next 5K walk in my town," or "I will attend three parties this month." Though these activities can also be seen as part of your marketing, work alone is rarely enough for a satisfying life.

Health goals are important. You have to walk the talk to be credible. How about something like, "I will do one trade for massage each Friday through the year 20XX." We easily forget how much stress we carry just being a human, much less operating a small business where the focus is always on the care of others. Make sure to set goals in this area. Only by keeping yourself in optimum health will you be able to provide the best service to those who seek out your care.

And finally, *Education.* Even if you are required to do continuing education, this may be the last thing you want to think about as you approach graduation from acupuncture school! Still, if you love your work you should want to improve upon your current skills. How about something like, "I will study and master one Blue Poppy distance learning course in the first quarter of next year," or something really ambitious such as, "I will attain my doctoral degree in OM by the summer of 20XX."

➤ A final note about goals

The more often you write down your goals, the better you will get at it. You will also find that you meet more of your goals more often. Remember, as you write your goals, that there is no shortage of patients out there and no shortage of money. Think about what you want, put your mind to the necessary work to achieve it, and you can make the magic happen.

Take some time and look at the seven areas for goal-setting listed above. Write at least one goal for each area. Maybe get a small, attractive notebook to write down your dreams and goals every day. Then see if you can write five specific, measurable, attainable, realistic, and time-bound goals for your clinic or your professional life. Don't worry if you think they might sound crazy to anyone else. This work is to help *you*. It's also okay to write down the same goals day after day until you reach them. Trust your crazy dreams and remember, whether you think you can or think you can't, you're right.

POINTS TO PONDER FROM CHAPTER 2

- Goal-setting is a powerful tool you can use to help you plan for and then create your own success.
- People often don't set goals due to fear of failure.
- Good goals are S*M*A*R*T: specific, measurable, attainable, realistic, and time-bound.
- It is effective to have short-term goals (one week to six months) and long-term goals (more than six months).
- There are at least seven areas for which it is useful to have goals. These are family, financial, spiritual, work, social, health, and educational.
- It is useful to keep a small notebook or scrapbook for writing your goals. Write as many goals as you can every morning. Read them to yourself every day. After a few months, go back and read the goals you were writing then and see how they have changed and which ones you have achieved.

SECTION ONE: GETTING UP AND RUNNING

THOUGHTS FROM SUCCESSFUL PRACTITIONERS

Brian Mears, L.Ac. (Mountain Spirit Acupuncture)

In practice since: 2008 in Westminster, CO

Nature of his practice: Sees anything and everything, 50+ patients per week. "I have three treatment rooms and book on the hour and the half-hour. With three young children in addition to my clinic, I'm stressed but happy with my practice!"

Other experience: Pharmacy school, but "I never met any happy pharmacists, so decided to rethink that choice!"

Charges: $150 for one-and-a-half hour new patient appointment; $75 for a regular treatment. "We also sell packages, which are prepaid and save both my time and patient money, and we give referral incentives as well."

Marketing methods: "We have a good website and I pay for regular search engine optimization (SEO), but by now it's more word-of-mouth, with fewer new patients coming through internet marketing. We also do charity fundraising clinics one Saturday each month. That brings in lots of folks, usually some new ones. I put up chairs and we do community acupuncture style treatments for these. I tried some print ads at the beginning, even though my practice management teacher said not to! She was right; we never got a single call from these."

Current projects: "I want to move our records from paper to digital, but I'm not happy with any of the available software. We are building our own EMR application so we can move toward paperless."

Quotes:

"I wish schools would help us explore what it means to be more professional, and I wish there were discussions about being passionate about the medicine and learning how to share that passion with our patients."

"As a business person, it took me time to learn to manage cash flow, to pay attention to all the details and make them into user-friendly systems."

Best advice to new grads: "To be a success, you only need two things: patients and patience. Don't give up!"

Website: www.mtnspiritacupuncture.com

What Could You Be Doing While You're Still in School?

The transition from student to new practitioner can be a bumpy ride. In this chapter, we suggest a wide variety of projects that, being done now, may ease your workload and your mind during the first weeks and months out of acupuncture school. The more groundwork for success you have laid in advance, the closer you will be to the practice you desire the day after graduation. You will also experience far less stress.

First and foremost, get the most out of your education! Do the work, be curious, be serious, and get a firm grasp on the theory behind the medicine. Don't just go through the motions. Consider that if you think school is hard, being in private practice is *much, much harder.* Each new patient is a challenge, and you have to take care of everything for yourself, every day, including chart notes, research, marketing, bill paying, your patients' needs, and yourself! Also, as we will discuss in later chapters, *you* will be your best marketing tool. Thus, the better you know this medicine, the better and more self-assured your treatments and your marketing efforts will be.

Second, start thinking about and visualizing your life after school. Make these visualizations as real, detailed, and concrete as you can. Write them down, as discussed in the previous chapter on goals. Keep a planning/brainstorming notebook of all your ideas and dreams, networking contacts, phone numbers, sketches and photos, and leads for patients or marketing opportunities. Then think about the first concrete steps you will need to take in order to manifest your "dream" clinical practice. Some of these will very likely include the following:

▶ Create your roadmap

One of my favorite American icons, Yogi Berra, said, "You've got to be careful if you don't know where you are going, because you might not get there." So, even if you are not entirely sure of where or how you want to practice, some work done now will help ease the transition from student to practitioner. Homing in on possible places where you may want to practice is a good first step. Start with the cities, towns, or at least region(s) of the country that most appeal to you. This leads to some tasks.

1. Look up the statutes and regulations regarding acupuncture and the use of herbal medicine in the state(s) you are considering (see Important Web Tools & Links). While all but a few states now allow acupuncture, there are still one or two that require treatment to be performed by a medical doctor or under a doctor's supervision. Once you know the regulatory climate in the state in which you want to practice, you can start to look at other factors.

2. Check out the demographics of various cities and towns. There are many websites that will give you a wide variety of demographic information for areas all over the country. Call Chambers of Commerce (CoC) or visit their websites to get an even better idea about the places you are considering. This is always a good first step in setting up any kind of business in a new town. These organizations want to attract business to their area and are able to give you all kinds of statistics regarding population and expected growth, median income, primary industries, major medical facilities, educational and cultural climate and opportunities, average price per-square-foot-per-year for different types of business rentals, going rates on home and apartment rentals or purchases, and the median age of the population. They can advise you on getting a sales tax license or other required paperwork, the best business banks to deal with, and a variety of other useful resources. All this information will help you determine the

size and nature of the potential market and possible practice specialties that would be fruitful.

3. What is the feel of the community you are considering? Any area you decide to move to should first and foremost be one where you can be a happy and active participant. What's the political climate and does it fit with your personal beliefs? What religious affiliations are possible and does your preference have a presence there? Is it a supportive environment for raising a family if you so desire?

4. Begin taking a serious look at the amount of capital you will need to start up your practice and consider possible sources of funding. What pieces of equipment and furniture do you already have? What more will you need? Based on your research from #2 above, how much will you need for signing a lease for the approximate size of clinic you want? Contact area insurance companies about the cost of basic business insurance. How much is the state license fee, how much for installing a phone, practice management or insurance billing software, printing forms, and initial marketing? What will you need in reserve to pay personal bills for the first six months? How much do you have and what sort of family or personal financial support structure will you have in place when you graduate? Be as realistic as possible. (See Section 2, Chapter 3 for more on this subject.)

▶ Competition or allies?

You also need to know who's there already. You can begin with yellowpages.com or do Google and Bing searches to see where most practitioners are. Also visit the NCCAOM site and do a practitioner search for the relevant towns or zip codes. Write down all names and contact information you find. You may wish to contact them all (you should look at all their websites at the very least!), possibly get some part-time work from them, rent space from them, ask for referrals for a specific specialty you plan to pursue, and otherwise try to create a nice working relationship before you move into the area. There may be some sort of support or study group already in place. Some practitioners won't be happy about your move into "their" area, but don't let that disturb you too much. Others will be supportive and more helpful than you may think. They might even offer you a job (I've seen this happen!) or place to practice.

Other resources include **aaaomonline.org, acufinder.com, acupuncturetoday.com**, and the website for the licensing authority for the state in which you want to practice.

This exercise is designed to do three things. One, it lets you see where everyone is located. If a preponderance of acupuncture clinics are on one side of town, consider another side. Two, you may find that the little town of 15,000 people that looked so attractive already has 50 acupuncturists. That's not likely, but you may not like the numbers you see. Finally, you'll be able to research established practitioners in the area and check their rates, which helps you determine your own rates and whether or not you can make the living you need and desire.

▸ **How will you differentiate your practice?**
If you choose to settle in an area where there are other acupuncturists (or even if you don't), you can help yourself greatly by finding and serving one or more niche markets. This means specializing. While this may feel like a limiting factor for you in the beginning, it can produce patient interest in the community and referrals from other acupuncturists who are not as proficient in that specialty. Remember that there is no lack of human suffering with almost any condition, specialty, or body part. And, it is much easier to know a lot about one area than a little about a lot of areas. If you get really, really good at one thing, people will find out about it and refer to you when appropriate. (See Chapter 12 of this section.) I once had an arm

surgery from an orthopedist who *only* did surgery on arms, and he had more than plenty of patients! So give specialization some serious thought.

If you decide while still in school to specialize, use the resources available to you now to get some extra training in your area(s) of interest. The reason we mention specialization in this chapter is that it may be easier to get that training while you are still in school. Do some special research; talk with your instructors.

What's in a name?

Start doing some research on possible names now! Your clinic name represents you to the community and potential patients, appearing on your signage, letterhead, business cards, and website. A good name can help build a positive patient flow and bottom line; a poor one can have the opposite effect on your success.

As the basis of your brand identity, your name announces who you are and what you do and can lump you in with or raise you above your competition. When selecting the name of your business, here are a few questions to keep in mind:

- Does it make my business easy to market? The more information your business name conveys, clearly and concisely, the fewer explanatory words you need in ads, on signs, etc. In other words, if the name of your clinic is *Skin Care Acupuncture Clinic,* any ads you create do not need extra lines of type to tell people what you do. It's already in the name.

- Is it easy to remember, spell, and pronounce? *Whole Family Health Center, Boulder Herbal Medicine Clinic,* and *Orange Park Acupuncture Clinic* are all pretty easy to remember, right? They are short, concise, and can be pronounced by anyone who drives by your clinic or sees your website, brochure, or card somewhere. Why is this important? Hundreds of people may drive past your clinic sign every day, but, if the name is weird or hard to pronounce or remember, you may lose that future patient to the guy down the street. We do not suggest you use Chinese words like *An Shen* (calm spirit) or *Jin Shan* (golden mountain). These may sound exotic and have meaning for those of us "in the club," but they mean nothing to and may even put off the average American patient.

- Does it convey a clear understanding of what you do? *Womencare Acupuncture Clinic* and *Athletic Edge Acupuncture Center* are good names that communicate to your patient population both that you do acupuncture and that a selected group of people would benefit from your services. Look for ways to add the words "acupuncture," "Chinese medicine," "herbal medicine," etc. to convey your purpose.

- Does it market you to the specific niche you want to serve? Again, this is a great way to separate you from the average. Niche marketing can fill your clinic more quickly. Every athlete who sees *Athletic Edge Acupuncture Center* will have a pretty good idea what you do!

Once you select a few possible clinic names, try them out on friends and family and see what their reactions are. Can they spell the names without seeing them? Do they understand immediately what happens at a clinic with these names? If not, keep working on it.

Check name availability

Now that your mind is brimming with ideas, go to the website for your Secretary of State (SoS) and check name availability. Whether you are planning to be a sole proprietor, an LLC, or a corporation, you need to choose a business name that no one else in your state already has. Most of these websites are either www.sos.XX.us, with XX replaced by the initials of your state, but a few are www.ss.XX.us.

If your chosen name is available, you can usually register it right there online, but you may want to see if domain names are also available for your website as well. Also, while you are at the SoS website, find out what the reporting/renewal requirements are for maintaining your business name. Typically, renewal is once per year or every other year. You could register a business name before leaving school and then print business cards with your cell number and give them to all your friends and family for future reference. If they want to come to see you now, bring them to the school clinic.

> **POWER POINT**
>
> Before you register your business name with the state, check to see if that URL name (or some version of it) is available!

▶ Get a job

First of all, I need to say that most of you will not find jobs unless you want to work in a hospital; more and more of those positions are opening up across the U.S. Still, the overwhelming majority of acupuncturists work for themselves or perhaps with one or more colleagues. That is just the reality at the time of this writing. Still, there are some jobs out there. Here are some opportunities to research if you are intent on finding one.

- Pain specialty clinics are certainly aware of acupuncture, and multidiscipline treatment centers may be more common in the future, especially as acupuncture has been included as part of basic benefits under the new healthcare act in five states at present (2013) and more may do so in the future.* I'd contact

---

*At the time of this writing, CA, NM, MD, WA, and CT as an add-on rider, include acupuncture as an "essential health benefit." AK and NV are expected to approve benefits as well. Implications of this are both good and challenging; it may mean more patients, but it also means being inside the third-party payer system and learning to be proficient doing insurance billing.
http://www.nytimes.com/2012/12/06/health/interest-groups-push-to-fill-margins-of-health-coverage.html?ref=acupuncture&_r=0

every such center in my area and float the idea that my services can improve outcomes, shorten treatment times, and reduce dependency on opiates. There is research out there that you can print out as part of your presentation to any center or MD decision maker.

- There are also a growing number of jobs available in community acupuncture style clinics. If this interests you, join POCA at pocacoop.com and check the job postings regularly. This might be a good way to decide if the CA model is right for you.
- The U.S. Military and Veterans Administration have acknowledged the efficacy of acupuncture for pain, PTSD, anxiety and depression, and certain head injuries. They have not, however, chosen to hire L.Ac.'s and include us in their bureaucracy (and are instead training their own MDs to do this work). This could change, but will take time, persistence, and passion on our side to keep knocking on this door.
- In 2010, 40% of American Hospital Association member hospitals offered some type of CAM therapy. Massage therapy and acupuncture are the most common. As stated above, this is a growing opportunity for anyone willing to knock on enough hospital doors. If another acupuncturist is already working at a hospital(s) that interest you, drop off your resume and get on the list of interested practitioners should that or another position become available. Keep your malpractice insurance up to date.
- Infertility clinics are well aware of the power of Chinese medicine/acupuncture to improve the odds of their high-tech treatments being effective. If this is a field of interest for you, join ABORM for extra training in this field.
- If you are no shy violet, consider sitting down with your phone and computer and calling every practitioner within a 50-mile radius of where you live and asking if they are looking for another practitioner in their clinic, and under what conditions. You never know what will happen until you try.
- If you are single, outgoing, and not sure where you wish to

settle, consider the cruise ship jobs. If you work hard and don't spend money on clothes or partying, in a year you could pay down a considerable amount of student debt and have your living expenses covered. This is hard work and not for the introvert, but can be profitable for the right personality.

This is a fairly large subject and I won't cover more on this here since we have given it some in-depth attention in Chapter 8 of this section.

▶ Paperwork is easy

Something that is very easy to get out of the way while you're still in school is creating the various forms you will need to use as a practitioner. There are some forms samples on the companion website for this book, but don't let that limit you in designing your own. Look at the forms used in your school clinic as well. Maybe you can get some examples from recent graduates who were your friends during school. Just remember that they need to be easy to read and understand for you, your future front desk staff, and anyone else who may be reading them, such as insurance companies or lawyers.

There are many forms that you will need to run a clinic, communicate with patients and insurance companies legally and effectively, and perform and properly record patient care. From patient intake and follow-up, to patient information and clinic policies, to HIPAA and financial policy forms, you can begin filling a computer folder with these immediately. It will actually give you some peace of mind to know that you can start practicing effectively and legally on the day after graduation. Once you have your clinic name and address, you can place that information at the top of the forms. Below is a list of forms you will need; examples of many of these are on the companion website. Depending upon the subject of the form, many are also discussed at more length in other chapters.

Patient management forms
- patient personal information form
- patient health history
- liability waiver
- insurance forms
- notice of privacy policy (HIPAA)
- acknowledgment of receipt of privacy policy (HIPAA)
- individual rights for authorization (HIPAA)
- mandatory disclosure form (some states)
- informed consent (HIPAA)
- fax log (HIPAA)
- sign-in sheet
- new patient FAQ
- clinic policies (financial, cancellation, etc.)
- follow-up care (report of findings)
- herb instructions (bulk, granules, ready-made pills/capsules)
- referral information sheet

Business/legal examples and forms
- hardship waiver form
- INS form 9
- IRS forms W2/W4/SE/S4

▶ **Write some text for your website and brochures**

Your website is your clinic's second voice and image (you yourself should be the first). Brochures are another way to extend your reach into your community. People will judge you by your website before becoming patients. A brochure they may take home from an event or your office, put it up on their company bulletin board, or give it to a friend or family member. To be most effective, a brochure should contain just enough information to get people interested in acupuncture and Chinese medicine and its ability to treat a certain disorder but not so much technical jargon that they feel lost, bored, or stupid. See Chapters 2, 5, and 7 in Section 4 for more suggestions on this subject.

CHAPTER 3 | What Could You Be Doing While You're Still in School?

➤ **Business cards**

Once you have decided on a clinic name and a general location, you can create a "beta-test" business card. You may not be able to accept patients yet, but you can start generating interest by letting people know the business name, maybe a location (or city), and when you expect to begin your practice. Use your cell phone number to start (but get a land line when you open for real!). Remember, business cards are cheap; just get another box when you have an *actual* clinic address and phone number.

You can see that the example to the right is a beginning business card. While not perfectly complete, it tells people what you are, when you are going to be opening, a website for more information, and a phone number for questions. Having cards and a simple website will help you hit the ground running. You could actually have a few patients the first week you are open if you work at getting these out to everyone you can find!

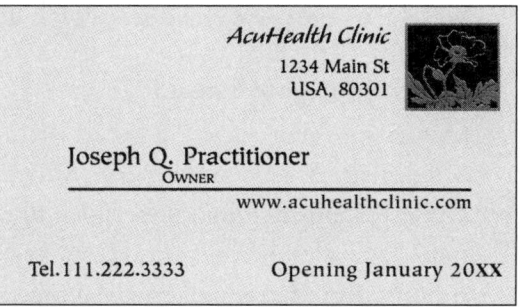

Once you are really in practice, you will get new cards with other pieces of information. Don't worry about that now. When you are ready to get your "real" business cards, see Section 4, Chapter 5 and Supplies & Equipment Links in the Weblinks section of the website. ●

➤ **Logo or no logo?**

A logo is a visual symbol that tells a story to potential patients. It is also something you could begin working on before you graduate. You may also decide to start without one, which is fine. It may take you awhile to decide how you want to describe yourself pictorially. When you do decide to create this image, you may want to enlist the help of a professional. One idea is to

25

call the art department at the local college and talk to the graphic arts instructors. See if they have a really talented student who would like a side job for their portfolio.

When working on this project try to think like a layperson who knows nothing about Chinese medicine, culture, language, or art. Make sure the picture that represents you is attractive, not confusing or off-putting to anyone. If you decide to use a Chinese character, for example, it may be wise to put the English translation in small italic type below the picture or on the back of your card. Also, the yin/yang symbol is so overused that if you use it, I hope you'll come up with a really new look.

➤ Equipment you'll need

One major financial outlay when setting up a clinic is physical equipment. As an acupuncturist, you are going to need two types: 1) items required to perform the duties of acupuncture (tables, needles, herbs, moxa, etc.), and 2) those required for running and managing a medical practice of any kind (computer, printer, fax, phone, etc.). As a student, money may be tight, but a little can go a long way on eBay and other online auctions. Another aid in checking these things off your list is family. How many birthdays or gifting holidays are there before you graduate? Use them to your advantage. Here's some stuff to ask for:

- **Computer:** You probably already have one, but it needs to be stated here and definitely on your list if you don't!

- **Printer:** Get a color, all-in-one printer-fax-copier-scanner. For the little extra money, the extra usage is incalculable.

- **Phone:** Even though online appointment software is improving, some patients still want to call the clinic to set up an

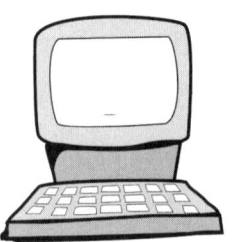

appointment. They want to be greeted by a friendly person, scheduled patiently, or leave a message if needed. You also want caller ID (and as many other bells and whistles as you can afford). Inevitably a new patient will call after hours, request a call back, but leave no phone number!

- **A good sturdy table** for each treatment room is obvious. Really nice ones may have shelves underneath or attachments for table paper, or even mechanisms to raise and lower them. Nice ones send a good message to your patients.

- **Desk(s), chairs,** waiting room furniture, carpets, decor, and shelving for herbal products. This is getting to be a long list(!), but it's better to know the reality in advance. In addition to online auctions, cruise local yard sales regularly and stay in touch with Staples and similar retailers for seasonal sales.

These are just a few recommendations. For a more complete listing of suggested business equipment and acupuncture supplies, see the supplier section on the companion website. One caveat: eBay can be great for discounted-but-new products, but I don't recommend buying old computer equipment. A used acupuncture table, desk, chair, work table, or shelving could be fine to recycle into your practice, but buying a used computer is a crap shoot. Printers, if they are good brands, have a longer life, but take care when buying used computing equipment.

▶ **Check out online scheduling software**
Choices in this type of product just keep proliferating (they may also come and go, making the list below inaccurate). While you are in school, try out online demos and read reviews. There are lots of differing opinions out there. Here are the ones with the best reviews at this time.

    Cliniko   Appointy
    Genbook   Schedulicity

POWER POINTS

What other things could you do while still in school?

- Choose advisors such as an accountant, attorney, banker, and computer consultant, if you don't already have them.

- Look into answering services, email blast services, online appointment-making software, and other ways for you to stay in touch with patients and potential patients quickly and conveniently.

- Shop for business liability and malpractice insurance.

- Find out worker's compensation regulations, levels of reimbursement, and paperwork requirements in your state.

- Check out computer sign-painting companies. (Signs may be on a door, window, car, or on wood, plastic, or metal.) Prices may vary widely, so shop around before you buy.

- If you like computer software systems for running your practice, take a look at what is out there for acupuncturists' offices, perhaps download a "test drive" copy or visit their websites.

- Take a look at OfficeAlly or find a service to file insurance forms for your clinic for a cut of the income.

- Will you need janitorial services, snow removal services, laundry services, grounds maintenance, medical waste disposal? You could get them all lined up and budgeted before you graduate.

- Will you need appointment cards, telephone message pads, preprinted super bills, prescription pads, or other printing services? Again, prices vary widely, so shop around.

- Planning a community style clinic? Join www.pocacoop.com at a student rate. This membership is a must.

Planning your herbal pharmacy

A pharmacy is a huge financial asset to your clinic. There are so many things to discuss here that this topic has its own chapter in Section 2. Fundamentally, think of your pharmacy as a profit center that can make money even when you are out of the office. Whether you choose a bulk herb, granule, or ready-made pill/capsule line of products, it will make your path to prosperity easier and give you another option for helping patients when acupuncture is not quite what the doctor ordered. Start researching product lines and companies now.

Where could you teach a class? What could you teach?

When you think about all that you have learned in school, what in all those skills and all that information could be something that you make into classes and lectures to promote your clinic? If you know where you are planning to practice, do some research on places you could offer classes or lectures. Is there a YMCA/YWCA, a lifelong learning center, community college, or other venues where classes are offered? Is there a free library or hospital lecture series, or corporate lunchtime lecture series? You can make a plans for these while you are still in school.

> **POWER POINT**
>
> Make a scan of both your state and national license and diploma before you have them matted and framed for the wall. Keep these in a digital folder. Then, when you apply to an HMO to be certified or when you need to show an herb company that you are who you say you are, you don't have to take them down off the wall and struggle to get another copy made.

Wait until the last minute for . . .

These final tasks you'll do only a few weeks before you are ready to open your practice:

- Call to have all your utilities and phone turned on by a specific date.

- Start accepting appointments from those friends who have been waiting.

SECTION ONE: GETTING UP AND RUNNING

- Place an announcement about your opening in all the local papers and on your Facebook page, blog, other social media.

- Take your brochure and other forms to the printer. I recommend using a local printer instead of an online one if you can. It gives you another opportunity to market your services and it's great to support other local businesses the same way you want them to support you.

- Order some needles! And maybe some herbs, too. (For more information on setting up a dispensary, see Section 2, Chapter 15 and Section 3, Chapter 6.)

- Mail out announcements to local physicians, chiropractors, health food stores, hospitals, HMO groups, human resource departments for all local companies larger than 50 employees, friends, stores or services for any specific niche market you plan to serve.

- Start planning your first open house celebration!

Finally, you can make all this work fun if you want to. Think of all this research, writing, and equipment prowling as the foundation of your success and stepping stones toward fulfilling your dreams. This is your own personal journey toward your chosen goal. So why not enjoy each day and each task as much as you can?

> **PRACTITIONER POINTER**
>
> "My best advice for new grads: START creating and building your practice. Now. Even before you graduate. Develop a buddy system of 3-4 people and work together to help each other stay accountable. Touch base weekly. When you commit to someone to do what you say you will, you're more likely to make progress, overcome your fear, share advice."
>
> —Elizabeth Healy
> New York, NY

CHAPTER 3 | What Could You Be Doing While You're Still in School?

POINTS TO PONDER FROM CHAPTER 3

- Don't wait until you graduate to figure out your next move. You can complete lots of stuff now to help you hit the ground running, such as:

- Find a home for your practice and research the demographics online, at the library, and on the phone.

- Determine a niche market that will keep you interested for years to come and figure out how to find and best communicate with patients.

- Find out if there are other practitioners (acupuncturists, MDs, DCs, or others that you could work for part-time).

- Decide on a name and logo, and write promotional brochure text for your practice.

- Forms, letters, HIPAA compliance paperwork, and other patient records paperwork can be created while you're still in school.

- Start searching for and collecting equipment for your practice.

- Take notes on what things you want to carry in your herbal dispensary.

- Create a list of friends, media contacts, MDs, DCs, PTs, L.Acs, human resources directors, insurance company executives, stores, and other service providers that you will want to contact when you open your clinic.

Dealing with Your Student Loan Debt | 4

Student loan debt in our profession has reached frankly epic proportions and is the subject of much consternation and worry, not to mention blogs, articles, and anger. If you are one of the lucky few who did not have to borrow or who did not borrow much, good for you. You can skip this chapter! If you did borrow, I'm sorry this is so large and possibly scary.

It's inappropriate for me to discuss the politics of student debt, but you can chime in on the subject through various blogs, Twitter feeds, and chat groups, and perhaps you already have! That said, below are some ideas for tackling and managing the student loan beast. Some readers will have already done all this homework and know more on the subject than I do. Still, I hope there may be one new idea here that helps make this less painful an ordeal than it may otherwise be.

▶ Start with what you know

- Gather your information. Make a list or a spreadsheet of all the lenders you owe money to along with the outstanding principal, interest rate, and contact information.

- Decide what your goals are with your loans. Do you want them paid down fast and furiously with the least possible amount of interest? Do you want the maximum amount of time to get your business up and running before you have to begin to pay them back? Do you want to seek maximum loan forgiveness? Knowing your goals, as in any other aspect of life, will help you determine how to proceed with your loans.

- Some repayment options will mean more paperwork, phone calls, and time to get your ducks in a row. Stafford and Direct

PLUS loans have the most options, so if you have other types of loans, check with your school loan/finance office for more information about available options.

▶ Deferment and forbearance

If you are trying to put off the first payment as long as possible or if you are having difficulty making loan payments in your first years in practice, ask each lender if you qualify for a forbearance or deferment. In some cases, this may reduce interest payments as well as penalties.

- A **deferment** is where your loan payments are temporarily suspended for certain situations like economic hardship, unemployment, military service, or enrollment in school. If you are granted a deferment, your interest will be suspended on subsidized Direct or FFEL, Stafford Loans, or Federal Perkins Loans.

- A **forbearance** is a temporary suspension of loan payments because you are experiencing economic difficulties but are not eligible for a deferment. With a forbearance, interest will still accumulate on the loan.

To keep your payments low for the life of the loan, consider an income-based repayment (IBR) option. This is a payment plan whereby your payments are based on your income and family size, not your loan amount. Personally, I suggest most of you apply for an IBR or Pay-As-You-Earn plan as soon as possible if your loans qualify. I have put links with more information about this on the website, in the Web Tools and Links section.

For example, a family of four with an income of $40K and debt of $88K will pay $60-90 per month depending upon the interest rate. When you make payments under the IBR plan and your payment isn't enough to cover your student loan interest on federal Stafford Loans, the government will pay the difference for up to three consecutive years. Any remaining amount due on the loan after 25 years of payment is canceled, which could add up to huge savings if you have a large student loan. To apply for IBR, contact your student loan servicer. More details are available at http://www.ibrinfo.org/.

- Research the consolidation options available to you for each lender. Most student loan lenders like Sallie Mae and Nelnet offer loan consolidation programs whereby you are able to combine your loans into one loan and make a single payment, but they do not have forgiveness programs for steady long-time payers such as Stafford and Direct loans do. Interest rates vary from program to program, so compare the interest rates offered by each lender to the current interest rate you are paying on your various loans. Based on where you can get the best overall rate, choose a lender to consolidate your loan and then fill out the necessary paperwork. Some lenders make a loan consolidation application available online.

- If your student loan debt is high relative to your income, you may also qualify for the Pay-As-You-Earn Repayment Plan. This option gives you the lowest possible monthly payment and can be used for Direct Loans of varying types. For details about which loans are eligible, check out http://studentaid.ed.gov/repay-loans/understand/plans/pay-as-you-earn.

- Make your payments on time to avoid penalties. Consider setting up an auto-pay from your bank account so you don't have to think too much about this each month.

A school official interviewed for this chapter stated that one major reason why costs for school are so high is that the process of getting and maintaining accreditation, which is what allows students to get government loans, is so expensive! If she is right, what a cruel irony that is.

CHAPTER 4 | Dealing with Your Student Loan Debt

POWER POINTS

1. You may pay more interest with an IBR because of the extended payment period. In general, if you have a large loan debt and small income, IBR will result in interest savings for you. However, if you have a small debt and a larger income, you may end up paying more interest. (If this is true, you should probably just pay the thing off as quickly as you can in any case). Ask your lender for details about how much interest you will be paying before signing up for IBR.

2. If you've already decided to apply for IBR, make sure your lender has updated income information for you before the annual anniversary of your enrollment in the program so they can determine your payment for the next year. A missed deadline can result in a much higher payment not taking your income into account. At the time of this writing, lenders aren't required to notify borrowers about this deadline. Borrowers using this program have reported that it can take up to three months to process the paperwork, and processing delays can also trigger a high payment.

If you're unsure about your anniversary date or what type of documents you have to submit, contact your loan servicer for more information.

More resources

www.eriseducation.com has a nice chart breaking down various types of repayment plans based on your personal repayment goals.

http://www.student-loanforgiveness.net/public-service-student-loan-forgiveness-program.html This site is full of information on debt forgiveness, consolidation, and all types of repayment plans. This specific page discusses the new loan forgiveness options for people who have Federal Perkins loans and Federal Direct loans, which are treated the same as Stafford loans.

www.ehow.com:how_12086368_rid-student-loan-interest-penalties.html This page has some very detailed, easy-to-follow instructions on how to manage your loans intelligently and when to use which type of payment plan and schedule.

Legal Stuff You Need to Know and Do | 5

Papers you need to start with

Operating a business takes ambition and perseverance. It also takes some start-up capital, a good location, and some required pieces of paper, the number and variety of which depend on the state where you practice. Some of these must go on your wall; others can be filed until you need them.

Your diploma

All states in the U.S. that offer a license to practice acupuncture now require you to have graduated from an accredited school of acupuncture/Chinese medicine and have a diploma that says so. Depending on your state, your diploma could be needed for a variety of things, but definitely for state licensure and malpractice insurance. Therefore, I recommend that before framing your diploma for display in your office, first make a digital scan and then make a half dozen paper copies to keep in a file. When you get to the last paper copy after a couple of years, you have the digital one to make more when/if needed.

National certification

Many states require you to be certified by the National Certification Commission for Acupuncture and Oriental Medicine (NCCAOM). If this is true for you, contact them as early as possible. There is an application process for taking the written exams for acupuncture, foundations of Oriental medicine, Chinese herbal medicine, biomedicine basics, and Oriental bodywork. Depending upon which ones you take, this is a few thousand dollars. So call early and be prepared mentally and financially.

> Visit them at www.nccaom.org or call (904) 598-1005.

Business license

If required at all in your state, this license is obtained through your local government. Contact your city government and ask. There may or may not be a fee or renewal requirements. It is usually straightforward and inexpensive since most cities and towns want new businesses, even small ones like yours.

Resale license

If you live in a state or city with sales tax on either services or product sales, then you need a resale permit. This allows you to act as a middleman for the city and/or state, collecting sales tax and sending it to them on a scheduled basis. Find out how to apply for this license in your state by searching Sales Tax + Your State and follow the links. For $99 (at this moment in time) you can get legalzoom.com to do all the paperwork for you!

➤ What pieces of paper must go on your walls?

When you have completed all of the above, you will have some items that should go on your walls, either in your waiting area or in your history-taking or treatment room. Anything that must be visible to everyone visiting your office will state "must be posted" or "must be visible." Usually your state license to practice, a business license if you have one, and your resale license if you have sales tax, need to be out where people can see them. In addition, you will of course want to put your diploma and certification from the NCCAOM where patients will see it.

Remember, no matter how far away from a Western medical practice style you think you want to be, your patients expect to see some things that echo an MD's office. These diplomas and certificates help them feel safe, confident in your abilities, and foster placebo effect. When it comes to the matting and framing of your certificates, get it done professionally. Not only can it last for years, it shows pride in your achievement and in your profession.

Where can you practice?

As of this edition, there are only a few states that do not have some type of acupuncture statute: Wyoming, Alabama, North Dakota, Oklahoma, and South Dakota. However, not having an acupuncture statute does not necessarily mean that you cannot practice there. For example, the laissez-faire state of Wyoming has no statute and does not regulate acupuncture at all, but you can practice there if you keep your nose clean and stay out of trouble. South Dakota and Oklahoma also have practitioners, but they stay under the radar and practice quietly.

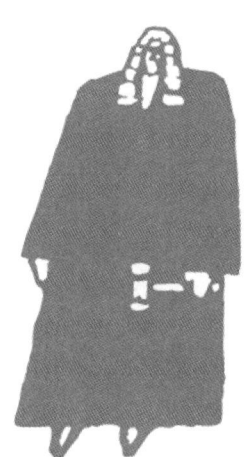

The Kansas law will allow you to practice only under the supervision and referral of an MD, DO, or DC. Of particular note is Louisiana, which does have an acupuncture statute but only allows practitioners to work directly for a physician.

Please note that laws are changing all the time and may be changing as I write this. NCCAOM.org, Acupuncture.com, and Acufinder.com keep reasonably up-to-date lists.

What can you call yourself in your state?

For most states, your title is some version of "Acupuncturist." It may be Licensed Acupuncturist (L.Ac.), Registered Acupuncturist (Reg.Ac. or R.Ac.), Acupuncture Physician (A.P.) or Certified Acupuncturist (C.A.). The following is a list of states that fall outside the lines of this conformity:

Florida: There is some confusion about acupuncture titles in Florida. Evidently you can be an L.Ac., A.P., or a Dipl.OM. A lengthy review of the Florida State Licensure website has given me no more clarity on these titles than when I started. Their state association, FSOMA, may be helpful if you plan to move there.

Louisiana: Acupuncture Assistant. You have to actually work for a physician.

Nevada: Here you are either a DOM (Doctor of Oriental Medicine) or an Acupuncture Assistant. You become a DOM by practicing for four years either someplace else or graduating from a four-year school. You become an Acupuncture Assistant by working under a DOM in Nevada. If you are interested in practicing in Nevada and have been working someplace else for four years or more, please contact the Nevada Department of Regulatory Agencies before moving to make sure you meet their requirements. (702) 837-8921.

New Mexico: Doctor of Oriental Medicine

Rhode Island: Doctor of Acupuncture

▶ How to get licensed in your state

The licensing authority in each state varies. In some states it is through the Department of Regulatory Agencies (DORA), in others the Department of Health. Each state requires different items with your application. Usually a copy of your diploma, in most states your NCCAOM and Clean Needle Technique certificates, often proof of malpractice insurance, and always a check. Every state has a license fee, but the cost varies widely from state to state. Both NCCAOM and Acupuncture.com have a link to every state agency on their websites.

▶ Why you need malpractice insurance

With continued growth of our profession along with changing views of acupuncture across the U.S., Canada, Australia, and Europe, more and more people are seeking our services. This is good for the growth of our profession, but also means that more of us will get sued. According to Michael Schroeder, Chief Counsel and Vice President of the American Acupuncture Council since 1986, lawsuits against acupuncturists have remained statistically flat over the last 15 years (1998-2013), increasing only at the same rates as our professional numbers increase. That's good news. Still, malpractice insurance is a relatively inexpensive way to protect your personal assets and your patient population if you are sued for a mistake or involved in a "nuisance" suit. This could happen to any of us.

In many states malpractice insurance is required for licensure. And if you wish to work in a hospital or any type of Western medical healthcare setting, or if you wish to bill third-party payers (insurance of any type), malpractice insurance will be a requirement whether your state asks you to have it or not.

The point is this—none of us thinks we could ever do anything harmful to another person while practicing within our scope. Even were that true, it does not mean that you won't ever make a mistake or that a patient will not make something up. When that happens, malpractice insurance is a saving grace. As long as you were within the guidelines of your abilities, training, and professional scope, your malpractice insurance will be there to cover your losses and to prevent you from losing everything you have built.

Malpractice insurance, whether or not it is required for licensure by your state, is really a cost of doing business that all of us should maintain. Every other medical provider you can name carries it, neither because they are negligent or sloppy, nor because they are fearful of false claims being brought against them. They maintain coverage because it is the professional thing to do and it protects their practice and their families as well as their patients.

> **PRACTITIONER POINTER**
>
> "Twenty years ago, I was accused by my state's Board of Medical Examiners of practicing medicine without a license. The charges were dropped, but what a nightmare! I can't recommend too highly hiring a top-notch lawyer to protect you from frivolous lawsuits and having a good malpractice policy to protect you from your own mistakes."
>
> —Bob Flaws
> Boulder, CO

As insurance coverage and access to Western medical treatment facilities with more seriously ill patient populations grows around the world, rest assured that we will be scrutinized, both our individual abilities and our profession as a whole. While our medicine may be rooted in an ancient tradition, we live and practice in modern times. As such, we need to be professionals that conform to the expected standards of our culture. That includes carrying adequate malpractice insurance coverage.

▶ Where to get malpractice insurance

The number of companies offering malpractice insurance for acupuncturists has grown over the past decade. At the time of this writing, there are at least eight companies out there easily found with a quick web search, and there may be more. There are important coverage questions to ask, the answers to which vary by company. You need to know whether they cover (either in the policy itself or as a policy rider): injection therapy, direct moxibustion, obstetrics-related acupuncture and whether it must be directly supervised by an obstetrician. You need to know if the policy is "claims made" or "per occurrence" and what that implies. Also, some companies offer less expensive policies for part-time or first-year practitioners, so be sure to ask about that as well. The companies (in alphabetical order) are:

    American Acup. Council – www.acupuncturecouncil.com

    Eastern Special Risk – www.easternspecialrisk.com

    Healthcare Providers Service Organization – http://www.hpso.com

    MIEC Insurance Cooperative – http://www.miec.com/ (available in California and Hawaii only)

    Norcal Mutual Insurance Group – http://www.norcalmutual.com (available in California only)

    OUM Healthcare Professionals Program – https://www.oumhealthcare.com

CHAPTER 5 | Legal Stuff You Need to Know and Do

Scott Danahy Naylon Co. – http://scottdanahynaylon.com

Wood Insurance Group – www.woodinsurancegroup.com

➤ General liability insurance

Any business with people walking in and around it is ethically and economically advised to carry general liability insurance to cover trips and falls or other accidents that may occur on your property or the property you are leasing. Almost every insurance company can give you a quote for this coverage. It is usually not expensive. Find a good price and a company you trust.

➤ HIPAA (Health Insurance Portability and Accountability Act of 1996)

Unless you read long government documents in lieu of counting sheep, the only thing about HIPAA that matters is knowing which practitioners it applies to and what they must do to comply. Some sources used to say that HIPAA applies only to healthcare practitioners who transmit a patient's pro-tected health information (PHI) electronically for various insurance purposes. It isn't true. Even if you don't (yet) bill insurance or transmit patients' PHI electronically, all of us collect a certain amount of protected health information from our patients in the normal course of practice. For that reason, we all fall under at least the privacy and accountability part of the HIPAA law. It is not that difficult to comply.

First, you must tell the patient *in advance of* their first treatment how you will both protect and use their PHI. You must protect all computer records (*i.e.,* password-protected databases and computers, a firewall if connected to the internet), and you must try to prevent unauthorized access to paper medical records (*i.e.,* keep them behind the front desk and in locking medical file cabinets). You have to note in the patient's chart each time you disclose any information (*i.e.,* faxing records to their MD or insurance company) and in some cases get their permission.

43

SECTION ONE: GETTING UP AND RUNNING

On your clinic's patient information forms you must ask:

- what phone number and address is okay for you to use to contact them.
- for their permission to send out newsletters and postcards, and give them a way to opt out of the mailings.
- permission in advance to send appointment reminders.

Patients need to be given a privacy practices notice to read and sign, and they are allowed to read your clinic's privacy policy whenever they want to or take one with them if they so desire, which means you must have such a policy written down. If your clinic has a website, your privacy policy must be on that as well.

All of this is done to protect patients' rights to privacy. However, it does not apply when trying to secure payment for services, normal clinic operations, or anything done for the care of the patient. This means that if a patient owes you money, you need not ask permission to send the bill to their house or to try to contact them by phone. You can also share their private information with a collection agency, but we hope you never have to do that!

There are a few other parts and pieces to HIPAA compliance, none of them very scary. For a more detailed description and how to comply, see Section 2, Chapter 9.

POWER POINT

What is the definition of PHI?
A patient's PHI is anything that "relates to the past, present, or future physical or mental health or condition of an individual, the provision of health care to an individual, or the past, present, or future payment for the provision of health care to an individual." [Public Law 104-191, August 21, 1996 – Health Insurance Portability and Accountability Act of 1996. http://aspe.hhs.gov/admnsimp/pl104191.htm.

CHAPTER 5 | Legal Stuff You Need to Know and Do

▶ Maintaining patient and financial records

Tax returns, financial receipts, and patient information must all be maintained for a certain number of years. The IRS says that financial documents, such as credit card sales receipts and deposit slips, need to be maintained for three years, or for two years after the taxes they support have been filed, whichever is longer. The best bet is to keep all supporting documentation for at least three years after the taxes have been filed. An IRS audit can go back three years unless you are found guilty of a crime, in which case they can audit your tax returns as far back as they want (so don't cheat). These records shouldn't take up yards of space. Keep them all together in a large envelope or folder labeled with the year. Also, legal eagles suggest keeping all original receipts, not scanned digital versions; these may not be acceptable if you are audited.

Where patient medical records are concerned, laws about their maintenance vary from state to state; there is no federal guideline. However, each state's statute of limitations is a good guideline to follow. Your state's requirement should be easy to find online.

Your malpractice insurance company will tell you to keep the records forever since patients have two years from the discovery of a problem in which to file a suit. It might be difficult for a complainant to prove malpractice 5-6 years after seeing you, but you never know what crazy case a lawyer will be willing to take! Thus, some sources say medical records should be maintained indefinitely. This is as easy as a back-up drive, the cloud, or a labeled CD if your records are digital. If you have only paper records, keep them at least as long as the statute of limitations (2-3 years for medical claims in most states). These need not be kept at your clinic. At the end of each year you can pull all paper charts of patients who have not come in for two years. Place them in a box in alphabetical order, label the contents as

Inactive Patients, and store them in a safe, dry location. Type a list of the charts contained in each box; keep one copy of this list inside the box and one at your office. When/if that patient returns, you know right where the old chart is and can easily retrieve it. If you keep your patient information digitally, this job is unnecessary.

If you use a patient sign-in sheet (not required but good if you bill workers' compensation), keep them for at least five years. Scanned and digitized is fine, or maintain all of one year's sheets in a binder, labeled with the year on the spine. There is a statute of limitations for a worker to file a claim, but lawsuits about these claims can go on for years in the courts.

In the case of the death of a patient, maintain the chart either indefinitely or for the term of the statute of limitations set by your state (typically 2-3 years). In the case of your death, your clinic records were your property and, as such, they are part of your estate and must be handled by whomever is settling it. Your will should state how such records will be handled. Typically, patients will be notified of their practitioner's passing by the obituary in the local paper, general word of mouth, or through a mass mailing to the practitioner's patient roster. The records can be kept long enough for people to claim them if they so desire, say 60-90 days. Then the remaining charts can be destroyed.

▶ Patient charting requirements

Always remember the golden rule of medical charting: *If you didn't write it down, it didn't happen.* Write down everything that occurs with patients, including phone conversations as well as any referrals to other practitioners that you may suggest. In paper charts, each page should contain the patient's name, age, sex, the date of service (or other interaction), and the initials of the practitioner. Your writing needs to be legible and in blue or black ink. If you need to add something to a chart-note after the fact, write it on a separate piece of paper with the date the information was added and sign that page.

While taking notes, if you have to make a change or if you write something in error, line it out with one straight line and write your initials indicating you are noting a change or error. The information must still be legible. Don't scribble or erase and don't use white-out.

> **POWER POINT**
>
> While many pracs still maintain patient records on paper, more of us are moving to electronic medical records (EMR). For any of us who work in a state that now recognizes acupuncture as an essential health benefit and are not operating a community-style clinic where no insurance is billed, EMR is going to be a requirement for participation in the system. In fact, if you bill third-party payers of any type, you will, at the very least, need to be able to use an electronic billing system of some type even if you don't maintain electronic records. For a lot more detail on EMR, see Section 2, Chapter 8.

If you are using a computer-based system for maintaining patient records, the software itself should have systems for these situations.

POINTS TO PONDER FROM CHAPTER 5

- Put your school diploma, any state or national certifications, and your tax license on the wall in your clinic. The tax license is a legal requirement; the diploma and certificates give your patients confidence.

- Check one of the websites we reference to learn about your state laws, what paperwork you must send to your state regulatory agency to practice there, and the amount of the application or annual fees.

- You cannot practice acupuncture legally in Alabama, Oklahoma, North Dakota, or South Dakota, and only directly under an MD in Louisiana and Kansas.

- Even if not required in your state, we suggest malpractice insurance. There are many good reasons to get it.

- For HIPAA, basically you must make every effort to keep your patient records confidential and you must tell your patients how you are going to do that. See Section 2, Chapter 9 for more detail.

- Maintain patient records for the period of time that is your state's statute of limitations or as long as your malpractice insurance company requests.

- Keep your patient records neat. No scribbling, no white-out, date and patient name on every page.

- Electronic medical records will be required with the changes coming under the Affordable Care Act. If you want to work inside the system or bill third-party payers, you'll need to be using some type of electronic recordkeeping system or at least have access to an online billing system such as OfficeAlly.

The Best Business Model for Your Practice | 6

▶ **Food for thought**

You may not be ready to think about what type of legal structure is best for your future business. While you read this chapter, however, know that the information here is to help you learn the ramifications of this decision or to help give you a nudge toward one or another model. Furthermore, while most new business owners begin as sole proprietors, you may decide to change at any point if another form of doing business becomes more appropriate. The information in this chapter will help you understand the pros and cons of each business model as well as the tax and legal implications.

▶ **Taxes we all must pay**

The structure of your business will determine the way you and your business are taxed. We all pay taxes—  perhaps to our city, county, and state, but definitely to the IRS. Additionally, we pay Social Security and Medicare, and possibly workers' compensation and unemployment insurance. It's best to set up an easy system for keeping track of it and do it with goodwill because, to some extent, it is unavoidable. While there are many things as a business entity that you can write off your taxable income quite legally (more on that in Section 2, Chapter 1), you should actually hope you make a lot of money and that you will be able to pay your taxes easily! We all grumble and gripe about taxes sometimes, but if you want to be in business, at the end of the day (actually the end of each month or quarter), you will be sending a check to Uncle Sam and possibly a few other government entities as well. The way you pay these taxes will vary depending upon the type of business structure you choose for your clinic.

49

Robert Kiyosaki, author of the *Rich Dad, Poor Dad* series, suggests we think of ourselves as being "in partnership with the government." We need road maintenance, schools, public parks, police and firefighters, all of which are supported by our tax dollars. Since this is not a book on radical politics or tax evasion, I encourage you to live within the system with as much intelligence as you can. I hope this chapter helps.

▶ Sole proprietor

A sole proprietor is the simplest business model. Although often a business of just one person, a married couple working together can form one sole proprietorship as well. Otherwise, if two people combine to run a business, they must form some other business entity or have two separate sole proprietorships.

In this model, the business and the person operating it are one entity from a legal and tax point of view. You get all of the profits from your business, but you are also *personally* responsible for all debts and liabilities, legal and financial. If someone sues you and you lose, both your personal and business assets are in jeopardy, so malpractice insurance is even more important for practitioners using this business model.

The main advantage of being a sole proprietor, and why so many people start out that way, is that it is the simplest and least expensive business model. You register your business name, get a bank account with a DBA, and a tax license and that's it. If the business needs to be dissolved, you close the bank account, remove any internet access, and the business is gone.

All profits from a sole proprietor business are reported on the owner's personal income tax form 1040. Along with that, you need to file a Schedule C: Profit or Loss from Business. Also, since there is regular income, you must file quarterly self-employment taxes (Schedule SE). This prevents you from having one huge tax payment on April 15. The IRS rule is that, if you will owe more than $500 in annual taxes, you are required to make quarterly self-employment tax payments or you'll be hit with a penalty.

Some disadvantages to being a sole proprietor include:
- Not all of your expenses will be deductible, especially those pertaining to employee benefits such as health insurance.
- Above a fairly low amount of income, you are likely to pay more taxes to the federal government.
- There is nothing to limit your personal liability in a lawsuit except a good malpractice insurance policy.

Partnerships

Legally, a partnership means two or more people combining business efforts with the same benefits and disadvantages as a sole proprietorship. There is no protection of personal assets, nor a legal distinction between the owners and the business. Partners should have a legal agreement setting forth how decisions will be made, profits will be shared, disputes will be resolved, how future partners will be admitted, how they can be bought out, and what steps will be taken to dissolve the partnership when needed.

As with sole proprietors, profits of a partnership model flow directly to the partners' personal income tax returns, and self-employment tax payments must be made on a quarterly basis. At the end of the year, each partner receives a Partnership Return of Income (Form 1065) and a Partner's Share of Income, Credit and Deductions (Schedule K-1). Again, not all employee benefits are available as deductions to the partners.

I don't suggest this type of business for acupuncturists! If one of your partners borrows money, signs a contract in the name of the business without your knowledge, or does anything illegal, you are also responsible! While working with others can be beneficial and satisfying, there are other forms of business that allow you the benefits without the shortcomings.

▶ Corporations

A corporation is considered by law to be a unique entity, separate from those who own it. A corporation can be taxed, can be sued, or can enter into contractual agreements. The owners of a corporation are shareholders, who elect a board of directors to oversee major policies and decisions. The corporation has a life of its own and does not dissolve when ownership changes.

Creating a corporation for your business gives you some legal protection against lawsuits. However, as described above, anyone can be held liable for personal actions, whether they happen at work or not. That being said, a corporation/LLC model may at some point be better for you than a sole proprietorship.

Should you decide to set up a corporation, there are many books available on how to form one and tons of online companies that help you to do so inexpensively in your state. Your corporation will have to be formed and recorded in the state in which you intend to practice. Most states perform this function through the corporation division of the Secretary of State's office. Below is a short breakdown of the various types of corporations and their tax and legal implications.

1. C-Corporation

The original "big-boy" corporation, all other corporate entities are based-on or scaled-down versions of the C-Corp. Usually applicable only for large companies, this structure provides personal protection to the shareholders and the benefit of being able to go public to raise capital. A C-Corp, however, has the notable drawback of double taxation, which means that corporate profits are taxed first and then any dividends paid to the shareholders (you in this case) are also taxed. You can look up requirements for your state if interested, but this is rarely a logical choice for small medical clinics.

2. S-Corporation

An S-Corporation, legally, is mostly the same as a C-Corp. The difference is that the S-Corp has "pass-through taxation," thus avoiding the double taxation mentioned above. Instead, dividends (called distributions in the case of an S-Corp) are recorded and taxed only on the shareholders' personal tax returns. The best thing about this is, while you have to pay yourself some salary, you can pay yourself partially in distributions in addition to the salary, on which you do not pay any Social Security or Medicare (FICA). This is a 15.3% savings on those distributions! (LLCs, discussed below, have the same benefit if they choose to file as an S-Corp.)

An S-Corp has the same requirements for organizing as a C-Corp. Annual meetings, annual reports, and an elected board of directors/officers are required, and at least one shareholder. Forming an S-Corp usually requires some legal assistance, but is far less expensive and complex than a C-Corp. Look online for companies who do this for reasonable rates in your state.

3. Professional Corporation (PC)

The Professional Corporation was invented for private practitioners in the health industry. At one point, it offered the same types of benefits that an LLC now offers. However, since its inception, the cost and effectiveness of a PC has been surpassed by the LLC (discussed below). The PC offers its owner-members personal protection from the liabilities of other members of a group office as well as allowing for the flexibility of operating as an S-Corporation.

This type of corporation is restricted to those in the professional world: doctors, accountants, architects, acupuncturists, etc. In California, it is your only option besides an S-Corp (LLCs are not allowed). All persons operating under a PC must be licensed in the field in which they are practicing. A PC must have a board of directors/officers, is required to hold recorded annual meetings, and must establish bylaws for operation.

4. Limited Liability Company (LLC)

The most flexible model of all, an LLC allows you to operate as a partnership if necessary, but gives owners the protection of a corporation. An LLC can be taxed as either a corporation or a partnership, though this must be declared at the time of organization. Like a corporation, an LLC can own property or enter into contracts. However, since the company may or may not dissolve when ownership changes, most contracts include the name of your LLC as well as the individual names of members.

The LLC is now permissible in most states, but not for acupuncturists in California. Less expensive and requiring less paperwork than a corporation (no annual meetings or reports), LLC owners are called members, not shareholders. As in a partnership, members share profits as well as losses from the business. Shares of the company are divided among members based on percentage of ownership since each must put actual assets into the LLC to be a member. An LLC can be taxed like a partnership, each member reporting their share on personal income taxes, or like an S-corporation with members receiving part salaries and part distributions from company profits. This decision must be made when filing for your Employer Identification Number or EIN (use IRS Form SS-4 to do this).

If an LLC chooses to be taxed as a partnership, the same tax forms as for a partnership are used. Members are paid their share of the profits in lieu of salaries, reporting quarterly to the

IRS on a Schedule SE with an estimated tax payment. The main difference is that most employee benefits are deductible from the profits of the company so members won't pay taxes on them. In a partnership or sole proprietorship, they are not deductible. At tax time, members receive a copy of the form 1065 and a K-1, which shows the division of the profits or losses from the company at the end of the previous tax year.

An LLC protects its members from double taxation but, unless members chose to file as an S-Corp and take some of their pay as distributions, they will pay more taxes in the form of Social Security/Medicare, as discussed above in the section on S-Corps. With less paperwork required for an LLC than the other corporate choices, this is a good one to consider if you are opening a clinic with one or more partners.

4. Non-profit corporations [501(c)3]

This corporation is different from all the others in that it is not taxed at all! The corporation itself does not pay federal, state, property, and often not even sales taxes. Regular payroll taxes and FICA, however, are taken from the salaries of the people who work for a non-profit (you). Acupuncturists form non-profit corporations in order to obtain grants to do research, treat underserved populations, and otherwise do good works in the world. There are several models for this in our profession doing all sorts of interesting work both in the U.S. and abroad.

If you have this interest, you need the help of a lawyer to file the paperwork (extensive), good writing skills for grant writing, and a clear idea of what you wish to do in order for the IRS to say "yes" to your application. At the time of this writing, the fee for a 501(c)3 application is $850 to the IRS, $50 to most states. As a member of the Board of Directors, you have some limited liability protection, but not for your acupuncture practice, so get malpractice insurance as well.

SECTION ONE: GETTING UP AND RUNNING

▶ A word about being sued

From the descriptions below, you can see that a corporate structure or LLC provides you with some level of personal protection; a sole proprietorship does not. However, while a corporation may protect your personal assets from a legal judgment against you or your business, it does nothing to keep you from being named in a lawsuit. If someone wants to sue you, they can. Of course being named in a lawsuit, though a bummer and a hassle, does not mean there will be a decision against you, but anyone *can* be named.

The protection granted to a business operating as a corporation (or one of the corporate variations) is for your personal assets only. That means if you are sued and there is a judgment against you, your malpractice insurance and company holdings can be gone after, but not your home, savings accounts and investments, your brand new Harley, or your condo at the beach. Especially if you are going into business with a partner or two, a corporate structure or LLC will provide protection for your personal assets if or when you or someone in your business makes an inadvertent error.

Also, it is important to be aware that this protection is only applicable to actions for or within your business, within your scope of practice, and without malfeasance or negligence. That being said, let's take a look at the pros and cons of each business model.

▶ What's best for you?

You may not be ready to think about business model options when you first start a practice and are

> **PRACTITIONER POINTER**
>
> "My business has been set up as an S-Corp from day one. Is it the best way? I really don't know, but accountants have advised me to do this for the greatest tax benefit. They leave the medicine to me and I leave the business/taxes/legal stuff to them."
>
> —Susan Schiff
> Delray Beach, FL

more concerned with getting patients in the door. That's why most practitioners start out as sole proprietors and may never change business models over the life of their practice, which is fine. Questions to ask yourself include, "Do I have personal assets that I want to protect more than my malpractice insurance will? Do I wish to have partners in my business? Am I making enough that the impact of Social Security/Medicare (FICA) tax would be less with an S-Corp or an LLC filing as an S-Corp?" Depending upon the answers to these questions, another model may be a better choice, and we think it is wise to have knowledge about your options. We also advise that you discuss these options and any questions you might have about them with an attorney or tax accountant or both as your practice grows and develops.

POINTS TO PONDER FROM CHAPTER 6

- Because there is much to think about when you first start up as a business, most practitioners start as sole proprietors without thinking about other business models.

- Taxes for each type of business are assessed differently and each offers a different level of legal separation between the owner's assets and the business's assets.

- As a sole proprietor, there is no separation between your personal assets and your business if you are sued. You are also personally responsible for all debts and liabilities of your business. However, closing your business is as easy as locking the door, unplugging the phone, and taking down your website.

- Partnerships require a great degree of trust in that you are legally responsible for each other's business

"Points to Ponder" continue on the next page

conduct. In a partnership you create a contract specifying how to share the profits or losses experienced by your business. Otherwise . . .

- Partners should make sure that their business charter or contract clearly delineates the financial terms when the business is dissolved.

- There are three types of corporations, an S-Corp, a C-Corp, and a PC or Professional Corp. Most private professionals who wish to incorporate for legal protection or tax advantages should consider either an S-Corp or a PC.

- An LLC provides almost the same level of legal protection as a corporation and avoids the problem of double taxation. It also has some of the same features as a partnership. For people wanting to open a group clinic with a clearly defined financial and legal relationship between and among themselves, the LLC is an option to consider seriously.

- There are lots of books and websites on the pros and cons of each business model. Beyond the basics, it's a good idea to consult either an accountant or attorney when setting up and filing papers for anything other than a sole proprietorship.

Working with Others | 7

Owning your own business is not for the faint of heart. Being the *sole* manager/owner/operator is, at least for many people, even more challenging. While working alone does have advantages, it is also accompanied by challenges that, for some, are easier to manage if they can be shared.

Working alone gives you ultimate decision-making power, with no one else's opinions or feelings to complicate anything. There is also the benefit of not having to share the income that your business generates. However, working alone means you are the sole source of energy, income generation, creative juice, and marketing efforts.

Having a partner that you trust (irrespective of the legal form of your business) can be of benefit to you and to your patients, providing additional "qi" and giving you the peace of mind of knowing someone has your back. For example, during a family emergency or at other times when you need to leave your business for a few hours or a few weeks with very little notice, or when you take a vacation, you cannot just close your doors for a week or more without losing current or potential patients. A clinic partner who can take care of your current patients and keep your doors open for new ones is invaluable in these situations.

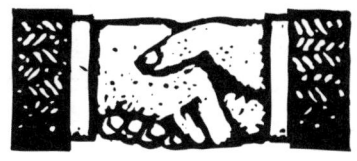

In addition to covering each other's patients when needed, a clinic partner can spark your creativity, be another voice in your community, give you a reality check when needed, and generally share the work load. Sharing ideas with someone who has just as

59

much at stake in the business as you do can take the smallest idea and transform it into something profitable for you and for your patients. Two minds are usually better than one, especially if your relationship allows honest give and take and is based on respect and goodwill.

Sharing educational costs is another possible benefit of a clinic partnership. (I'll reiterate that I'm NOT talking here about the legal term "partnership".) With hundreds of educational events each year, having a colleague to share this potentially vast pool of information is a huge benefit to both practitioners as well as the patients. The information from any class can be shared with the partner who kept the clinic running while the other was away, and you can both learn something new. The next time, it's the other partner's turn. You can also share a clinic library, but be sure to label which books belong to each of you!

More practitioners (especially energetic ones) mean more income for each/all of you. Thinking that having partners will mean you make less money is an inaccurate assumption. Having two or more 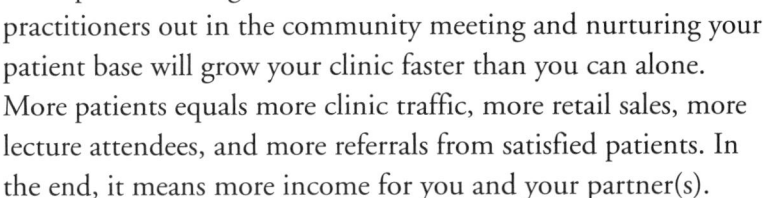 practitioners out in the community meeting and nurturing your patient base will grow your clinic faster than you can alone. More patients equals more clinic traffic, more retail sales, more lecture attendees, and more referrals from satisfied patients. In the end, it means more income for you and your partner(s).

Another good reason to have a partner is the benefit to all your patients. In your career as a health professional, there will sometimes be patients who are not a "fit" for you or your treatment style. Instead of referring that person to some other clinic altogether (though occasionally that may be the appropriate response), there is another practitioner right there in your office. When this works, you don't lose that potential income to your business. Another situation that happens is the patient whose improvement plateaus–they just stop getting better. Before they lose faith and leave your care, you can, if appropriate, refer this patient to your partner. This gives the patient a new treatment style that may help them continue to improve without your clinic losing the income. You can say something like, "Nancy, I'm going to have you see my colleague, Sarah, next visit. She can give your condition a fresh look and she uses treatments that are not part of my training. I think she can help you continue to improve." Let your partner read your chart notes, ask questions about the diagnosis, and discuss further treatment options. In this way, the patient wins and so do you.

➤ Take a look in the mirror

Before you begin your search for a colleague to share your business, take a deep and realistic look at who you are and your style of business management and patient interaction. Be as honest with yourself as you can about your strengths and weaknesses. This will help you find a good match for your clinic partner and avoid the possible pitfalls of trying to work with someone who is not a good fit.

Start by assessing your own social or people skills. Are you a people person or a quiet type? Having at least one partner who is good with crowds, can socialize easily with folks from all walks of life, and is not shy about promoting your services is a huge asset if that is not your strength.

Also, one of you needs to be comfortable with number-crunching. Many new practitioners begin with something like QuickBooks to keep track of income and expenses, which is pretty easy and intuitive. Still, being able to work with numbers, being comfortable with math skills, careful with the recording of accounts receivable and payable, and understanding basic accounting terms is really helpful. Even when your business has grown enough to hire a bookkeeper, you will still need to keep track of some basic daily, weekly, and monthly financial information to operate securely and profitably.

The fundamental idea here is to find someone who is skilled in areas of running a business where you aren't as strong. Working with someone else can be a way to improve every area needed for business success: marketing, finances, operational systems, and patient care and education. This is good for you as practitioners and for your patients and community as well.

▶ Management and systems

Whether you form an LLC, a Non-profit Corporation, or are two Sole Proprietors, someone has to be the ultimate organizational brain of any company, creating clear business structures and systems that allow for smooth day-to-day operations. If that is something you feel comfortable creating, then find a co-worker or colleague who is a little less organized and who likes clear direction and systems within which to work. Otherwise, try to partner with someone who's had some managerial experience or perhaps owned their own business in the past. Even if he or she was not successful in their first business, sometimes those are the best lessons a businessperson ever learns.

▶ Operating agreements

When working with one or more other practitioners, as many operational details as possible should be in writing and signed by all parties in advance of opening your clinic (*i.e.*, a contract or operating agreement). Sit down together, perhaps with an attorney, and draft a contract or operating agreement. This agreement may seem unnecessary in the honeymoon stage of your new business, but will be an invaluable asset when and if the time comes to part ways.

POWER POINTS

Areas where you may need operational procedure guidelines:

- Herbal company choices, markup to patients
- Inventory management
- Profit-sharing agreement
- Hiring and firing procedures
- Confidentiality of all patient information
- Record-keeping and patient management
- Marketing activities
- Holidays and holiday/vacation pay
- Conflict resolution procedure
- What happens when one party wants to leave the business
- What happens if one partner dies or is incapacitated

No matter how well you get along now, things can happen that alter how you feel about each other. Additionally, circumstances change in life: marriages, children, divorces, ailing family members who need our care. It is under these circumstances that you will both be very happy that you have a contractual guideline for dealing with whatever has arisen.

You may be able to find a standard agreement on legal software available at an office supply store, or you can download forms from a company like Legalzoom.com. Regardless of the origin, format, or changes and additions you make to your contract, it is highly recommended that you have an attorney look over the document before all parties sign it. By using an online service or a legal forms software and the above list of topics, you may be able to write the lion's share of your agreement, but you don't want it to have "holes" that cause problems later. A small legal fee for gettiing it checked over is worth the money.

Please note that this is not a "partnership" agreement in the legal sense unless you are operating your business as a formal Partnership (see the previous chapter). It is simply the wise thing to do to create a contractual agreement with anyone you work with as an equal, regardless of the legal form of the business. If you have a corporation, for example, you already have corporate by-laws that govern behavior where the company is concerned. This is different in that you are establishing a working agreement to hammer out the legal/systems details of working together in the most collegial and clear way possible.

What should be in my operating agreement?
An operating agreement is very similar to an employee handbook, except that this one is for the owners. The best ones include as much as possible about the optimal operations of your clinic. You can start with how profits and losses are to be divided, a procedure for selling one's interest in the business (if that is relevant), everything about using the phone and computer for business or private purposes, who owns the herbs and other product lines, who is responsible for what activities (cleaning, marketing, signage, ordering of products and supplies, banking), vacations and sick days, what behaviors neither of you will tolerate, and, most importantly, conflict resolution. How will disagreements about any problem be resolved? If you do not specify and agree about this now, it can be very expensive and painful later on.

Capital, profits, and losses
Everything with regard to money needs to be as clear as a newly washed window on a sunny day. Whether the capital to start your company comes from one or both of you equally or from an outside source, be sure to state how capital is brought into the company. If you both have an equal share/stake in the company, you should share profits and losses equally; if the stake is not equal, then the division will be different. This is

most important where losses are concerned, especially if those losses are incurred from the normal operation of the business. An example of such a statement is:

> The profits of the business shall belong to the (members/owners/whatever you are called) equally (or at a certain percentage if relevant). All expenses incurred in the course of operating the business and any losses arising therefrom shall be paid out of the earnings of the business, or in the case of a loss, the losses shall be paid by the (again members/owners, etcetera) in equal shares.

This point needs to be absolutely clear between everyone concerned. If you go out of business for any reason, this section will be your guideline for handling any losses you may have incurred. Also, you don't want a business partner who is happy to share the profits equally but balks at sharing losses. Anyone who wants to be an owner must agree to the risks as well as the benefits of ownership.

Accounting
This section of the operating agreement, based on your business model, states how your accounting will be done and how you will pay your taxes. If you are a corporation, for example, then you receive paychecks throughout the year and taxes have already been deducted from those. Also in that case, you must pay quarterly estimated taxes on any corporate distributions that you took when there were profits to be shared between or among you over and above your salary.

What you all agree not to do
This section of your agreement, the list of prohibitions related to the owners' behavior specifically regarding the business, may be the most important. First, no partner may borrow money or use the business as security against a loan in the name of the business without the agreement of the other partner(s)/

member(s). And that's just the first item. This section can include anything you need it to. If you operate as a corporation, at least some of this will be covered in your by-laws. However, there are still areas that may not be. For example, you may wish to restrict each other to this one business at least for a time or not until the profit/loss equation of your agreement is amended to change the percentages. This may seem unnecessary, but if your partner decides to work full time in some other trade, leaving you to run things alone but still expecting a share of the profits, you will have a guideline for changing the agreement!

You should also have a section stating that the one partner cannot sell (or lease, trade, donate) their interest in the company without the other partners' agreement. This section can also describe a procedure for evaluating the worth of the business so that a share price can be agreed upon. If this is a corporation, this item will be addressed in your by-laws, but it will need to be written if you have some other business model.

Who owns the company name?
If one partner decides to leave the company but you started it together, the remaining owner typically keeps the name, but this needs to be stated clearly in your agreement.

First right of refusal
If one partner decides to sell their interest in the company, this concept requires that they first offer their interest to the remaining partner(s), with a set number of days for a decision to be made. If the other partner(s) don't buy, the leaving partner is free to sell to whomever they wish (unless you include specific requirements such as the new partner must be a licensed practitioner of specific healthcare professions [acupuncturist, naturopath, physical therapist, etc.] with so many years' experience and no outstanding lawsuits or malpractice claims against them and at the same or higher price than agreed upon

in this document). If the departing partner wants to lower the price, they must offer that price to the remaining partner(s) before it can be offered to someone outside the business.

Option to purchase on death or incapacity
Should one of the owners/partners perish or become disabled or unable to work, this section specifies the rights of and process to be followed with your partner's family or heirs. This section also helps you avoid someone from your partner's family wanting to help run your business. Make sure that this section includes specifics such as:

1. The surviving owner/partner(s) can purchase the interest/shares from the deceased or incapacitated owner/partner.
2. A price may be specified for this purchase. If it was not, then the matter shall be arbitrated or based on a professional valuation of the business.
3. The surviving owner/partner(s) keeps the business name if they keep the business.
4. If the surviving owner/partner(s) has no further desire to maintain the business, its assets are divided equally between the surviving partner(s) and the family of the deceased or disabled partner.

Arbitration or mediation
Settling a dispute outside of litigation in a courtroom is less expensive and less time-consuming if a serious disagreement should arise. It will help you keep the business operating smoothly and even may allow an agreeable resolution of the conflict.

If you and your partner cannot agree on a specific mediator, then you must hire three, one that each partner selects and a third selected by these two mediators. The decisions of the arbitration or mediation must be final and binding upon all parties and their respective heirs, executors, or assigns.

Amendments

The final section of your operating agreement covers how the document may be changed or amended as needed in the future. If you decide there is a reason to edit your contract, this section gives you the authority to do so without having to rewrite the entire thing!

You can see from this chapter that there are many things to think about when deciding to work with other people, irrespective of the business model you have chosen. It's worth the time to get this right before you open your doors. Skipping this work is a definite way to lose friendships down the road. This document allows everyone to understand what is expected of each other and what the group rules and regs are to keep your business operations smooth and your personal relationships alive and well. In the Letters/Contracts section of the website, there are examples more details as well as a contract example to give you a place to start.

CHAPTER 7 | Working with Others

POINTS TO PONDER FROM CHAPTER 7

Group working environments can be very satisfying and advantageous for a variety of reasons. Companionship, stability, group intelligence, shared responsibilities, expanded services to your clients, coverage of your practice when you go on vacation or if you have a personal emergency.... Those are just a few.

- Before entering a group clinic arrangement, however, consider what you bring to the table as a partner and what you want from the other party or parties to balance your strengths and weaknesses.

- Once you decide to open a clinic with one or more partners or friends, make sure you have a clear-cut, written agreement about everything you can think of. This helps you keep those friends. You may prepare an agreement using legal software, but getting it checked out by an attorney is not a bad idea.

- For more information on business models, including Partnerships in the legal sense of that word, see Chapter 6 in this section.

Getting a Job in Another Practitioner's Clinic | 8

While discussed briefly in Chapter 3, I feel this subject deserves more thorough treatment. Statistics from the world of chiropractic medicine show that new chiropractic graduates who take employment for a year or two with an experienced doctor before going out on their own grow their practices faster and easier when they do eventually go solo. This is logical. Getting experience with how an office is managed, how patient records are kept, how to successfully bill insurance companies, how problem patients are dealt with, how to manage a front office staff, hiring and firing practices, HIPAA record-keeping, and all the many details of running an office can only make any practitioner's transition to private practice easier.

This type of situation, while far less common in the world of Chinese medicine except for community acupuncture clinics, has advantages for the established practitioner as well as the new graduate, discussed below. I also encourage more practitioners with experience to provide these "mentoring" opportunities if their offices have the space to do so. This is a great boon to our profession as a whole!

> **PRACTITIONER POINTER**
>
> "When I got out of school, my most powerful experience was working directly in the clinics of two practitioners who very generously took the time to teach me many things. This included information about how they ran their clinics as well as how to handle difficult patients and avoid legal or interpersonal problems. I believe that if every experienced practitioner shared their knowledge in this way, many more young practitioners would succeed and prosper."
>
> —Laura Freeman
> San Rafael, CA

If this sounds attractive to you, here are a few strategies to find a practitioner who will allow you to get your feet wet in their clinic. Since it is the exception in our profession, finding such a job requires persistence and a little luck, but if this is what you want, here's how I would seek to make it happen.

▶ How to find a practitioner to hire you

You should begin your search during your final year of school. You don't want to find that someone-to-hire-you too many months before graduation, but you need to put together all the possible ways to find them early enough not to miss deadlines on any publications in which it might be useful to advertise.

1. Can you access your school's alumni through the administration or is there an alumni association that you can contact? Explain what you want to do in either case. They may not give you the list because of privacy concerns but may be willing to send your postcard or email if you pay any associated costs. If your school has an employment placement office, they may be able to help with this project.

2. If you cannot access your alumni directly, is there an alumni newsletter sent out from your school or through an alumni association? If so, find out the upcoming publication deadlines and if you can place a classified ad in the next issue. You want to place your ad in the issue that will go out 3-5 months prior to your licensure (so pretty close to the time of graduation).

3. Is there a state association newsletter and/or email list or chat group in your state? Most states where there are schools do have a state association. Similar to #2 above, find out their advertising deadlines and place an ad in that newsletter as well. We'll talk about what your ad might say below.

4. Join every Facebook and LinkedIn practitioner group and post what you are looking for on these groups as well. If there is no response, wait a month and do it again. Private message anyone whom you believe may be able to help you or spread the word to their groups.

5. If you wish to work in a community-style clinic, join POCA and watch their job listings weekly.

6. If you have no other possible way of getting to practitioners, go to the NCCAOM website and look up every practitioner in the state or city or area where you wish to practice. Those practitioners may not have graduated from your school, but you never know where opportunities will arise. Check out their websites, blogs, or Facebook pages, and contact all of them by whatever method you can.

7. If you are open to moving anywhere in the U.S. for a short period of time, you can place a classified ad in a national publication as well. With *Acupuncture Today*, for example, you can advertise in their paper publication as well as their web publication. This goes for Acufinder.com and any other similar online bulletin boards and resources you can find. Why not a Craigslist ad while you're at it?

I suggest you create a file for this project, in which you keep info about publications, websites, deadlines, (e)mailing lists, copies of the letters you sent or ads you placed, notes on phone conversations, and any "nibbles" you have received from your efforts—everything pertaining to this project. If you keep a calendar, put notations to yourself about follow-up phone calls, newsletter deadlines, or any other work that you need to do to make this job that you seek a reality. Be as organized as you can; this is no different from any other type of job search.

So, what should your ads, postcards, letters, or emails say to spark the interest of one or more practitioners to hire you? Below are some possible scripts you might use.

➤ Classified/Craigslist ad or web bulletin board posting

"Hey, practitioner! Too busy to file paperwork, manage forms, do outbound calls to patients, or market your practice as much as you'd like? I can help with all this and more. July 20XX graduate seeks full- or part-time position in established practice. Will work in reception, pharmacy, or clean bathrooms. Will trade work for use of clinic during evening or weekend hours. I am motivated, flexible, and creative. If you are interested in discussing this with me, call 111-222-3333 or email me at newgrad@acuweb.edu."

➤ Postcard or email copy

Email tends to be informal and you could use either similar text to the classified ad above or the postcard copy below. The postcard copy is a little more structured because it's on paper:

> Dear Practitioner,
> Too busy to file paperwork, file insurance forms, do outbound calls to patients, or market your practice as much as you'd like, I can help with all this and more. I am graduating from XYZ Acupuncture College in July 20XX and looking for a full- or part-time position in an established practice. I am happy to work as a receptionist, in your pharmacy, or clean bathrooms if that is your need. I will work for money or a partial trade for use of your clinic during evening or weekend hours. I am motivated, flexible, creative, and open to your ideas. If interested in discussing this with me, call 111-222-3333 or email me at newgrad@acuweb.edu. Help is just a phone call away!
> Thanks for your consideration. I look forward to hearing from you.
> Sincerely, Sally Jones

➤ Letter copy

For a letter you might want to be more formal and thorough. You could include a photo of yourself (a photo can also go in emails or on postcards), a copy of a research paper you did in school or other writing if you are good at it, or a curriculum vitae (CV) if you have an impressive before-acupuncture-college resume. If you have already created a business card, include that as well. If you have a Presentation Folder, you could offer to follow up with one if they want to see it. A letter you can download and rewrite to your own specs is included on the companion website in the marketing section.

> **POWER POINT**
>
> **While you are in school, consider:**
>
> Your online presence goes with you everywhere, and for a long time. Any practitioner who is looking at you as a potential employee will be checking you out wherever you have an online profile. You may want to limit what others may post on your Facebook page and be circumspect about what pictures you post. Your private life should be just that, private. Don't let it keep you from getting a job you might very much want!

▶ **How to negotiate your situation**

This can be tricky, especially if you have never negotiated for pay or perks or trades in the past. The first thing to figure out is exactly what you want from the situation in terms of money, space, business and patient management experience, and clinical experience. Make a list of your goals and desires for this position and tape this list to the inside front of the file where you keep all your other notes. Next, make a list of all the work that you would be willing to do and feel capable of doing in order to secure such a position. That's where you start. Then:

1. Remember one important secret of negotiation is that whoever is the most willing to walk away with no deal usually gets the most from any negotiation. While this does not put you in a great position if you really need the work, try your best not to feel desperate for a job or behave or speak as if

you are. If you are talking on the phone or by email, keep your list of goals and your list of job capabilities in front of you. Be as flexible as you can, but don't give your services away for nothing in return. Your work has value.

2. Decide what you need to make per hour in cash or trade for this to work for you. While a great deal less than what you can earn as a practitioner, it might be worth your while to accept $13 per hour for work as a receptionist/pharmacy operator/janitor/office person position 20 hours per week if you also have free use of the clinic rooms during evenings, weekends, and/or the practitioner's day off. If you are starting from scratch, you don't have any patients yet anyway, and a rent-free clinic or at least one room with all the equipment you need (tables, phone system, TDP lamp, etc.) could be a great leg up. It'll give you time to get your feet wet while having a little safety net.

3. Any practitioner with brains is going to want a minimum 1-2 year commitment from you. It is very disruptive to have practitioners or office staff coming and going from your clinic every few months. Don't even think about trying to find a job like this if you are not in a position to work for someone that long.

4. If the deal is to be for an off-peak hours rent trade only, but you really like the clinic and want to work there, decide if it would be preferable to simply rent space for a year or if there are very specific jobs you could do for a minimal number of hours that would be worth it to the practitioner and to you. This gives you more time to be out there building your practice.

5. You will need to have a clear-cut arrangement concerning product sales and profits, use of computers, file cabinets, and other office equipment, access to supplies such as table paper, cotton swabs, etc., who is allowed to turn the heat up or down, and as many details of the clinic operation as possible.

All agreements that you make with the practitioner, LLC, or corporation must be in writing.

6. If you are selling medicinals that belong to the practitioner from whom you rent or the clinic in general, try to negotiate at least 10% of the profits for yourself for any sales to your patients. This gives you the incentive to sell them and creates more profit for the clinic as well. Offer to create a system that allows everyone to easily keep track of office sales. This will help with inventory control in any case, no matter who gets the profits.

7. Consider having a clause in your contract stipulating that you want to use your own line of herbal products after a certain number of months and that you will create the space or carry the products around in your car if space is not available. Cumbersome, yes, but this may be your only real option if the clinic space is very limited, the clinic doesn't sell herbs at all, or the practitioner(s) use products that don't meet your needs, *e.g.*, if you are doing a completely different specialty than anyone else who works in this clinic.

8. Go meet the practitioner(s) in person. This is important for both of you. I don't advise taking a job in a clinic you've never seen or with a clinician you've never met.

9. Consider a three-month trial period at the end of which the final contract will be negotiated between you or you go your separate ways.

10. If this is happening in the town where you plan to locate permanently, consider specializing. Practitioners will be more open to your offer if you are planning to specialize in a specific niche different from their own. For example, if you

want to do dermatology and skin care, it might be a nice addition for a practitioner who specializes in gynecology, and it will not be in direct competition with them.

> "If opportunity doesn't knock, build a door."
> —Anonymous

For practitioners reading this chapter and feeling skeptical, we offer the following thoughts. If you are in practice but do not have an office staff or receptionist or anyone to put together formulas for your patients, consider making an offer to create a job like this for someone from the next graduating class at the closest acupuncture college. The advantages are greater than they might appear to be on the surface of things:

1. Instead of just part-time office support, you get that support from someone who understands Chinese medicine and can knowledgeably answer your patients' questions.

2. You get someone to manage your herb inventory and put together powder or bulk orders who understands Chinese herbal medicine and who is less likely to make mistakes or require extensive (and expensive) training.

3. You get someone to see your patients, answer the phone, fill prescriptions, and generally hold down the fort while you are on vacation without sending patients to another clinic.

4. You are freed up to see patients and not have to run the front desk, request payments, answer the phone, or manage herb inventory at least for a certain number of hours per week.

5. If your new assistant sees patients during hours you are not there, your clinic is open more hours with more phone and foot traffic to buy products and spread the good word about your services. More traffic makes more business for everyone.

6. If you collect most of the profit from increased sales of herbal or other products, after a few months this could cover most if

not all of what you pay your assistant. Then all the rest of the advantages they bring to your clinic are gravy.

7. If you hire someone whose specialty is different from yours, you have added new services to offer your patients without competition between you. This can increase your clinic's word of mouth buzz.

8. You are offering an invaluable service to the profession by helping train a new practitioner in how to run a successful clinic. The more successful practitioners there are, the more political clout we have, the more public support we have, and the stronger all of us are as a group.

> **PRACTITIONER POINTER**
>
> "I started out working in a chiropractor's office that is 650 square feet. The office has a good location. His receptionist made all my appointments, and the bathrooms were always clean! I worked when he didn't, which was Fridays, Saturdays, and evenings as needed. I had the option of using the space during other times if a patient really needed to be seen immediately. I paid him $400 a month, which was more than paid for by doing *tuina* for his patients on Thursdays from 4-8 (he paid me for this). Doing the *tuina* worked out well and always brought me acupuncture patients."
>
> —Elizabeth Liddell
> Philadelphia, PA
> elizabethliddellacupuncture.com

So as you can see, such an arrangement can be profitable and satisfying for all involved. We encourage both students and practitioners to create such mentoring partnerships. Depending upon your situation, and if both sides have integrity and work together, everybody can win with this one. You can use some of the suggestions in the previous chapter to create a contract for this arrangement or see the basic sample on the website in the Letters/Contracts section.

CHAPTER 8 | Getting a Job in Another Practitioner's Clinic

A WORD ABOUT NON-COMPETE CLAUSES

Commonly seen in contracts is a non-compete clause stating that for so-many-years-and/or-so-many-miles from the clinic where you worked you will not set up practice after you leave. The legality of these varies widely by state (and even from one judge to the next!). However, a one year term is frequently enforceable if the agreement is enforceable for other reasons. Reasons for allowing enforcement vary but often are tied to the protection of trade secrets. Thus, if an employee does not know company secrets (which clearly includes customer data), the agreement is not going to be enforced if it comes to a court battle. Some states don't allow non-competes at all in the medical area; others do, so find out. If presented with such a clause in a contract that seems excessive, it's best to seek legal advice.

POINTS TO PONDER FROM CHAPTER 8

- Statistics show that practitioners who are able to work under the wing of another practitioner are more likely to survive and prosper than those who do not.

- Contact your school alumni and others practicing in the area where you want to work. Place an ad in the alumni newsletter, state newsletters, national publications, and all web resources.

- Create a nice letter or postcard to send to every practitioner in the area where you'd like to practice.

- Before you negotiate, make a list of what is and is not negotiable. Beyond that, be as flexible as you can.

- For practitioners already in practice, there are some advantages to creating an "internship" job in your clinic. Check out my list.

Working in Hospitals or Integrated Clinics | 9

Working in a Western medical environment of one kind or another is becoming more common in our profession. Hospital jobs are increasing and there are probably more MDs interested in hiring an acupuncturist to work in their clinics than we know. Although we have no specific evidence of it, this may be especially true for MDs who have some training in acupuncture but not in Chinese herbal medicine or, having done training in acupuncture, realize they don't really have the time to make it work financially if they do most or all the treatments themselves given the realities of Western medical care. There are also some specialties that may be more amenable to combining your services with theirs than are some others, notably orthopedic surgeons, rehabilitation specialists, neurologists, "holistic" general practitioners, and infertility specialists. (Do a search for members of the American Holistic Medical Association in your area as a place to start!)

While there may be some complexity when negotiating to work in such an environment, if we want to really be accepted in the mainstream of medical care in this country, such arrangements need to become more the norm than the exception. It may take some persistent networking to find a sympathetic MD to hire you or take you on as a clinic partner. However, from what we have found with practitioners who are working in hospitals or multidisciplinary clinics, it is always a question of making yourself known as a credible resource, offering to do hospital in-service talks, or otherwise putting yourself continually in the path of MDs in as many ways as you can. If you persevere in your search and show people that you can communicate in a way that makes sense to them and that your services are valuable to their patients, you can succeed.

CHAPTER 9 | Working in Hospitals or Integrated Clinics

▶ Why should an MD hire you?

There are at least two factors in our favor. First, MDs outnumber us more than 20-to-one, DCs by more than four-to-one. Second, MDs are being asked regularly by more and more of their patients the same question, "What do you think, Doc, should I try acupuncture for this problem?" That being the case, if a reasonably open-minded MD has any extra space in his or her clinic, they might be quite open to the idea of having an on-staff acupuncturist at least renting space in their clinic and having the office staff schedule the appointments or even do the insurance billing.

▶ Variations on a theme

In calling several practitioners who are working with MDs or in hospitals, we hear variations on a similar theme. One practitioner found her position because she joined a Women's Health Discussion Group that included two gynecologists interested in complementary alternative medicine (CAM). When one of the gynecologists joined a multidisciplinary clinic, she asked the group to bring in her fellow group member as the on-staff acupuncturist. As such, she was paid a pro rata share of her patient visits; the remainder covers overhead costs such as full-time receptionist services. She receives regular referrals from her clinic partners. She keeps proceeds from all herbal product sales.

Another practitioner made a conscious decision that he wanted to work in a Western healthcare environment even if it took him a few years to create that reality. His strategy involved several steps, including hiring a resident at a nearby hospital to work in his clinic doing basic Western diagnostic intakes in conjunction with his acupuncture services. Patients were charged extra for this service. The resident made a little income "on the side" besides his hospital salary and the acupuncturist had something more than most to offer his patients. This acupuncturist had two such residents work for him over a three-year period. In the

THOUGHTS FROM SUCCESSFUL PRACTITIONERS

Jeannette Painovich, DAOM, (Jeannette Painovich Acupuncture)

In practice since: 2000, now in Los Alamitos, CA

Nature of her practice: Internal medicine; an emphasis in women's health

Other work: Participated in a 2-year research study at Good Samaritan Hospital to see if acupuncture helped with heart disease and reduced the overall costs of care. Unfortunately, due to billing practices, there was no real way to determine if opiate usage was also reduced for these patients. Also worked at Good Samaritan Hospital in Los Angeles doing acupuncture rehab with stroke patients and conducted research at Cedar Sinai Medical Center examining acupuncture's effectiveness in both heart disease and menopausal symptoms. A 3-year effort was needed to get credentialed to work in Good Samaritan Hospital!

Marketing methods: Has a membership in the American Women's Medical Association, open to all types of medical practitioners. She networks a lot with that group and has gotten referrals from various MDs in the group.

Current projects: Submitted a research training grant from NCCAM to conduct research at the *UC Susan Samueli Center for Integrative Medicine* to do research on acupuncture effectiveness in treating heart failure. (This foundation also pays for acupuncture at Children's Hospital of Orange County.)

Quotes:

"To find/create work in a hospital, an inside mentor or champion is an absolute requirement. They will help you gain access to the people who make decisions and help you understand the culture of the institution."

"To work in an integrative way, we must show research-based evidence for what we can do. Otherwise, we don't get any respect or belief."

"Due to ever-growing medical costs, hospitals are trying so hard to cut any and every possible expense from their system. We have to prove our financial worth to get inside."

Best advice to new grads: Be armed with the evidence needed to network with those in the field of your choice. Be prepared for all types of questions and practice quality persistence because it may take you longer then you think to get their trust and referrals.

Website: www.drpainovich.com

CHAPTER 9 | Working in Hospitals or Integrated Clinics

meantime, he arranged to do talks and in-service trainings for the hospital at which these residents were employed. Due to his friendship with one of these docs, he was later offered a salaried position at a hospital special services satellite clinic.

A third practitioner in California became an active player in his city's Chamber of Commerce. By attending events, working on fundraising committees, and networking with all types of people, he has developed a practice almost completely based on orthopedic surgeon referrals.

A fourth practitioner in Minnesota works full-time in a satellite clinic for a large city hospital doing mostly postoperative pain cases. He has to see three patients per hour, four days a week, but he has as many clinic rooms as he needs, all his supplies purchased, sharps disposed of, malpractice insurance paid, appointments made, and billings done. He takes home $65K a year, has learned to work comfortably in this environment, and likes the regular paycheck.

My final example here is a practitioner on the East Coast who is an RN. She considered going back to a local hospital to get a part-time job while she grew her practice. During her interview process, she discovered that some of the people at the hospital were more

> **PRACTITIONER POINTER**
>
> "I believe that acupuncture is an idea whose time has come in the West. Emergency Medical Services here in Chicago has mandated safe, effective alternatives to opiates, especially in the treatment of chronic pain, because they see that patients are damaged by long-term opiate therapy. The Hospital Accreditation Association advised Stroger County Hospital, where we work, to implement an integrated medicine model and expand research in this area. Acupuncture will be filling a key role for both these areas."
>
> —Frank Yurasek
> Lombard, IL

83

interested in having her services as an acupuncturist than as an RN! At first, however, they were afraid that they would not be able to afford the "equipment" necessary for acupuncture care, but she was persistent with her phone calls, gave them needle and other product cost information, and at the time we last spoke, she was negotiating her salary to work as many hours as she wants at this hospital.

Let's break down this process in a bit more detail.

▶ Working in an MD or DC clinic

The most common specialties of doctors who are open to offering acupuncture through their clinics include infertility, women's health care/gynecology practices, oncology clinics, pain clinics, and chiropractor offices. One might also think that orthopedists and allergists would be interested, but I have not heard that from practitioners so far.

If you are negotiating for work in a Western medical or multi-practice clinic, there are several ways that you might make it work. You could simply pay rent, collect your own fees, and charge whatever you want for services. Or you can pay a flat fee to the clinic for each patient seen if they are scheduling your

> **PRACTITIONER POINTER**
>
> "In 2007 I was asked to join an integrated group practice with doctors and nurse practitioners. The opportunity really fell in my lap, and it's been a great job. I rent my space for a flat fee, work six days a week, and have full reception services. I get many referrals from the MDs, and practicing there gives me excellent credibility. I also have learned a lot from working with MDs. To work well in this situation, you need confidence in our medicine and your skills as a practitioner, but you need to respect the doctors and know that we have a lot we can learn from our Western medical colleagues. If you can be a diplomat for Chinese medicine, this type of work is really fun!"
>
> —*Anonymous*
> *Austin, TX*

appointments and collecting your fees for you. However, for the most credibility, it is best to actually be a salaried employee.

Recently, a practitioner who had been approached to work in an MD's office called me to ask what salary package I thought he should try to negotiate. I suggested he consider what he would want per hour if he did not have any overhead other than malpractice insurance, annual CEUs, and professional association dues, which would actually be the case in his situation. We agreed that if all his supplies and insurance billing were to be included in the package, he would be quite happy with $50-$55 per hour for the 25-hour week contracted for. Although unable to use herbal medicine, that came to over $65,000 before taxes for working four days a week, six hours a day. Not too shabby for someone only two years out of school. However, why not see if you can get the doc (or hospital) to subsidize your malpractice insurance as part of your pay package and agree to another full day of work if the deal goes well on both sides?

When trying to get in the door, remember that you bring value to any MD's clinic, offering services they cannot and increasing the foot traffic to their clinic, with your referrals bringing them more patients as well. Send them a professional, informational/promotional packet about you and your services plus some research about acupuncture. There are samples of cover letters for these folders on the website for this book. Also see the chapter on Presentation Folders in Section 4, Chapter 5.

I suggest you deliver this packet in person. You might even bring something nice for the front desk staff, such as a coffee mug or two with your name and contact info printed on it, filled with Hershey's Kisses or your clinic pens. Tell the front desk people you are interested in offering your services at their clinic and hope they will see that your information gets to Dr. So-and-So.

▶ Getting your foot in a hospital door

If you know prior to graduation that this is something you are interested in, find ways to get involved with at least one local hospital now. Volunteer on a fundraising committee, or attend brown-bag inservice lunches or special events at the hospital. Introduce yourself to everyone you can. If you pursue this, you can make connections within the hospital system and structure, possibly with doctors who have private practices outside the hospital; these folks can be of tremendous help to you when you work inside these complicated bureaucracies. Use any opportunity to connect to administrative folks, because these people can either make or break your success working in a hospital setting.

If you are moving to another area, you can at least cruise the websites and find out who is doing what in the hospitals there. Is there someone in charge of CAM programs or research? Do they already have an inpatient or outpatient acupuncture program? If they do, it's worth calling to see if you can reach the administrator of the program and the acupuncturist(s) who work there to get your name on a list of people being considered for work if the program expands or someone leaves.

See if you can find out whether the hospital has office space available for doctors private clinics (many do) and if any of this space is empty. I know of one hospital-based acupuncture clinic that operates like this. Who is in charge of leasing the space available? What hoops would you have to jump through to be considered for a lease? An office inside a hospital gives you tremendous credibility, tons of exposure to potential patients, and possibly easier access to MDs who also have offices there.

Search local newspaper archives (2-3 years back) for articles about the hospitals. Who raises money for them and how, what sort of problems have been in the news, and what special things

CHAPTER 9 | Working in Hospitals or Integrated Clinics

happen at this hospital? What names do you find doing this research? What ideas does this search generate? Once you have gathered as much info as you can, start putting together your pitch. This needs to include:

1. How can you solve a problem for the hospital? For example, in your cover letter, site the Bravewell Collaborative Report in which major U.S. integrative hospitals were surveyed. This report showed that acupuncture was the most useful CAM therapy the hospitals could add to their services. It also showed that patients were often willing to pay for acupuncture themselves when it was available through the hospital itself, which means it can be another profit center. Hospitals are always looking for more income.

2. Create a mini business plan. At least you can present some numbers about costs (with the exception of their cost per sq. ft. to have you there). Include a per day salary, needles, basic supplies (probably no moxa or herbs), and throw in your malpractice insurance cost just for grins. You never know what they might cover if you are able to create a position.

   On the income side, list what is reasonable for billing standard acupuncture codes (97810 and 97811 for regular acupuncture; 97813 and 97814 for electro-acupuncture), say $40-$50 per code. Most treatments require one each of the paired codes, so about $80-90 per treatment, though they likely won't be reimbursed for the full amount. List a 10-15% smaller amount for time-of-service payments where no billing has to be done (yes, that's legal), say $60-$68 per visit. They may not give you extra money for diagnosis or patient assessment, but you can ask.

3. Include a discussion about the growth of acupuncture in the U.S. over the last 25 years, the respect acupuncture now has from the U.S. Army, the conditions you feel you can treat most effectively, and how acupuncture helps with post-

operative pain, post-chemotherapy nausea and fatigue, and stress-related and functional disorders of all types. You might also find some support on the NIH website or in articles at the National Hospital Association website about the damage that excessive opiate-for-pain use has been shown to do. Certainly the U.S. military is interested in acupuncture as an alternative.

4. Mention that, with adequate space, you can treat 3-4 people per hour. They can do the math.

5. Avoid Chinese medical jargon. No one can translate the word "qi" so don't use it. Don't discuss TCM diagnosis. A hospital only wants to know what type of patients you can treat, how many you can treat in a day, and whether this will make money for them. If you are successful with this effort, you might get to discuss Chinese medicine down the road when your program is producing money for them!

6. If you can find or create an insider champion to support your effort here, it will make all the difference. If you are staying in your own town, start with your family physician. See if he or she is willing to introduce you and recommend your services to the right folks at the hospital. If you were able to participate at the hospital in any capacity prior to graduation, see if the contacts you made during that effort can now help you in some way (introductions, invites to events, letters of support). Dress nicely, smile, and don't give up at the first "no."

7. Don't try to work in this environment if you have a low frustration threshold, as it may take you awhile to win the cooperation and respect of everyone involved. Don't try to do this if you have a problem with Western medical terminology or a chip on your shoulder about Western medicine. This will require you to pay attention to what's going on around you, be flexible, know how to think bi-modally (Chinese and Western medicine at the same time), work as part of a team,

show up on time, bring your A-game, and work hard every shift. But it can pay well and be very rewarding.

8. Know that with each of us who works "inside" the system, we are paving the way for greater and ongoing access to these situations and patient populations. How excellent to be a leader and ambassador for our wonderful medicine to a larger population!

> **Things to consider when creating a work agreement with a hospital (and in some cases with an MD clinic)**

These questions need to be at least discussed, and better yet written in your contract or work agreement with any hospital or other public health facility.

1. How much should you charge? If you had no overhead at all, how much would you need to make per patient or per hour to be comfortable? That's where you might start. If most of your patients will be billing insurance, discuss how much you will be reimbursed for various codes.

2. Who will order supplies and who will pay for them? How will needles and other biohazard materials be handled? If you are required to pay for these items, could you be reimbursed?

3. How many treatment spaces do you want or need

> **PRACTITIONER POINTER**
>
> "I work three days per week at Kaiser Permanente as an independent contractor. The credentialing process was pretty comprehensive and took some time, but it was worth it. I feel the compensation is very good, and all I have to do is show up and treat. They do the scheduling, accept payments, and pay for supplies. Although I am not able to prescribe herbs or burn moxa, I see a variety of patients that I'd never see in my private practice."
>
> —*Nancy Bilello*
> *Denver, CO*
> *www.denveracupunctureandherbs.com*

to work efficiently? If you need more than one treatment space at a time to be efficient or make an adequate living, will that always be available?
4. Be collegial and neither arrogant nor intimidated. If you value what you do but start from a position of building a positive relationship with the other practitioners and administrators on the hospital team, trust is likely to be easier to build. Also remember that, to get along most effectively, you need to dress in professional medical style and speak medical-speak comfortably.
5. How will your services be marketed; who will be responsible for doing it? Will you have access to other departments to put out brochures, put up signage, give in-service lectures, attend meetings, and meet others who are potential referral sources? Will you be allowed to use the hospital name on your card to help you market outside the hospital?
6. How long will you work there before your contract is up for renewal? Under what conditions can you terminate the contract legally? Is it transferable to another practitioner? What can be renegotiated if you wish to renew?
7. Are there any other duties for which you will be responsible in addition to doing acupuncture? Do any of these require training?
8. Will you be permitted to prescribe herbal medicine in appropriate situations? If so, how will it be paid for?
9. Will you be salaried, an independent contractor, paid by the hour or by the patient? Will you have any benefits such as health insurance or paid vacation? If not right away, when might such benefits begin and how do you apply for them?
10. If most or all patients are billing insurance for your services as well as other services in the hospital, how will that billing be handled and how does it relate to what you are paid.

There are more articles being written about practicing in integrated environments all the time in state and national publications. Check out the archive at *AcupunctureToday.com*, especially those by Kristen Porter, Beth Sommers, and Christian Nix. Ask on Facebook and LinkedIn for friends of friends who are doing this type of work and would be willing to have a conversation with you. You'll be surprised how many there are and what they'll share.

We hope these stories inspire you to go out and put yourself in as many situations as you can where you get to show and tell about East Asian medicine, acupuncture, and your services in particular to the Western medical community. The opportunities are there. It is up to you to go and find them.

POINTS TO PONDER FROM CHAPTER 9

- It may take some persistent networking to find a sympathetic MD to hire you or to find a position in a hospital. However, from what we have found with practitioners who are working in these settings, it is always a question of making yourself known as a credible resource, being a good communicator, and doing that often enough to be in the right place at the right time.

- This is a good time and place to use a presentation folder as described in Section 4, Chapter 5 on Marketing. You can include everything you want to present to a doctor or a hospital in one neat package.

- Consider creating a relationship with the hospitals in your area. Join the auxiliary fundraising committee, attend inservices and events, teach a class, and generally find ways to get involved. Meet as many admininstrators and doctors as you can in these efforts. Let them know about your interest.

- If there are already people working in the hospital, get on a list of people who are interested should the situation change or the current practitioner move.

- Create a mini business plan showing the hospital how they can make money by adding an acupuncture clinic.

- Be prepared for setbacks, smile, dress nicely, and keep knocking on doors!

Your Community Acupuncture Clinic | 10

The phenomenon of community acupuncture (CA) has changed the landscape of what it means to be an acupuncturist for a growing number of practitioners all across the U.S. and now in Europe and Australia as well. At the time of this writing there are several hundred community acupuncture clinics (difficult to get an exact number as it's always changing), and the number is growing by the week. As described on the community acupuncture co-op website, www.pocacoop.com, this model "is based on many of the traditional community styles of treatment often practiced in Asia. In setting up the first CA clinic, the founders asked some simple questions: What were the barriers to people getting acupuncture? What is really necessary for acupuncture treatments? How can acupuncturists make a sustainable income providing treatments to more people? The result is the CA model, which includes some fundamental re-imaginings of what acupuncture is and can be, and many helpful systems that help clinics run smoothly."

➤ The basics

Researching community acupuncture clinics and talking to owners, I find that there are a variety of hybrid clinic styles out there in addition to the standard one-room-with-many-recliners-and-a-rolling-treatment-cart model. Many have private rooms available for patients who are contagious, or for small children, or for people who just want more privacy. Still, the basic model for all real CA clinics is that simple acupuncture treatments, delivered as often as patients can afford, get good results at prices that are comfortable for the average person. At the same time, many CA clinics see their role as also offering a community-based place of comfort and ease (and often lots of other services) in their neighborhoods.

> **POWER POINT**
>
> **Facts about the community acupuncture model**
> 1. The focus is on providing access to affordable alternative care to everyone as well as communitarian values.
> 2. One motto is "more treatments more frequently." No insurance is billed and people pay what they can afford.
> 3. Treatments are done in a group setting, with simple diagnostic and charting processes, and lots of operational systems to keep your focus on the patients.
> 4. POCAcoop.com offers all types of systems, advice, mentoring, and support for clinic members. Membership cost is on a sliding scale.
> 5. Lower prices; simplify everything; build community are three fundamentals of a good CA clinic.

The proof is in the pudding. This model is successful for people who follow the program, especially those who use the tools and advice that are available from the People's Organization of Community Acupuncture website. Easy? No, but starting any business is not easy. Rewarding? Yes, clearly, and especially for people with a communitarian, participatory, let's-do-it-all-together, acupuncture-is-a-job-like-any-other-job, attitude.

Some fundamentals of operating these clinics include:

- Patients pay what they are comfortable with between a given range, typically $15-$40, no questions asked. No insurance is billed.

- Online appointment booking is used for many if not most clinics. This is easier for many patients and allows the practitioner to spend time treating, not answering the phone.

- Treatments are kept simple, straightforward, and as often as possible. Many clinics do not prescribe herbs.

- Most practitioners are, ideally, treating 5-6 patients per hour and do not have time for moxa, cupping, or tuina. Effectiveness is based on frequency of treatments.

- Full integration into one's community and neighborhood makes for a more successful clinic, with a variety of possible ways that people participate. This may include things such as:

  - being a drop-off/pick-up point for a local food co-op

  - holding a farmer's market in your clinic parking lot

  - maintaining a community bulletin board for all types of local events

  - using your space after hours for community meetings

  - offering trades for volunteers to work in your clinic in various capacities

- Treatment work shifts are 4-5 hours and clinics may be open seven days a week in some cases.

- Systems for managing many business aspects of CA clinics are vital for profitability.

- Acupuncturist is a job like any other, without elitism or "specialness."

- All treatments can be done in the main clinic room; private rooms are not required for anything.

PRACTITIONER POINTER

"We wanted to bring affordable acupuncture to our town. Not only have we done that, but our patients love it here and love the people who work here. They feel cared for and heard by all of us.

The hardest part for us was learning that you don't get paid for all the hours you work as an owner. Second was getting comfortable with the message about frequency being the key to acupuncture success when working with new patients."

—Lisa Lowe and Karen Marks
Arvada, CO
www.oldetownacu.com

▸ Does this sound good to you?

As far as I can see, community acupuncture is an idea whose time has come and the number of clinics following this model will continue to grow. In my personal opinion [HW], the best things about CA clinics are that they offer job opportunities to many new graduates and offer access to care for average working people earning average wages.

CA removes the "boutique specialty" feeling/reputation of some acupuncture clinics and creates a variety of ways that people can build both real community and a sense that acupuncture is normal, everyday healthcare, available to all. By doing that, we may actually experience a serious increase in the percentage of our population who are receiving acupuncture. That alone is a recommendation for any of you who find this model of work attractive.

That said, this is clearly not for everyone. If it does not feel right for your personality, there are many other possibilities, as we have presented in other chapters.

If this does sound appealing, I [HW] strongly suggest that you join POCA (www.pocacoop.com) as soon as possible. It is not expensive and the Wikis alone are worth far more than the price. These will help you with every imaginable aspect of starting and running your business. The forum discussions cover every topic you can imagine such as:

- Product reviews of all kinds, down to what hand-cleansers are best as you go from recliner to recliner with your rolling cart

- What online appointment software people are using and why they like it or not

- Marketing efforts that have or have not been effective for members

- Spreadsheets for tracking your treatment numbers and income. Free and downloadable.

It is truly a gold mine. Additionally, POCA members have access to many well-priced continuing education courses and an annual POCA conference with all kinds of useful courses and discussions. There is a lot more that could be written here, but the POCA folks have it all on their website already.

POINTS TO PONDER FROM CHAPTER 10

- The community acupuncture (CA) movement has grown rapidly since its inception in 2002, now with over 250 clinics that conform to POCA guidelines and probably another 100 doing various hybrid variations.

- Community acupuncture has revolutionized acupuncture availability in the U.S., making it affordable for regular folks earning regular wages.

- Based on the idea that "more treatments more often" makes the most difference in acupuncture care, CA clinics allow people to pay what they can afford, $15-$40 per treatment.

- Very organized systems allow practitioners to treat 4-5-6 people per hour in a one-room environment with simple treatment protocols.

- CA clinics also work to become community centers for all kinds of neighborhood activities besides acupuncture.

- If this is your interest, join POCA Coop, a gold mine of information, resources, training, and support for acupunks!

Going Where Your Skills Are Needed | 11

This topic could be a paragraph or two in another chapter, but I feel strongly enough about this to give it its own chapter heading, even if it is only two pages. Consistently and repeatedly, I have heard the same things from practitioners who have had the largest, most successful practices the most quickly. There seem to be two major categories of practitioners who do the best. First are those who specialize in a very specific area of practice. If they are clever enough to decide on a specialty prior to graduation, they can often have several job offers, clinic partner offers, or referral networks put in place weeks and months before they have their diploma. The other ones are those who have the courage to go where no practitioner has gone before.

Those who are willing and able to take their skills to smaller cities and towns and who make the effort to connect with the community where they settle seem to do better faster. This does not mean no marketing effort. It means that their marketing efforts have been more effective more quickly. Depending upon the situation, we have heard of people with very full practices in less than one year. One practitioner we spoke to from a relatively rural

> **PRACTITIONER POINTER**
>
> "My advice is, move. This is a tough one for many people who are rooted in the community where their school is based. But it is worth thinking about. I moved to a small to medium-sized community where I am the only one around and I was previously known. My weekly patient load has been consistently high since I opened my practice. This would not have happened had I stayed put after graduating."
>
> —Daniel Schulman
> Prince Edward Island, Canada

CHAPTER 11 | Going Where Your Skills Are Needed

area was advertising for a new graduate to come and work for him, his patient load was so large. He had been in practice less than one year. Another, who moved back to his family's small hometown, had an average of 30 patients per week within six months of opening his practice.

In Section 1, Chapter 3, we discussed the need to do demographic research on the town or area in which you think you might like to practice. If possible, we encourage you to include some small cities and towns in your search and to take this medicine to places where there are few, if any, practitioners. There are, at the time of this writing, about 23,000 practitioners of acupuncture and Chinese medicine in the U.S. There are over 70,000 chiropractors and over 300,000 practicing MDs. Ten years have elapsed since the first edition of this book and with still only about 5% of the American public currently using our services, we are not yet even close to saturation of the market except in cities where there are acupuncture colleges. So do your homework and get out of town!

Think About Specialization | 12

This subject has also come up in other chapters. However, I feel it is important enough for you to think about it again, and carefully. There are several possible specialties within Chinese medicine that are effective clinically and could bring you success financially. I suggest you consider the following:

- Gynecology
- Pediatrics
- Dermatology
- Geriatrics
- Sports medicine
- Oncology
- Psychiatry
- Workers' compensation injury management
- Assisted reproductive technology
- Diabetology
- Chronic pain specialist
- Headache specialist
- Male urology and sexual dysfunction specialist

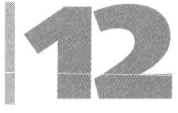

"Specialist"

It may seem that you're limiting the number of patients who come to you if you specialize, but consider that there is no lack of people with any given condition. If you become very skilled at treating a specific group of disorders, everyone in our professional community will know of it eventually. I know one practitioner who specializes in oncology only, especially cancers of the breast. She has a waiting list of three months to get in to see her! Another friend of mine is well-known for his skill as a gynecologist. He gets calls from women all over the U.S. who want to come to see him, and referrals from other L.Ac.s near and far.

CHAPTER 12 | Think About Specialization

Being a general practitioner is the hardest of all "specialties," requiring you to be reasonably competent in the treatment of almost every ailment since you never know what is going to enter your door. It is far easier to become really, really good at treating a smaller, finite group of conditions, where there are only so many symptoms and patterns routinely involved. The material you need to have memorized cold is far less. You can even get to a point where you know most of what you will do for a patient by shaking their hand and watching them walk in and sit down in your exam room.

This does not mean you never take a patient with an ailment outside your specialty. But you might not ever have to. And if you worry that being a specialist is not a "holistic" approach, I say this: Chinese medicine is, by its inherent nature, a holistic approach to diagnosis and treatment no matter what disease you are treating. It is built into the system because we base treatment primarily on pattern discrimination, not on disease diagnosis. Patterns always describe the whole person, taking into account body, mind, and spirit.

> **PRACTITIONER POINTER**
>
> "In my thriving practice, Watsonville Acupuncture, I specialize in treating musculoskeletal conditions and see about 70 patients a week. I must say that nothing I learned in my OM program of study prepared me for what it would take to start a practice of this magnitude: creating a marketing program, establishing referral sources in the medical community, and most of all providing the professional presence that patients want. My goal has been and continues to be to bring OM to all those who have no idea that it exists. This brings me great joy."
>
> —Eric Meyer-Reed
> Watsonville, CA

POINTS TO PONDER FROM CHAPTER 12

- There are several distinct advantages to specializing.
- There are no drawbacks (in my opinion).

SECTION TWO
Working on Your Own

Business Basics | 1

"It is easier to go down a hill than up, but the view is from the top."
—Anonymous

This chapter is an introduction to some basics you'll need to determine no matter what type of business you are starting: your business name, business cards, supplies and equipment, software for running your business, how you keep records, managing needle inventory, and more. Some of this nitty-gritty information is also included in Section 1, Chapter 3 for students. For those of you already in practice, or if you are ready for the next steps, this information is far more complete.

▶ How to pick a name for your business

Since close to 90% of acupuncturists have their own businesses, choosing a name is one of the more important early decisions you must make. The name you choose can be excellent marketing for your business, or it can confuse or even put off potential patients. So, when researching names for your business, there are a few important questions I want you to keep in mind:

- **Does it make my business easy to market?** The more information your business name conveys, clearly and concisely, the fewer explanatory words you need in ads, on signs, etc. For example, if the name of your clinic is *Skin Care Acupuncture Clinic,* your Craigslist or Yelp ads do not need extra lines of type to tell people what you do. It's already in the name.

- **Is it easy to remember, spell, and pronounce?** *Whole Family Health Center, Boulder Herbal Medicine Clinic,* and *Orange Park Acupuncture Clinic. . .* are all pretty easy to remember. They are short, concise, and can be pronounced by anyone who drives or walks by your clinic. Why does it matter? Hundreds, perhaps even thousands of people may pass your clinic sign every day. If the name is weird and hard to pronounce or remember, you may lose a future patient to the clinic down the street. Also, I suggest you avoid Chinese words like *An Shen* (calm spirit) or *Jin Shan* (golden mountain). These sound exotic and may have meaning for you, but they mean nothing and may even seem "strange" to the average American patient.

- **Does it convey a clear understanding of what you do?** *WomenCare Acupuncture Clinic* and *Athletic Edge Acupuncture Services* are good names that communicate to a prospective patient both that you do acupuncture and that your services are for a specific group of people. Use words such as "acupuncture," "Chinese medicine," "herbal medicine," etc. to convey your purpose if possible.

- **Does it market you to the specific niche you want to serve?** Again, this is a great way to separate you from the average. Niche marketing can fill your clinic more quickly. Every athlete who sees *Athletic Edge Acupuncture Services* will have a pretty good idea what you do!

Try out your list of possible names on friends and family and see what their reactions are. Can they spell it; do they understand it? You might even try it on the barista at your favorite coffee shop. Who knows? You may just score your first patient!

Check name availability

When you get some ideas, go to the website for your Secretary of State and search name availability. No matter which business model you choose, you will need to select a name for your clinic that no one else has. See Section 1, Chapter 3 for a full discussion of this process. Also check URL availability for the names you are considering.

▶ Business cards

Your business card is a constant marketing tool. Both a calling card and appointment card, you will use it for numerous purposes, even more during your start-up phase. Whatever your plans, a good business card with a good design is a good idea.

Business cards work well when used like confetti at a 4th of July parade. Print 1,000 and see if you can hand them all out in four weeks. If you have the courage to do that and you have a user-friendly card, your patient load could double in two months! For a thorough card checklist, see Section 4, Chapter 5 on things that must go into a presentation folder. Here's a short list to consider for now.

Fonts: Keep them simple, easy to read, and no smaller than 11 point type. Two font styles on a card is enough.

Name: Your name should be easily seen, before any other information on the card.

Internet information: If you have a website, put it on the card. No website yet? ... at least put your email address.

Phone: After your name and website address, the phone number is the most important thing on the card.

Business information: Include the name and address of your business somewhere. If not, then a QR code so they can visit your phone-friendly website on their phone right now.

Logo: If you have a logo, its location should balance the text in some way. Consider using the logo as a watermark background to the text. Watermarks should be printed in a lighter color than the text at no more than a 10% density or screen.

Material: Use a nice quality card stock. Your business card represents you when you meet another medical professional or prospective patient, and a business card that wows is less likely to be thrown away.

Color: No neon or shiny stuff! It's way too difficult to read. No more than two colors unless it's a color photo of you.

The Back: This is valuable real estate; don't let it go to waste. Use it for a map to your clinic, or a "next appointment" note. If you live in a small community, print one of the following on the back: a schedule of the town's important events, *e.g.*, "5/25: strawberry festival," the high school football team schedule, or an inspirational message. The more uses your business card has, the more likely it is to be kept.

> Consider putting a QR code on your business card! This takes users directly to a smart-phone friendly website or landing page with info on how to connect with you online.

Old cards: When information changes (a new phone number, your married name, a new website, a new football season [see above]), get new cards. Do not scratch out the old information and handwrite the new. It looks unprofessional.

Photo: A card with a photo makes it easier to associate that card with the conversation or encounter that led you to get the card, making it a more powerful marketing tool in the long run. To do this right, I recommend you get a professional photograph of yourself. You can also order paste-on photos the size of a postage stamp. These can only be made from a digital photo, but are not otherwise expensive. Try Photo.Stamps.com Zazzle.com, or similar services.

▶ Logo or no logo?

A company logo can be a thing of beauty that sticks in people's minds. However, starting without one is fine. When you do decide to create this image, enlist the help of a professional unless you did such things in your pre-acupuncture life. One possibility is to call the art department at the local college and speak to the graphic arts instructors. Graphic arts students need to assemble a portfolio, and getting their designs used by a real business is good for them and could be inexpensive for you. Ask for a recommendation to a talented student. You might also try Elance.com, a website for artists to compete by bidding on your job. I've had good luck with this service.

A logo is a visual symbol to represent what you do and who you are. When creating it, think like someone who knows nothing about Chinese medicine or language. Once you have a logo, put it on everything you print. See Section 1, Chapter 3 for more details on logo design.

Your USP

"Drivers wanted." "It keeps going, and going, and going." "Are you in good hands?" "Because you're worth it." Did you already identify the products or companies that these lines represent? They are all good examples of a *unique selling proposition,* a phrase that states what distinguishes you from your competitors and gives people a reason to do business with you.

If you decide to write a USP for your business, try to come up with something that is immediately understood in one line, a clear, concise statement that conveys a benefit to the people you wish to serve. Put it on your stationary and letterhead, business cards, sign, and website. A USP can be a mini-commercial when introducing your clinic.

Here are a few examples of acupuncture-related USPs:

- Athletic Edge Acupuncture Services: "Enhanced performance for every athlete"

- WomenCare Health Center: "Because healthy women make a healthy world"

- Skin Care Acupuncture Clinic: "Because beauty is more than skin deep"

Creating a good USP can be fun. I think the best way to do it is to throw out ideas one after another without thinking about them too much; don't edit yourself. The more you come up with, the more creative you may get. Enlist the help of a clinic partner or friend to write them all down. This exercise may help you to envision what you really want your business to be about.

➤ Software needs

To run an effective business today, all of us use computers loaded with software of all kinds as well as access to the internet. There are lots of programs out there to operate both the business side and the acupuncture side of your clinic.

1. Generic business software:

    Accounting software: There are all shapes and sizes of programs available, but the most well-known is **QuickBooks.** This very intuitive, user-friendly bookkeeping program has both a professional and home version. The professional version, **QuickBooks Pro**, is well worth the money if you are planning to do your own bookkeeping for months and years. The help and tutorials sections are very useful during set-up, but if this is completely intimidating for you, it may be worth it to hire a bookkeeper to set up **QuickBooks** for you and give you a short lesson in using the software. Could this be a good opportunity for a trade or barter?

    Scheduling: Allowing patients to make appointments directly on your website is getting easier all the time and there are lots of software choices (see page 27). You can print out a daily paper copy and do a daily back-up to refer to later, but a digital version of your schedule is nice since you can also take it with you anywhere if you have a smart phone or tablet. This is handy for those new in practice and out of the office regularly doing marketing. You can even schedule an appointment from your phone for a new patient if you are giving a lecture or working an event and someone requests it.

2. Practice-specific software:

Medisoft: Available for years, this software is the top of the food chain for electronic medical records (EMR). Version 18, new at the time of this writing, keeps track of patient appointments, has smart phone add-ons, does superbills, electronic billing, can be modified (with effort) to keep herbal dispensary inventory, and can bill for multiple practitioners.

People like this software despite thenecessary adaptations. The pricetag of $500-$1,300 depends on which bells and whistles you want.

Medical billing services: If your practice is going to have a sizeable number of insurance patients, you'll need to be able to do electronic billing. This is how the insurance industry is moving, and to participate in the Affordable Care Act, it will be a requirement. Go to EZclaim.com (fee-based) or OfficeAlly.com (free) for information if you need something like this now. If you don't get to this point in your practice for a few years, search for these services when you are ready. You can also hire a company to do your online billing for you such as Acupbilling.com, Acuclaims.com, Accuclaim.com, or a local service in your area. These services take a small percentage of each claim, but your billings are not likely to land

> **PRACTITIONER POINTER**
>
> "I am a sole proprietor who treats pretty much every type of condition in my practice. It took me four years working with a business coach, taking business and self-development classes to get my practice where I wanted it to be. In that time I learned all sorts of things, but two important ones stand out. First, create systems. Systems are the basis for how successful companies operate. They provide clarity. Systems for: financial records, administration of the clinic, marketing, quality assurance, history and intake process, and patient communication. Second, your commitment has to always be to the patient's health. If patients know that, they more easily become committed to treatment."
>
> —Bertram Furman
> San Diego, CA

in the questionable file on an adjuster's desk. You can search on LinkedIn or Craigslist for people who do this type of work in your own area.

Acupuncture practice software: Specific to our profession, there are a number of options available, although fewer than there used to be. Some programs are able to do billing and keep track of herbal inventory. Unlike *Medisoft,* they have acupuncture-specific info already loaded. Some programs not only offer billing and patient management tools but boast educational information on points, herbs, and herbal formulas. Some also come with pre-loaded vendor information for ready-made formulas. Prices and service contracts vary, but are not cheap. Product tours are available at the websites. Here is contact information for some acupuncture-office-specific software available (in no particular order):

AcuBase: http://www.trigram.com
TaoClinic Professional: http://www.taomedic.com/html
ClientTracker: www.ginkgosoftware.com
AcuPartner: www.acupartner.com
Practs.com: Your secure data lives on their server/cloud; you pay based on the number of patients you see. Nice idea and you don't waste $$ on buying software updates.

▶ Business equipment

The two types of equipment you'll need are generic and trade specific. All health service companies have a front desk and a computer but not all of them have needles and TDP lamps!

1. **Computer:** With endless options available, how is a person supposed to decide? It used to be that upgrade-ability was the holy grail. Since the life of a new computer is longer now than it was a decade ago, it is probably true that in 5-7 years (it used to be 1-2 years!) your system will be outdated and unable to run much of the software then being developed. If I were in the market, I'd buy a laptop with the largest CPU,

most memory, and that is indefinitely upgradeable (whatever that means these days). Then I'd spring for the newest versions of every software I want to use.

2. **Printer:** You'll need one for all sorts of things: superbills, office forms, herb instructions, letters to MDs. With a high-quality color printer and a good warranty, you're set for a few years. They are not that expensive, so buy a good one or you'll spend money on repairs that cost more in the long run. FYI, an all-in-one printer-copier-fax-scanner could be a great birthday present from Mom!

   Having the ability to copy a list of suggested exercises, a self-massage routine, or a piece of research for a patient on the spot is very nice. Also, when and if you start billing insurance (see Section 3, Chapter 2), you have to photocopy patients' insurance cards to keep on file. How will you do it without a copier?

   Almost every computer with a phone line can send a fax with a cheap piece of software. But what if what you want to send is not on the computer? With a scanner, you could import and just email it.

   If you plan to do any flyers or educational pieces for patients, having a scanner can be really helpful. Scan a nice photo for your herbal information page, website, or put a picture of your clinic on a postcard you are sending out.

   Even if you don't see a need for some feature of an all-in-one today, in six months you may find that feature indispensable and you'll be happy you don't have to drive somewhere to get it done.

3. **Phone:** While it's doubtful that I need to talk anyone into buying a phone, I do need to state clearly that I think it unwise to try and run a business from your personal cell phone. A dedicated landline phone, aside from any features

of the phone itself, gives your clinic credibility. I personally would not leave a message on someone's cell if the outgoing message is a personal one with the addendum "You can also leave messages here for XYZ Acupuncture Clinic." I admit I'm a Boomer and maybe Millenials have a different take, but I think it's a good idea to have all aspects of your business as friendly to as wide a group of people as possible.

That said, you could hire a local service to install a full professional phone setup. Otherwise, buy the best generic phone you can afford, with voicemail, speakerphone, and caller ID. I also recommend hiring an answering service because some people don't like to leave messages on a machine, especially if it's their first time to call your clinic. If you are not ready to hire a receptionist, this is the second best option. If you can only have an answering machine, keep your answering recording on silent mode when treating patients. Your outbound message should tell people you will call them back in a *guaranteed* amount of time; that way you are more likely to get a message rather than a hang-up. More on receptionists in Chapter 10 of this section.

Caller ID is a wonderful creation for business owners. Sure as the rain in Seattle, people will call up and leave a message requesting a call back, yet forget that while you may know all about Chinese herbs, you cannot call them back if they don't leave a number. Hence, the usefulnees of caller ID.

Lastly, set up your clinic phone to forward calls to your cell when you are out of the office so you don't miss patient calls and so you can update your schedule from anywhere!

4. **Office furniture:** This topic is covered at length in Chapter 6 of this section: The Look and Feel of Your Clinic. The computer, printer, phone, and credit card machine require a desk and a chair. You may also need a work table or counter area. Lamps and lighting for your reception area and treatment

rooms will make work easier and influence the overall feel of your clinic.

Another requirement for HIPAA is a locking file cabinet for patient charts (unless they are kept on a computer). As we discuss in the chapters listed below, the question is not really *if* you store your patient charts, it is *how* you store them and keep them secure. For more about HIPAA compliance, see Section 2, Chapter 9, on HIPAA and Section 1, Chapter 5, on Legal Stuff.

5. **Treatment tables:** You need a sturdy table in each treatment room. You may be able to find good quality discount tables by calling massage table companies and asking to buy a tradeshow demo table. Also check your local paper and eBay for practitioners selling equipment. Just make sure the tables you purchase carry a decent amount of weight and and are made for professional, not home, use. Discount stores also sell tables. The price may be right, but the patient who is on the table when a leg snaps off is unlikely to return for another treatment!

▶ Paperwork ●

To run an efficient, legal acupuncture clinic, you need specific forms. From patient history and charting to HIPAA privacy requirements, this book's companion website has forms for you. Included is an example of each of the forms listed below that you may need to operate your clinic. Feel free to use the forms as they are or modify them to suit you. More about forms and their legal ramifications is in Chapter 5 of this section.

Forms on our website:
- intake forms
- patient health history
- liability waiver or permission to treat form
- insurance Assignment of Benefits form

115

- notice of privacy policy (HIPAA)
- acknowledgment of receipt of privacy policy (HIPAA)
- individual rights for authorization (HIPAA)
- disclosure form (HIPAA)
- informed consent (HIPAA)
- fax log (HIPAA)
- sign-in sheet
- patient private information form
- clinic financial and cancellation policy form
- follow-up care (Report of Findings)
- herb instructions (bulk internal and external, patent)
- referral information sheet

▶ Office supplies

Day-to-day operation of your clinic requires basic supplies. Still in school? Start on a stash of supplies in advance by asking for these as stocking-stuffers this year!

- **Stapler and staples:** Get a good one; cheap ones break or jam.

- **Paperclips, biz-card holders, plexiglass sign holders**

- **Paper:** Buy it by the box. Office Depot and Staples always have deals: a box of 6 reams for the same price as 4-5 individual reams. Check their websites and weekly ads.

- **Packing and invisible tape**

- **CMS 1500 forms:** We will be moving to online billing in the coming 2-3 years, so you may want only a few on hand if you're going to bill insurance at all. Check online for the best pricing and buy as few as you can (maybe get several practitioners to share one box). HIPAA regulations have made this form the standard. *Don't copy them and send them in in black.* They must be in red, just as they come from the printer. Better yet, go with OfficeAlly.com and start billing online now.

- **Printer cartridges:** Always keep at least one extra on hand.

- **Pens:** Unless you take patient notes directly into your computer, chart notes must be done in ink (preferably black). You'll be amazed at how quickly pens disappear from the front counter, a marketing opportunity you can use to your advantage! Get your clinic info printed on decent pens and give them away to patients and people everywhere you go. Do some shopping around before you buy as there are lots of choices.

- **Postage and envelopes:** Even a small office can produce a lot of mail. Buy #10 envelopes in boxes of 500 or, if you just signed, multi-year lease, consider envelopes printed with your address and logo. You can find good pricing online.

    How you do postage depends on your business: 1) Get a postage machine and pay the monthly fee plus postage (a must if you are selling anything mail order through your website), 2) go to the post office and buy 100 stamps at a time, or 3) buy postage online. The problem with stamps is that, if you want to send something larger or heavier than a regular letter, you'll have to go to the post office anyway. Then again, waiting in line could be a marketing opportunity; you could probably give away several business cards during a 10-minute wait! If you order stamps by mail, the post office delivers them to your mailbox. Go to http://shop.usps.com.

- **Tissue and TP:** Every medical office needs tissue in each treatment room and behind the front counter. In a building where the bathrooms are not inside your clinic, toilet paper is included in the rent. If your bathrooms are inside your clinic, try a discount store or your local EcoProducts store for TP, paper towels, tissues, and bathroom cleaning supplies.

▶ Ordering needles

We all have our own opinions about needles. By the time you are reading this book, you are likely to know your preferences. Thus, in this discussion we'll consider a system for inventory management and ways to get better prices.

Prices: Wherever you buy your needles, more boxes purchased means a lower price per box, an incentive to order for several months rather than by the week. Most companies will give a small discount if you buy 10 or more boxes, but at 50-100 boxes, the discount is considerable and may also include free shipping. Call a few distributors of the needles you like and compare prices and shipping costs and delivery times. Also, if you tell them you just graduated and are looking for a needle company to do business with, you may get an initial order discount. In that case, it may be wise to order what you think you'll need for a few months and to show your faith in yourself!

Your first order: At first it may be difficult to know how many needles you'll go through how fast. You can, however, guesstimate patients per week in the first month and multiply by the average number of needles you typically use per patient. (By the time of graduation, you should have an estimate of your needles-per-treatment number.)

I suggest you start with varying lengths of whatever gauge needle you prefer. The length needle you use most often will obviously make up the bulk of the order. If you can afford to order enough boxes to get a discount, do so. My own initial needle order might look like this:

   34 gauge (0.22) x 1" (25mm) – 8 boxes
   34 gauge (0.22) x 2" (50mm) – 8 boxes
   34 gauge (0.22) x 3" (75mm) – 4 boxes
   34 gauge (0.22) x .5" (13mm) – 4 boxes

36 gauge (0.20) x 1" (25mm) – 6 boxes

36 gauge (0.20) x 1.5" (25mm) – 21 boxes

This order is 50 boxes. A 40-50¢ discount per box saves you $20-$25. Free shipping would save another $15-$20.

Many needle and all herb companies require you to register at their website or email them a copy of your license. This is also true with ordering sharps containers. Be prepared with digital copies of your papers as discussed in Section 1, Chapter 5.

> Hint: If you typically use 32-34 gauge needles on every patient, perhaps get a few finer ones for children, elderly, diabetic patients, or other very sensitive people you may treat.

Inventory: When your needle order (or any type of order) arrives, before putting it away check the actual box contents against both the invoice and with what you think you ordered, which is easy if you sent the order by fax or email. Once checked for accuracy, this first order is the start of an inventory sheet (with *Excel* this task is easy, but can be done on paper as well). To help you maintain an adequate supply of needles at all times, here is one system.

The four parts to maintaining your inventory are: 1) date, 2) boxes on-hand, 3) level, 4) to order. The date helps you know how fast you are using needles but has no other importance. For example, I personally [HW] like to do inventory and place my order the last working day of each month.

First, you count the unopened boxes of each length and gauge of needle in each treatment room and storage cabinet or closet. (For inventory purposes, you only count unopened boxes.) You count each size and gauge of needle separately and write those numbers down (see sample next page). Adding the numbers across the page for each specific length and gauge of needle gives me the total boxes *on-hand.*

SECTION TWO: WORKING ON YOUR OWN

The next number is your *level,* which means the number of boxes of each type of needle that you like to keep on hand. For example, if you think 20 boxes of 34 gauge, 1" needles is adequate, that is your level for that size. These numbers will grow with your practice, so just start somewhere based on what you think you'll use and adjust your *level* as necessary over time.

Subtracting boxes-on-hand from level gives you what you need to order to bring inventory back to level. With needles taking several days to arrive, you are not likely to maintain your exact level, which doesn't matter as long as you don't run out of needles. Your basic inventory count sheet could look like the one below.

> **POWER POINT**
>
> There are new needle companies coming into the industry all the time. Don't assume the ones you used in school are all that is available. Call several suppliers and ask for some free samples of any new lines on the market that they carry. Between three or four suppliers, you could end up with a week's supply of needles absolutely free!

Hopefully you are using enough needles that you need to place an order after each inventory count! If you keep track of orders digitally, that's great; if you have an orders notebook, put any newly-placed order in the *pending orders* section. When the order comes in, check the box contents against your order and re-file it in the *completed orders* section. You

Date of inventory: Friday, August 21, 20XX							
Item	Rm 1	Rm 2	Rm 3	Other	On-hand	Level	Order
34 x 1	2	3	1	12	18	20	2
34 x 2	1	2	2	5	10	10	0
34 x 3	etc.						
32 x .5							
34 x 1.5							

might also note the check number used to pay this bill or that it was paid by credit card on such-and-such date.

➤ Hazardous waste disposal

Proper needle disposal means "sharps" containers, which are sold by most acupuncture supply companies. However, it is easiest to get a contract with a medical waste disposal company that includes a mail-in program for returning full containers. Such contracts are inexpensive, but look online to find a company with the right program for your needs. The style you prefer and the size of your treatment rooms affect the size and style of containers you order. Unless you start a community style clinic where you are moving from chair to chair with a rolling cart, I [HW] think wall-mounted containers are the safest, as they will not get knocked over by accident (a spilled sharps container is not fun). Second best from my perspective are the large-bottom countertop containers. If you get these, put them in a corner if possible to protect against accidental spills.

Whichever style and system you choose, make sure to keep records of your paid bills and how often you dispose of the containers. Some managed-care networks like to make sure you do, in fact, use disposable needles. These records are proof of your compliance.

➤ Basics of business

The basics of getting up and running presented in this chapter are the same as for most businesses, except for needles and sharps containers! If you start out right with these things, you've gone a few good steps toward your goal of a successful clinic. Next stop: budgeting your start-up. Let's keep going!

POINTS TO PONDER FROM CHAPTER 1

- Choose your business name carefully. One that helps you market your services, is easy to pronounce, and explains what you do will serve you best. Register your business name with the Secretary of State so that no one else can use it, and buy your URL to match.

- Keep your business card simple, clean, and easy to read. No fancy fonts, no small type. If you want to make it fancy, use glossy paper stock and put a nice photo of your smiling face on it!

- Only use a logo if you can design a really good one. Trite symbols of Chinese culture or medicine may not convey much. If a picture is worth 1,000 words, make sure the picture you use says the words you want to say to the market you wish to reach.

- Computers and software are a part of running most businesses these days. If you are still in the market, get a computer that can be upgraded easily with more memory, a bigger hard drive, new software, etc.

- You may want business software such as QuickBooks, appointment scheduling software, and medical records software, which is available both specifically for acupuncture offices and more generally for any type of medical office. This will be required by the Affordable Care Act if you want to participate.

- Look for deals on office products, furniture, and other equipment, but make sure to buy treatment tables that will hold all sizes of humans and hold up under the heavy use you are going to make happen in your clinic!

- You can download samples of forms that every acupuncture office needs from our companion website and redesign them for your own use!
- Keep a careful inventory of your needles to learn how many you use of what sizes over a period of months. If you can order in large quantities you'll get better pricing.

Setting Your Fees and Managing Your Budget | 2

▶ **Setting your fees**

Your fees can be just as important as your location, your business name, and your style of practice. If your fees are too high for your city or town, it may deter potential patients from considering your services. On the other hand, if your fees are too low, you will not survive long or at least not thrive in the world as we know it.

So, how do you figure out your rates when opening your first clinic? There are a number of factors you must consider when making this decision: the lifestyle and income level in your area, the going rates of other practitioners in your area, the amount of money you need and want to be comfortable, the type of clinic you are planning to run, and what you think the value of your products and services actually is.

▶ **What's the going rate in your area?**

First things first. Before you do anything else, find out what the going rate for acupuncture is in your area. In Section 1, Chapter 3, about building your practice while you're still in school, I mentioned that this task can and should be done before you ever get out of acupuncture college. If you will be the only acupuncturist in your town, find out the prices in two or three neighboring towns. This task can be largely done online. However, if you are ambitious and brave, I suggest you actually call every practitioner in the area. Introduce yourself as the new acupuncturist in town. Don't be shy. There are more than enough patients out there for all of us to share. One new practitioner only increases the number of potential patients who will benefit from our medicine. Be honest during these conversations; tell them that you are trying to figure out your fees, among other things. Ask what they charge and how people react to their prices. Are patients easily able to pay and continue with treatment, or do they sometimes balk at rescheduling for "financial reasons?" Do they have different rates for different payment types? Do they offer a time-of-service payment discount (which may not be legal in all states) or any other discounts? Are they operating as a community acupuncture clinic? Do they do any fundraising events or pro-bono services?

You'd be amazed and what you can find out from these phone calls, but if this is too scary, get a significant other or friend to call and simply ask for the rates at each clinic.

While other practitioners' prices may or may not factor in to how you set your rates, you still need to know this information. If nothing else, you have begun to introduce yourself to everyone else in the area. These practitioners are your colleagues and you may come to rely on them in the future for referrals, for covering your practice when you are out of town, or for a bottle of herbal medicine that you need for a patient but your clinic has run out.

▶ How much is too much? How much is too little?

What do you feel comfortable charging? If your fees are more than what you believe your services are worth, it will come through in your body language and your voice, and patients or potential patients will think them too high as well even if the rates are really quite fair. If you don't feel comfortable charging as much as the other practitioners in town, this may have nothing to do with the real value of your services. You do deserve to receive compensation for what you have learned and the effort you put into patient care! Although the community acupuncture movement has changed the discussion of pricing for our services completely, in some practice environments and depending upon your overhead and practice style, there is such a thing as charging too little.

Because we often assign value to things based on what they cost, it is logical that we believe something more expensive must be better. Take, for example, the experience of buying a new vacuum cleaner (or wash machine, or coffee maker, or whatever). You are standing in the small appilance aisle with 20 choices to consider. The various models have different features. After finding the ones with the features we are looking for, our decision usually comes down to price and brand, but here's what's interesting. Research shows that most people will discard the lower-priced models first. "Do I really want to buy the cheapest one?" "Why is it so inexpensive?" "Maybe it will break and I will be back here again paying for repair services." These are examples of the thoughts most of us will have.

Then we will look at the Mercedes and Cadillacs of the appliance you are purchasing, and the internal conversation may go like this. "Do I really need all of those bells and whistles? This one won't work any faster, and it's so expensive." Thus the two or three most expensive choices are crossed off and we make a selection from among the medium-priced items, often based on brand names.

This example suggests that, unless you are operating as a community acupuncture clinic, trying to compete based on low-end pricing may mean your services are suspect as too cheap and, therefore, possibly ineffective. If a new client who knows nothing about our profession is considering several practitioners, they may equate your low fees with something wrong about your services or skill. Thus they may ultimately choose a higher-priced practitioner because of the perception of value. In the end, most people make purchasing decisions based on perception of value, trust and word of mouth, not just on price.

Consider another example. Most of the people we know are not driving around in the least expensive cars on the road. Otherwise we'd all be driving Yugos and Kias. We buy a car based on a complex set of perceptions and beliefs that include a wide variety of issues. Price is certainly among those concerns, but is not always that high up on the list compared to many other issues. The same is true of how we purchase healthcare services. People don't necessarily want cheap healthcare. They want trustworthy, caring, reliable, and effective healthcare.

There is one other thing that I think we all need to consider. It is a researched fact that people who are not charged for or are charged less for the same pill rarely get well as quickly and completely as people who are charged more.* That means there is some relationship between placebo effect and money paid for services rendered! If your clinic is lovely, your treatments good, your customer service better than just adequate, and your bedside manner compassionate, you may actually get better clinical results if you are charging a little more for your treatments than if you are charging too little. It bears repeating that people don't necessarily want cheap healthcare; they want effective, compassionate healthcare from someone they trust.

▶ How much money do I need?

Have you ever thought about what it would be like to do, mostly, whatever you wanted, whenever you wanted to do it with regards to your finances? Pay all your bills on time, retire your student loans in half the time required, take those weekend trips without months of planning and saving, or repair your clinical equipment without having to forego a monthly

*http://healthcare-economist.com/tag/placebo-effects/

> **PRACTITIONER POINTER**
>
> "When working with a local fire department to get my employees CPR certified, I decided to pay for the cost of the training. My thought was that if there was no cost to the employees that they would have no excuse for not getting certified. What happened was a disaster. Of three classes offered at different times on different days only three of 80 employees showed up. The rest called in with stories of car problems, or 'I forgot.'
>
> "Two months later I posted sign-up sheets in the employee break room offering CPR classes for a cost of only $5 per person. As before, the classes filled quickly. To my surprise, I had a 100% employee turnout. Why? Because even though the class was only $5, that money meant something to those employees. They had a stake in their future, and had to reach into their own pocket in order to attend. They had assigned value to the class—monetary value."
>
> —*Anonymous*

paycheck. Who has not dreamed of living the life of the financially well-off or at least financially stable practitioner? So what would it take to get there? Below is an exercise you can use to determine how much money your clinic needs to generate per hour to grant you the paycheck you deserve.

Set aside any of the numbers you have come up with to this point, and now let's look at how much you need to make in order to live the life you want. For this exercise, we are going to use a few worksheets that you can find on the companion website in Budgets Worksheets. ● You can see an example of the last page of these worksheets on the next page, but we suggest you go and print these out and fill them in with pencil as we discuss this information. Or you may search and find one or another online budget worksheets to play with in digital form.

CHAPTER 2 | **Setting Your Fees and Managing Your Budget**

We're going to start with the desired end result. How much money do you need for personal expenses per month? Or how much do you want? $5,000? $10,000? What's your number? This has to at least cover your expenses *at home*, including any student loans, car payments, rent, heat and light, and the like.

Take your desired income and enter it on the money line for total personal budget. Now, take some time and fill in the other budget items: clinic rent or lease amount; general liability and malpractice insurance; needles and other supplies; utilities; phone/internet. Now add in the cost of front desk help. If you do not already have a clinic, then use the following figures to help you determine this number. The going rate for *beginning* reception help is $13-$15 per hour. For 30+ hours per week, then, you can expect to pay something between $430-$500 per week. On top of this, add 7.65% (FICA) and usually around 2-3% unemployment. If you are providing any employee benefits and workers compensation insurance, add that under their salary amount as well.

> "O money, money, I'm not necessarily one of those who think thee holy, But I often stop to wonder how thou canst go out so fast when thou comest in so slowly."
>
> —Ogden Nash

Now, add up all of your figures (including the front desk wages for a month) and fill in total business cost per month. Multiply that number by 12 months. The resulting number is your overhead for one year. High, isn't it? Don't panic yet! We are going to break this down into manageable bites as we go down the form. The next step is to divide your yearly overhead by 50 weeks. We say 50 because you do want some vacation, don't you? If you are planning to take more time off, then use the remaining number of weeks to divide into your yearly overhead. However more than two weeks off in your first year is a luxury you may not be able to afford.

Budget Summary

1. Money

Total Business	$ _____	
Total Personal	$ _____	
Sum: Business & Personal	$ _____	Total Monthly Budget
Multiply by 12	$ _____	Total Annual Budget
Divide by 50	$ _____	Revised Weekly Budget

2. Time

Hours Per Week [_____]

3. Money/Hour

Revised Weekly Budget Divided by Hours per Week = Gross $ Per Hour

$ _____ / _____ $ _____

This is what your clinic needs to generate per hour.

How many hours per week are you planning to work or do you presently work? Are you a part-time practitioner at 20 hours per week? Or do you work full-time 35-45 hours? Divide your weekly overhead by that number of hours per week. This number is the amount of money your clinic needs to produce each hour, by one method or another (treatments, rental of space, product sales, or classes taught).

Where does this number fit when compared to the results of the previous questions in this chapter? What portion of this needs to be made from treatments? Is this amount higher or lower than the average treatment price of other practitioners in town? Will you have to see two or three patients per hour to get there? The answers to these questions will also relate to how many treatment rooms you have available and how you prefer to treat. For example, if you do lots of moxa or tuina, you may only be able to see one patient per hour. If you have access to only one room, then you are definitely limited in the number of people you can see and your cost per treatment may need to be higher, you may need to consider moving, or you may need to make more income by other methods, which most clinics need to do in any case. You may have a room to rent out one-or-more days per week or during the evening. You should have product lines to sell, whether Chinese herbal medicine, skin care products, nutritional supplements, books, or something else. Just as it is difficult to balance on a chair with only one leg, your budget will be easier to balance with more than one source of income.

▶ Keeping to a budget

As your practice grows, it's wise to keep careful track of where you actually are financially in relationship to where you'd like to be. Keep a log of expenses, income, and cash flow each month or each week and compare it to your financial goals. Every day you should have in your mind how many new patients you need this week and how many bottles of whatever you sell in your clinic you need to sell to reach your goals. If you are short by a patient or two per week, take actions to bring them in. Visualize a full patient load. Call your inactive patients to see how they are doing or take some other marketing step to fill in your empty clinic spots. See Section 4 on marketing for other ideas on how to fill up your appointment book. The act of staying conscious of where you are in relationship to your "dream" budget will help you realize that dream. This requires some attention to detail, but you will be surprised that it will really help you reach your

SECTION TWO: WORKING ON YOUR OWN

financial goals to know where every cent you make is coming from and where each one you spend is going.

Any month that you are doing better than your budget, use the extra cash to pay down student loans, put money into savings, hire that person you've been wanting to manage your front desk, or buy something to help you grow your practice.

▶ What about a sliding scale?

Many public clinics, like Planned Parenthood or other social service style clinics, base their fees on a sliding scale related to the patient's income. This is usually tied to the federal guidelines ● for what is considered above and below the national poverty line for the size of a family. However, if you bill insurance, you must charge all patients who receive the same service the same fee. Otherwise, you may be prosecuted for insurance fraud. The only exception to this is if you decide to have a formal hardship waiver, ● which stipulates in writing at what income level a person qualifies for a reduced fee. (A payment at the time of service discount of 10-20% is also legal in many states). While this sounds straightforward, it means you will require a way of determining what a prospective patient's income actually is. Thus, if you are going to offer some kind of discounted services due to economic hardship or for any other reason, there have to be written guidelines which are equal and transparent to all. You cannot arbitrarily offer one patient a discount because you feel sorry for them and not offer the same discount to another patient in a similar financial situation. See Section 3, Chapter 2 for more detail about sliding scale fees.

▶ What feels right?

This is the last step. Having done your research, asked your questions, and added your personal figures, scanning these numbers helps you find your comfort level with treatment prices. This is extremely important. When you tell a new patient they need to come in twice a week for the next month, they need to sense that you are comfortable with your prices and believe you are worth that amount of their time and money. For a sensible, honest discussion about this issue, I highly recommend Matthew Bauer's book, *Making Acupuncture Pay*, which is full of practical advice on many subjects including setting your prices and is otherwise very different from this book.

> "By no means run in debt; take thine own measure. Who cannot live on twenty pound a year, cannot on forty."
>
> —George Herbert

If you have checked the local competitors and your pricing is someplace in the middle and it allows you to meet or exceed your clinic's income requirements, you can rest assured that your prices are fair for your market. This means the people you serve will not feel taken advantage of or gouged. In this way, you are more likely to feel and behave comfortably with the financial policies of your clinic. The knowledge that your pricing will meet your personal needs without gouging your patients will give you confidence that you are doing what is right, fair, and needful for both yourself and your patients.

THE COMMUNITY ACUPUNCTURE MOVEMENT

The community acupuncture (CA) clinic model is designed to make our medicine affordable for people who make modest, middle-class incomes and who are unlikely to seek our care if fees are higher. Offering basic acupuncture care in a group setting with efficient diagnostic procedures and simple treatment plans, prices are kept low ($15-$40 per treatment) and people are encouraged to get treatments frequently, similar to the standard of care in China. With the median family income in the US at about $50K for a family of 3-4, this is the only model to realistically allow the vast majority of Americans to experience the benefits of acupuncture. Please see Section 1, Chapter 10 for more detail on operating a community acupuncture clinic.

POINTS TO PONDER FROM CHAPTER 2

- First find out the going rates for similar services in your town or region.

- Decide how you feel about those rates and whether your services are worth more or less.

- When setting your fees, consider that most people want reliable, trustworthy, compassionate, and effective health care more than cheap health care.

- Do a realistic budget to decide what you actually need to create in income per hour to make your life work. Remember that you can and should have more than one income stream in your clinic to create the required amount.

- Until your practice is a word-of-mouth-marketing success and you can charge whatever you want, keep a budget so that you know exactly how many patient visits and new patients you need, how many bottles of herbal medicine or other products you need to sell, or what you need to charge another practitioner in part-time rent to make your budget work.

- If you cannot make the numbers work, consider getting professional help from someone who can help you figure out how to make it work. You might contact SCORE (www.score.org), an organization that matches up entrepreneurs with experienced retirees with all types of business knowledge.

- The community acupuncture clinic model allows middle-income people to afford our care. Depending on where you wish to practice and how you like to work with patients, this can be an excellent approach to business. See Section 1, Chapter 10 for details.

How Much $$ Do You Need to Get Started? | 3

Some people are blessed to graduate from school with very little student loan debt due to savings or family support for their pursuit of a new career. Most, however, are not so lucky. It is estimated that 75-80% of graduates have $80,000 or more in debt upon graduation. At 6.8% (the rate at the time of this writing) over 20 years, that's approximately $600 per month for an $80,000 loan! This certainly makes the idea of going out and borrowing another $10-$20K to start up a clinic seem daunting, if not downright depressing. However, there is always more than one way to access capital and, depending upon your personality, an additional $10-20K loan on top of what you had to borrow to go to school may not really make it any harder to sleep at night. In fact, borrowing the money you need may help spur your motivation to work hard and succeed in your practice. In this chapter, I'll discuss fixed and variable start-up costs and creative ways to raise the capital you will need during your first years of practice.

▶ **How much cash do you need?**

It is possible to start your practice on a shoestring, which I define as anything less than $10,000 during the first year. Please remember, however, that one of the main reasons for small business failure is undercapitalization. What that means is that a business did not have enough capital for the start-up phase when income is always unpredictable. In such cases, a really bad month or even a bad week can make it impossible to pay the rent unless you have a back-up line of credit or family assistance. In order to determine how much you will need for your new clinic, let's look at some real-world budget scenarios and see what it really costs to start and run a thriving practice.

Below are hypothetical start-up budgets for four ways a practice could be run: 1) out of your house, 2) renting space from another practitioner, 3) in a 1,000 square foot clinic space with one partner, and 4) in a 600-750 square foot clinic space by yourself. Figures are based on averages from speaking with practitioners all over the U.S. I have also included costs for equipment and furniture that you may need to purchase at the beginning if you have not collected any of these items during your years as a student. For all scenarios I am assuming a reasonable salary for front desk help.

➤ Practicing from home

Later on in this section I discuss the pros and cons of running your practice out of your house from a professional and logistics point of view. At this point I am only presenting hypothetical overhead for a home-based clinic. Please note that this is based on you owning, not renting, the space where you live. In this case, I am assuming a clinic with one treatment room and a small waiting/reception/herb area, which seems to be typical for home clinics (though I've seen much larger). This scenario also assumes that the business is being run as a sole proprietorship. So there is no corporation paying rent to you for the space, although that is another possibility to consider. Costs shown are annual. The cost of buying herbal medicinals is not included in any of these calculations because that is a profit center, not a pure expense, and everyone does it differently. The size of this clinic space is 500 square feet; I am figuring supply costs based on seeing 30 patients per week and also assume that any practitioner starting this way is buying furniture and equipment for their clinic somewhat on the less expensive side. Also, most people will already have a computer, some extra chairs or an extra coffee table, desk, artwork, carpets, or other accessories that may be pressed into service for a clinic. *I understand these numbers will vary widely.* Thus I have made some generalizations that you may add or subtract from your own calculations.

Annual operating costs (Fixed costs are in green.)

Lease (You can deduct pro-rata share of the mortgage from your taxes for the space you use, so you save here!)	$0
Salary 20-hr/wk front desk staff (annual). I suggest you hire staff as soon as you can. It will help you grow, but may or may not be part of your 1st yr.	$15,000
Heat & light (based on avg. mo. bill of $200 in a 2500 sq.ft. house & a 500 sq.ft. clinic in that house)	$500
Clinic supplies (needles, table paper, paper towels, cotton balls, alcohol swabs, moxa)	$1,050
Malpractice insurance	$850
Student loan payments	$7,200
Continuing education (do online when it's on sale or through your state association when it's low cost)	$200
Office and cleaning supplies	$250
1 phone line & high speed/wireless internet	$500
License fees (vary by state)	$150
NCCAOM recertification ($230÷4 yrs.)	$57.50
Equipment repair or replacement (includes possible computer breakdowns)	$400
Marketing (cards, brochures, pens, website)	$2,000
Bookkeeping and accounting costs	$500
Sharps disposal (one large box per year)	$35
State/national association fees	$300
Total Annual	$28,992.50

One time costs (you may already have some of these items)

Computer	$500-1,500
Printer/fax/copier machine	$150
Phone equipment	$150
Treatment table	$600
Heat lamp, TDP lamp	$150
Furniture (coffee table, two chairs, carpets, lamps, desk, office accessories)	$1,500
Total	$4,050

All this means that your annual costs in your first year if you are practicing at home might come to $24-$33K ($2,000- $2,750 per month) plus what you pay yourself as described above. Actual figures depend upon what things you have accumulated before graduation, what services you hire out (bookkeeping, IT), how many hours you hire someone to answer the phone (if at all), and the size of your student loan payment. If you have graduated with some nice new equipment for your clinic, then your first year expenses could be a few thousand dollars less than for those who did not. These figures will give you a place to start. Assume that in any overhead scenario in this chapter, I am including a student loan payment of $600 per month, which is the low side of average.

> **POWER POINT**
>
> If you wanted to take home $3,000 per month in your 1st year and your home-based practice is costing an average of $2,000 per month to operate for a total of $5,000 needed, you would need to see 22 patients per week at $56 per patient visit to get there. That's only 4.5 patients per day, five days per week at a very reasonable rate! (Good news: these numbers do not include any product sales in your clinic.)

▶ **Renting space from another practitioner**

Your annual costs in this type of scenario will obviously vary depending upon a number of factors, including how much space and time you use and how much equipment you do or don't need. If the clinic is fully equipped and you are just coming in with your black bag of practice supplies, you may pay a little *more* in rent, but it may cost you far *less* than if you are renting and equipping an entire suite of rooms for full-time practice. No matter what sort of deal you work out, you will still have some fixed costs such as CEUs, malpractice insurance, practice supplies, license fees, marketing expenses, and possibly student loan repayment as well as your rent. Let's talk about rent costs in this type of setting.

The average cost around the U.S. for professional rental space is $16-22 per square foot per year. Depending upon what part of the country you live in, how much of the shared clinic space you have access to, and how many hours per week you are using the space, a 150 sq.ft. room (10×15') used full time could cost you $275-$450 per month. You'll have to negotiate whether your appointments will be made online at your own website or by the clinic receptionist, access to herbal medicines in the clinic or bring in your own, use of common areas, and storage of your patient files (if on paper). Access to phone and internet, heat and light, cleaning service, sharps disposal, or other operating costs may also be included in your rent depending on what you can negotiate. Now go back to page 137 and add in some of the other costs listed there to figure an annual total.

If you are using someone else's completely equipped rooms and front desk services, you should expect to pay higher rent than if you are supplying all the furniture and fixtures, but such an arrangement can be helpful in your first year or so because it lowers your start-up costs. In such cases, make sure you have something in your contract for what happens if something breaks, you drop burning moxa on the carpet or the table and

POWER POINT

If you rent space three days per week and pay $500 in rent monthly, your *average* cost to run your practice will be around $15,000 per year. If you can see an *average* of 16 patients per week at $55 per visit your first year for 50 weeks of the year, your take home pay for *those three days* per week will be $45,000 before taxes. If you can see an average of 16 patients per week at $60 per visit, your take home pay will be $50,000 before taxes. (Note: these numbers do not include income from sales of any products and $55-$60 is a quite modest price per treatment around the country.)

cause a burn, or for any other possible source of friction that may arise when someone is renting someone's property in addition to the space. In all cases, do your best to care for things in this clinic as if they were your own.

▶ A shared clinic

So you're graduating and two of your schoolmates want to go in on a clinic space with you. Once you have agreed upon a location and name for the clinic, décor, designs for letterhead, biz cards, and marketing plans, you will have to decide how the space, time, and costs will be shared. My first suggestion is not to get too small of a space. The universe will not let your practice grow and expand as easily if there is nowhere for it to expand into. I think 800-900 sq.ft. is a minimum workable size depending upon the layout of the space and whether everyone wants to practice full time. That will allow three generous or 4-5 small treatment rooms, a waiting-reception area, storage closet, and a small pharmacy area. If the space costs $18 per sq.ft. per year, that's $1,350 (18×900÷12) per month (plus utilities and insurance) split three ways if everyone is paying an equal share. There will also be a damage deposit and possibly last month's rent to come up with in advance. In such cases, I suggest you either create a limited liability company [LLC] (see Section 1, Chapters 6 and 7) or that everyone in the clinic form their own professional corporation [PC] so that each of you is protected from the others' potential clinical errors.

Whatever business structure you choose, you still need a contract drawn up. You may be great friends and think you'll never have disagreements. Don't believe it. In my experience, a good contract protects friendships and it's worth hiring a lawyer to do this for you. To keep the legal fees to a minimum, sit down together and create a list of the things you want the contract to do or to prevent. Even if you create an LLC, there are all sorts of things that need to be decided and agreed upon in order for all of you to be happy and feel secure. This includes items such as which expenses will be shared and which will not, whose name(s) will be on the lease, what lines of herbal medicine or other products will be carried and how profits from sales will be tracked and shared, how disputes will be handled, who will be in charge of hiring and firing employees, how someone leaves the practice and under what circumstances others may join, and what to do if one person's practice gets off the ground faster than the others and he or she needs more space and time. This list could go on and on (see Section 1, Chapter 7).

Still, it can be wonderful to practice with others. In addition to moral support, you will refer patients to each other, cover each other's practices during vacations, share creative marketing and décor ideas, and help each other with clinical issues. It will cost you less than operating your practice alone and you could conceivably be open seven days a week! Your costs in this situation are likely to be similar to those of someone renting space from another practitioner or perhaps a little higher. See page 137 for a list of other common expenses.

➤ Your own private clinic

This situation is the most expensive in both start-up cost and continued operation cost. However, if you are moving somewhere you don't know anyone or are not excited about renting space or sharing space, you need to figure out the costs of doing it all by yourself. What I hear from around the country is that the average cost of running a clinic is $27-$40K annually or between $2,500-$3,500 per month depending upon what sort of space you rent, where you live, and what amenities you offer. As stated above, you may be able to control some of the variable costs of running a clinic, but the fixed costs are just that, fixed. See Chapter 4 of this section on negotiating a lease to help you get the best deal you can. I also strongly suggest that in order to thrive, you need two treatment rooms in addition to

SECTION TWO: WORKING ON YOUR OWN

your reception/pharmacy area. You may be able to get by with 550-650 square feet, but probably not less than 500 unless the second treatment room is *really* tiny. You want your clinic to look professional and comfortable, not cramped and dingy. Also, you cannot chop your marketing budget down to zero, although in the marketing section of this book there are lots of ideas that cost far more in time than money.

> **POWER POINT**
>
> Renting space in someone else's clinic with no separate landline for phone service? Accept client credit card payments by using a service like ROAMpay®, Square®, or GoPayment®. Patients can make appointments through online software at your website and keep in touch with you by email and texting. Once you get your own clinic, add a landline for patient convenience!

In any case, based on an annual practice cost of $30,000 and a take home pay of about $55,000 before taxes your first year, you'll need to see 30 patients per week at $58 per patient visit to get there. To just break even (overhead and student loan only), you will need to see about 12 patients per week at $58 per visit. That does not include income from product sales, renting out space, or anything else you might do to earn a living in your clinic.

▶ How to generate working capital

If you are lucky enough to have a working spouse, you may be able to start with the "break even" numbers listed above in all the scenarios we have discussed, not that you want to hang out there for very long! If you have to make a living, however, in addition to paying back your loans, you'll need to get patient visits up to 20-30 per week pretty quickly. See the marketing chapters (Section 4) for ideas on how to do that and *don't stay in a place that is over-saturated with practitioners*. In the meantime, if you have no money at all to start your practice, you will need to generate a few thousand in working capital and do it quickly. So what are the cheapest sources of money you can find?

- **Home equity**
  If you have not done so already, it might not be a bad time to refinance your house. If you are now paying more than 5% in mortgage interest (at the time of this writing), you could get several thousand dollars out from a refinance and still be paying the same amount in monthly mortgage payments. (If interest rates rise, this may not be a viable cheap money source.) Put it in an interest-bearing money market account and only use what you need. If your practice grows really quickly, you can use the money you borrowed from yourself for your monthly mortgage payments! Or, if you are really gutsy, sell your house in the city and move to a smaller town where life is less expensive. Use the money you have left over after buying a new, less expensive house to capitalize your start-up years. A third method might be to ask for a line of credit based on the equity in your home. Such credit lines can be quite inexpensive. Again, only use what you need and pay your minimums and as much more as you can each month promptly. Use any excess to pay down student loans.

  > "If you are going to worry, don't do it. If you do it, don't worry."
  > —Michael Nolan

- **Credit unions**
  Credit union loan rates are often an entire percentage point less than a regular bank. If you have a family member that is already a credit union member, you should look into the rules for joining as well as their loan and line-of-credit rates.

- **Family**
  This, of course, is one of the best ways to borrow money because there is often very low or no interest on the loan. There may, however, be other more complex "strings" attached to such cash, but depending upon your relationship with your family, it *is* a source of funding to consider. If you are worried about the potential effect on your relationship, write a simple contract for repayment and stick to it.

- **Moonlighting**
  When I started my first business, I had several house cleaning jobs to cover my bills while I got the new business off the ground. I made enough to pay my rent and modest living expenses. So the new business did not have to support me for the first year. This is a tough row to hoe in terms of personal time, but, if you are young and healthy, it can work.

- **Life insurance loans**
  If you have a life insurance policy, you can often borrow from the cash surrender value without any business plan or other qualifications. These loans also have very attractive interest rates in many cases. The same may be true with some types of retirement accounts.

- **Acupuncture birthday gifts**
  This is for anyone with a large family. Write your friends and family just before your birthday during the last year of acupuncture school. Tell them that you will need $7K, $9K, or $10K to start your practice and you are looking for pledges which can be paid back over the next three years or can be taken in free treatments. You may find that your family supports what you have been doing in school over the last 3-4 years and will pledge their support quite generously.

- **Venture capital/Angels**
  Private venture capital is not out of the question. If you are dreaming big and want to start something truly special in the way of a clinic, we suggest you get a book called *Finding Private Venture Capital for Your Firm* by Robert Gaston. He estimates that over 700,000 people commit over $50 billion in venture capital annually in this country. Ask your banker, lawyer, accountants, or other business people if they know anyone in this category, or look online at places like www.venturehacks.com or

www.ventureworthy.com. You might have to go and give a speech explaining and supporting what you want to create, but, if you have a big dream and a *good* business plan, you never know. You could also find an investor by posting a classified ad in the "Business Opportunities" section of your local paper or business publication. Remember that such people are looking for a good return on their money. That means your plan must be well-organized and designed to turn a solid profit within five years or less.

- **U.S. Department of Agriculture**
  This branch of the federal government oversees about 29 money programs. Their Business and Industrial Loan Program can help start almost any kind of business as long as it is in a town of fewer than 50,000 people. They want to foster economic growth in rural America. They will not loan you the money directly, but they will guarantee up to 90% of the principal for the local bank that does the lending. You can check out their website at http://www.rurdev.usda.gov

- **SBA micro-loans**
  The Small Business Administration has a program designed especially to help part-time or home-based businesses. These loans can be a few hundred to several thousand dollars and have reasonable interest rates. Call 800-827-5722 for more information.

- **Traditional bank lines-of-credit**
  If you have a good credit history, look into a line-of-credit at local banks. They require collateral, so this is easier if you have a house or other assets, even if they are not liquid. Ask for a bit more than you think you need. Of course, you don't have to use it if you don't need it, but it's there if you do. With interest rates at reasonable levels in recent years, this may be easier than a traditional loan. A business plan and application will be required.

- **Grants to fund research**

    If you are a good writer and have a specific area of interest or you plan to serve a very small niche market, you might be able to find grant money to fund a research project using acupuncture or Chinese herbal medicine. This would be a way to see lots of patients and get experience in a specific area in which you will become an expert. It might limit the type of patients you can see for a while, but it could be a very good way to get a clinic started and get a reputation in a specific field of interest. Your public library should have listings of foundations and corporations and the type of research they find interesting. Or, for more information on grant-writing, contact the Grantsmanship Center in Los Angeles. Ask for their article called "Program Planning and Proposal Writing," which is just for the novice grant-writer. This can be hard work, but if you can find a project that gets a foundation's interest, it would be a huge feather in your cap and a great item on your resumé. You can start planning for this type of funding before you ever get out of school.

- **Crowd-funding**

    This may require a Tom Sawyer level of persuasion skill, but it is worth a try. Kickstarter and GoFundMe have become popular ways to start a business, and writing up the required forms makes you really think about how your business will operate and succeed. If local people put in some green, offer them treatments in exchange if they are willing to allow you to contact them. (Some people prefer to remain anonymous.)

▶ Conclusion

You *can* find, create, borrow, receive, or earn the money you need to start your business. That is one of the things our country has always been about. . . new business growth. You'll even be surprised at who might help you. First you need to think about how and where you want to practice and do your homework about how much you will need over the first 6-12 months of your life as a practitioner. Once you know exactly what you need to generate, it is easier to figure out how you are going to do it. Also, consider that if you are in a certain amount of debt already, don't choke as you are rounding third base. If you do borrow money, 1) *do* create a business plan and a careful budget and 2) *don't* be wasteful or fritter away your capital on things that are not necessary.

POINTS TO PONDER FROM CHAPTER 3

- The typical one-person private practice costs somewhere between $2,500-$4,000 per month if you are practicing out of your own private office. Home-based and shared practices cost somewhat less.

- This chapter gives you some average fixed cost figures to use in order to determine what you will need and how soon after graduation you will need it.

- You may not need all the money immediately, but it will be difficult to start up with less than $10,000 in seed money during the first year.

- If you start your practice out of your house, renting space from another practitioner, or sharing a clinic with one or more other practitioners, your start-up costs will be less than if you start by opening your own private clinic in a commercial or professional leased space.

- There are lots of possible sources of funding including personal bank loans, private family loans, grants, home equity loans, your life insurance policy, crowd-funding, or your retirement accounts.

Finding Space and Negotiating a Lease | 4

There are several factors that go into negotiating a lease for your clinic space. With a little luck you will be dealing with a reputable, trustworthy person who is not out to cheat you. That being said, good contracts make for good relationships because everything is clear and down on paper. It is good to know who is responsible for what so that if a problem or question arises, there are no gray areas that may lead to arguments or even legal action on one side or the other. Here are the things you need to at least consider when negotiating a lease.

What does the ideal space for you look like?

I suggest you write down in advance what your ideal clinic space will have. Will the street be quiet or a high traffic and visibility area? Will there be public transportation nearby or a large parking lot? Will it already be zoned as business or medical office space? What build-out needs, such as sinks, railings, shelving, or extra treatment spaces, will you ask for? Do you require wifi? What square footage do you want? How many sinks or bathrooms will you need? If it is a multiple-use office building, who else is in the building and will they be sympathetic to what you do? Is the building ADA (Americans with Disabilities Act) compliant? What about using moxibustion?

Do you need broker representation?

A professional broker service is a nice option if you are busy and want spaces previewed according to your specifications before you take the time to look. Such services will also help insure that your lease is fair and they will be your negotiating agent for anything you want to request from the landlord such as build-outs, new carpets, and annual rent increase percentages. It is usually the person who owns the space who pays the broker's fees. However, if you use a broker, make sure that they have done some representation for people in some type of private medical or allied health practice so they have some idea what your needs are. If they have specialized in negotiating for manufacturing firms, they may be excellent at that but may not really have a clue what your needs are.

What is rentable vs. usable space?

Be sure you know how the space is being measured by the landlord. Rentable space means that the landlord is including that space in the square footage for which you are being charged. Usable space means it is the actual space you can use for your work. Rentable space for which you may be charged is common area space such as hallways, lobbies, public area bathrooms, elevators, or crawl spaces. This is often split on a percentage basis between all the tenants in the building and can be substantial. If you are to be charged for any rentable but not usable space, try to get a cap on the price and how much these expenses may be raised during each year of the lease (if at all).

Is the building in good shape physically and legally?

Make sure you take a look at the age and condition of things such as elevators, stairwells, and ramps for disabled people. If the building is old, for example, try to get a clause in the lease that excludes you completely from paying for improvements that may be mandated by city or federal codes. Such extraordinary items could cost you thousands in unexpected expense, such as replacing an old elevator or adding ADA required ramps. As a lessee, these should not be part of your financial responsibility.

Is the lease gross or triple-net (NNN)?

What do these terms mean? A gross lease is great, but more and more rare. It means that all the taxes, insurance, and maintenance of space is included in the total amount of the lease. Triple-net means that, over-and-above the square foot per year cost of the space, you will be charged a portion of 1) taxes, 2) insurance, and 3) CAM (common area maintenance, discussed above as rentable space). This can include repairs, gardening, lighting, snow removal, depreciation of machinery, security, resurfacing, and other expenses. Make sure you get in writing what is included in the triple-net and get a cap on annual NNN fees.

What is included in the term of the lease?
Term of the lease means how long it is and what your renewal options are. It's a good idea to make sure you have the right to extend or renew the lease and that you are clear about the required timing of giving notice to stay or go at the end of the lease.

Are you allowed to alter the space?
Unless you are walking into someone else's acupuncture clinic, it is likely you will need to alter some things about the space. You need to know if you are required to get permission for things like putting up paintings or shelving, making holes in the wall, moving walls or doors, or anything else you may want to do. Also, be clear in the lease about how major repairs will be handled during the last year of the lease; you don't want to repair something major on your nickel during your last year there.

Who is responsible for rebuilding after a casualty?
If there were a fire, flood, or terrorist attack, can you negotiate a "no rent to be paid" arrangement while repairs and rebuilding are being done? If not, you need to make sure you have an insurance policy for this and a "plan B" for where you would practice in such a case. This did happen to a friend of mine!

What is escalation of costs?
Most leases will increase by a small percentage per year over the life of the lease. If you can, try to negotiate this as an exact

figure or percentage not tied to the consumer price index or the current lease values in your area. This allows you to plan in advance what your costs are and what your income requirements are. As a new practitioner, try to start as low as possible even if it means a higher amount at the other end.

What is meant by breach/cure?

Breach/cure is a legal term describing what happens when you do something (on purpose or inadvertently) that is expressly a breach of your lease. The most important example of this is that you know how your landlord handles lapses in payment and eviction notices. For example, what if your check gets lost in the mail? Will he or she call you after X number of days instead of serving you with an eviction notice? This sounds like it should be simple good human communication skills. However, it is important to have it spelled out in your lease so that no misunderstandings arise.

What are your insurance requirements?

It is important to include in a lease what sorts of insurance your landlord requires. Make sure that, if he or she requires double (yours and his) coverage for liability insurance, that the companies have a mutual waiver of subrogation between them. That means they will not be arguing instead of getting the job done for you if there is a suit against the building for any reason. Try to negotiate this down to a simple renters property insurance policy. These are usually quite inexpensive unless you are using deadly chemicals or something. Also, get more than one quote; they can vary enormously. And understand what your insurance liability really is as a renter. If someone falls down in the parking lot, is that your responsibility or the landlord's and how much coverage should be required of you for various types of incidents?

What is your exit strategy?

Be sure you are clear about under what circumstances you may get out of the lease. For example, do you need to sublet but keep the lease in your name? Or can you transfer the lease to another party? Or will the landlord require a completely new lease? Be sure you understand this clause.

➤ Leasing space in someone else's clinic

Above are the basic items that you need to consider when you are signing a lease for your own clinic. If you are signing a rental agreement with another practitioner to use any part of his/her clinic for some part of each week, there are other things you need to negotiate.

How will your rent be figured?

If just starting out as a practitioner, try negotiating an arrangement whereby you only pay a percentage per patient. Such agreements do exist and are fine. However, we see a motivational problem with this type of deal. If you have to pay a flat fee per month, you are more likely to do what is necessary to fill up your hours with patients than if you only have to pay rent by the patient. Your attitude about your practice is paramount to your success, and I encourage you, even at the beginning, not to operate from a position of fear.

As a sub-lessee, the important thing to avoid is any responsibility for the specific items in the leaseholder's agreement with the landlord. That is to say, your rent should be a flat fee with no clauses regarding insurance, no responsibility for building up-keep, snow removal, etc. You should have a clause regarding an exit strategy, just to keep things clear, as well as specifics about when your rent is due, hours of access to the clinic, keys, management of HIPAA privacy rules for your patients and other practitioners' patients, any financial obligations concerning clinic-wide marketing campaigns such as open-houses, website costs, or Yelp/Google/Facebook ads, and guidelines regarding the clinic pharmacy usage and profits.

Who owns the herbs?

It is inconvenient for you to have to bring your own herbs with you if you are renting space in someone else's clinic unless you have your own shelves. On the other hand, it is inconvenient for your patients to have to write two checks on each visit (one to you for the treatment and another to the owner for the herbs). This is even more complex if the clinic uses credit cards. Then there is the issue of who gets what part of the profits on the herbs sold if they are not specifically yours and how inventory is managed. Who decides what lines of product will be sold?

The easiest way to handle this is to have your own herbs and phone-attached credit card processing method, such as Square®. Another possibility is a clinic-wide credit card payment log with a section for each person renting space in the clinic to track usage and perhaps get a 10% cut of all sales. In this scenario, there is an inventory sheet where any product that is sold is written down, so that product is replaced as necessary. This is cumbersome, if equitable, and requires practitioners to pay more attention to detail (more than some may be able to manage!) than other methods.

There are other, less cumbersome ways to handle this situation. One practitioner I know prefers a different product line from those carried where she rents space. She deals with this by having herbal products drop-shipped directly to the patients from her distributor on the same day as their treatment; the product reaches the patient within 48 hours of the visit.

> **PRACTITIONER POINTER**
>
> "Hire an attorney to check your contracts if you plan on renting space from another healthcare practitioner. Everyone says, 'It's just a formality, I just trust everyone.' But, if things go south, a little investment on the front end can save you thousands in dollars and headaches down the road. Take care of the details up front and avoid costly errors later. Good luck!"
>
> —Geoffrey Hudson
> Springfield, MO

Patients pay her retail for the product in advance. She pays one bill to the distributor at wholesale prices once per month, and makes a profit even though she maintains no inventory.

Another practitioner built her own shelves in the clinic so that she can have her preferred product lines on hand all the time, selling everything with her own phone-attached credit card processor. See what arrangement will work best for you and the person from whom you are renting. However you work out arrange-ments for herbal product sales, it is always better to have your specific deal in writing so that everyone knows what to expect.

> ### POINTS TO PONDER FROM CHAPTER 4
>
> - Write down your exact needs for your clinic space.
> - Consider hiring a broker to find your space and negotiate your lease. This does not cost you any $$$.
> - Make sure you understand all aspects of the lease from beginning to end:
>   - Term of the lease, required insurances
>   - NNN, escalation of costs, rentable vs. usable space
>   - Who pays for repairs? Can you put up shelving?
>   - How to get out of the lease if necessary!
> - When sub-leasing space in other people's clinics, make sure you are not responsible to the landlord, only to the leaseholder.
> - Get a flat rate and fill your hours!
> - Be sure you know all your responsibilities and rights.
> - Be clear about profits from herb sales and the handling of patient credit cards.

Creating a Business Plan for Your Clinic Can be Fun | 5

Wait! Don't skip this chapter! We know you don't want to do this, but we will hold your hand (see the website) and try our best to convince you that this is 1) doable, 2) important, and 3) fun. Yes, really! So, give this a look and you will see why it will help you be more successful. OK, here goes.

According to Joanna L. Krotz in an article titled "7 Biggest Mistakes of Business Startups" published on microsoft.com/business, the number one deadly sin of a start-up is *no business plan.* If you plan on opening your own private practice or clinic, we've got news for you: You are a start-up. As Krotz says, "There is no single omission that bodes worse for a start-up's future than the lack of a clear business plan. Fail to plan and you plan to fail."

Having a written business plan means that you've done your homework and you've carefully thought out how you are going to open and run your clinic and make a profit. *It is your own self-created road map to success.* It is a goal-setting document. It is a reference tool. It is, at the end of the day, a very encouraging piece of work that actually shows you how you are going to get from here to there, who your allies are, where any stumbling blocks or potholes in the road may be, and what you need to do to realize your professional dreams.

It is up to you whether you develop this plan for your own use or to share with others. But, if you plan to borrow money from a bank or other professional lender, they're going to want to see a written business plan. Why do lenders require a business plan? Maybe because they know that anyone with the energy and focus to do the work required here is more likely to do what they say they will and pay back their loan! It means you are a grown-up who has thought about what running a small business really takes. Think about it. If this feels too complicated and difficult, do you really think you are cut out to be in business for yourself?

It is my feeling that even if you're going to fund your new business from your own savings, it's imperative that you write out some parts of a business plan to insure the likelihood of your success. If you are lending money to yourself, you need to be able to answer the question, "Would I lend money to this person?" with an emphatic "Yes!"

A good business plan is a working document that helps keep you on track for success. It is both a planning tool and a reference that you can look at weekly or even daily to help guide you when you can't remember what you were going to do next. A good plan should focus on the following key issues:

- your capital (money) requirements and cash expenditures
- your market opportunity
- a marketing plan
- a competition analysis
- an operating plan
- projected earnings chart
- an execution schedule of milestones and deadlines

Although we have not been able to find hard data on this, contemporary wisdom suggests that up to 50% of graduates of American acupuncture schools are not in full time practice five years after graduation. While there are many possible reasons for this, one common reason is inability of many acupuncturists to earn an income that allows them to do what they love to do full time. One of the main reasons for this inability is not carefully thinking about the economics of what they are going to do before jumping into practice. Depending on how you write your business plan and then follow through on its execution, you can guarantee yourself an income of $100,000 per year or more *if that's what you really would like to do.*

No matter what you are trying to accomplish, the process of planning, setting goals, and then successfully following through on those plans is the same. The difference between a dream and a goal is a step-by-step plan which leads you to that goal. If you use the forms we have put in the companion website as a workbook, you will have many of the elements of a successful business plan. If you want to present that plan to a bank or other lender, all you have to do is print out the information you have written into the forms to have a finished business plan. If you fill in all of the forms and go through the suggested exercises for each section, you are very close to fleshing out the bones of a solid business plan. You will have basic information about every aspect of running your business. In the Resources for Going Further section in this book and on the website, there is a list of several books and pieces of software that you may wish to use to help you further.

As you go through this information, you will note that I [HW] typically talk about customers as opposed to patients. There is also the use of other standard business jargon, such as sales, marketing, publicity, competition, competitive advantage, etc. These terms may sound strange at first when applied to a healing art. However, these are used on purpose in order to drive home the point that, no matter how good an acupuncturist you are, if you want to succeed in private practice, you also have to be a good businessperson, and that means thinking like a businessperson. Hopefully, you will be able to separate and keep these two hats straight, but, if you're not willing to put on the hat of the businessperson when it comes to running your practice, you might consider being someone else's employee.

> ### What is included in a typical business plan?

> "Begin each day as if it were on purpose."
>
> —Mary Anne Radmacher

Business plans typically follow a pretty standard outline, especially if you intend to show the plan to a bank or professional lender. Business plans are meant to provide specific information about the starting up and running of your business to people who hold purse strings: bankers and bean-counters. The following outline is based on *Adams Streetwise: Complete Business Plans the Easy Way* (book and software) by Bob Adams published by Adams Media Corporation, 2006; *Business Plans for Dummies* by Paul Tiffany and Stephen D. Peterson, published by IDG Books, 2010; and information provided by the U.S. Small Business Administration. This outline has been expanded on the website with explanations and samples of what each of these sections might say.

1. Front matter
    Cover letter
    Nondisclosure statement
    Title page
    Table of contents

2. Summary
    Business concept
    Current situation
    Key success factors
    Current financial needs

3. Vision
    Vision statement
    Milestones

4. Marketing analysis
    The overall market and recent changes in the market
    Market segments and target market
    Customer characteristics and needs

5. Competitive analysis
    Industry overview
    Nature of competition
    Changes in the industry
    Primary competitors
    Opportunities
    Threats and risks

6. Strategic planning
    Key competitive capabilities
    Key competitive weaknesses
    Strategy and implementation of the strategy

7. Services (and products)
    Services (and products) description
    Competitive evaluation of services (and products)
    Future services (and products)

8. Sales & marketing
    Marketing strategy
    Sales tactics
    Advertising
    Promotions and incentives
    Publicity

9. Operations
    Service and product delivery
    Customer service and support
    Facilities
    Insurance
    Licenses

> **PRACTITIONER POINTER**
>
> "Best advice for new grads: Don't be in a rush! Make a business plan, don't take shortcuts on setting up your business. Get help if and where you need it. If we had it to do over again, I think we would not be so quick to jump into a bigger space, even though our growth looked like it could handle it. And I would feel more apt to get professional help in the beginning (with our lease contract, etc) rather than having to seek it out later."
>
> —*Lisa Lowe and Karen Marks*
> *Arvada, CO*
> *www.oldetownacu.com*

10. Financial management
> Equipment and supply list (start-up costs)
> *Pro forma* income projections (profit and loss statements)
>> Detail by month, first and second year
>> Detail by quarter, third year
>> Assumptions upon which projections are based
>
> *Pro forma* cash flow
> Breakeven analysis
> Balance sheet

11. Supporting documents
> Tax returns of principals for the last three years
> Personal financial statement (bank statements)
> Proposed lease or purchase agreement for office space
> Licenses and other legal documents
> Resumes of all principals
> Letters of intent from suppliers, etc.

Simply by thinking about each of the above things and then describing them or your plans for them on paper, you will have *radically* differentiated yourself from the majority of American acupuncturists. You will now have a much better idea of what you are getting into and how you are going to make a success of it, however you describe success.

The website includes samples of every single one of the above outline items! ● You can download any or all of these letters, statements, and forms, changing them as you need to reflect your situation. If you must present your plan to a bank or other lender, all you have to do is reformat and print what you have written to have a finished business plan. As a businessperson myself, I absolutely encourage you, with pom-poms, bullhorns, and 76 trombones, to complete this project, even if you've been in business for a while. You won't be sorry; I guarantee it!

POINTS TO PONDER FROM CHAPTER 5

What's in a business plan and why should I do one?

- It is an important planning tool that makes you really think about what you are doing.

- It helps you realistically focus on your current position, forces you to state your short- and long-term goals, and make decisions about how you will go about reaching your goals.

- It gives you an action plan against which you can check your progress.

- It helps you in borrowing money and/or finding investors.

- It radically improves your chances of success because you have done your homework and are not just winging it.

Consider the Look and Feel of Your Clinic | 6

Medical research suggests that placebo effect accounts for up to 40% of any clinical interaction. What this means for you is that every sensory impression received in your clinic–the ambiance, sights, sounds, smells, and smiles–is important! When a new patient (or an MD, newspaper writer, or local politician!) walks through your door, everything they absorb through all their senses will form their first, very difficult to change, impressions. That means every element of your clinic's look, feel, and operation will either improve or hinder your chances of both business and clinical success.

Style and design elements vary widely from clinic to clinic. Still, no matter how good you think your clinic looks (and runs), the opinions that matter most are your patients'. While I have no interest in being the style police, this chapter will help guide you through some of the decisions you'll need to make, prod you to think about your design choices, offer suggestions for interesting possibilities, and spark your creativity.

➤ Choose a feeling

Being a "complementary and alternative" care provider may allow you more options than an MD when it comes to creating the feel of your clinic. That being said, it is wise to make design choices that are likely to be appreciated by the community in which you practice. No matter your choice of overall ambiance–"Western medical," "it's-all-about-women-in-here," or "you've-just-stepped-into-the-exotic-Orient,"–you don't want to alienate anyone. Going too far in any direction is rarely wise, unless you have a *very* specific niche. Even in that case, it's important that your decor says "professional" above all else.

▶ Starting from the outside In

After your website or business card, the first thing a new or prospective patient sees is the exterior of your clinic. If you are in a professional building or retail space with mandated signage and lighting styles, and exterior care included in the lease, you need not worry about exterior issues further. If you own the property and it has lawn or green space, good outside upkeep increases your curb appeal. This may mean shrubs, flowers, or a labeled Chinese herb garden, but should at least be a tidy, weeded, and watered lawn.

Whatever your circumstances, make sure your building, outdoor signs, walkways, and porch or entrance areas are clean and free of insect nests, debris, and cobwebs. Take a brief but regular walk around your exterior. A weekly, 30-minute effort helps maintain a clean and pleasant exterior.

Each morning, check the main entrance area, waiting room, bathroom(s), and treatment rooms for cleanliness and readiness to receive patients. Westerners expect medical facilities of any type to be clean. This is also a chance to restock facial tissue, paper towels, and toilet paper, or take care of any other details such as airing out the rooms from yesterday's moxa smoke, wiping down your treatment tables, or a last minute vacuuming.

▶ Colors in a healing space

The colors you choose for your clinic decor affect each patient who comes for care as well as those who work there (you). Since we want our space itself to encourage placebo effect, using quiet colors that are soothing and relaxing are best, especially for larger areas such as walls and carpets. To keep things from being boring, however, use brighter, richer colors as accents. Art and signage on the walls, plants, retail displays, and a colorful chair or lamp, can be attractive and tasteful. You want an inviting and interesting, but not garish or overly-busy general feel.

If you need help with color combining, visit a local paint store or home improvement center to snag a few promotional brochures to get ideas. Your goal is to create a clinic that both enhances patient relaxation and looks professional. With that in mind, use your creativity and heart to create a beautiful healing space where you will enjoy working and your patients' response to treatment is enhanced. Make your space so interesting that patients will want to talk about it with their friends.

▶ Your waiting area

A well-designed waiting room can be a centerpiece of your internal marketing. First, the presence of other patients in the waiting room tells new ones that your services are in demand, which has positive placebo effect. Second, educational information in the form of signage, brochures, or flyers about classes, new services, products, or community events can be one main feature of this space (discussed in detail in Section 4). Third, product displays can and should be interesting, well lit, and rotated regularly in this space. Finally, no matter how good you are at running on time, there will be days when you cannot stay on schedule or you may have to add an acute emergency patient into an already-full schedule. When this happens, a pleasant and interesting waiting area helps keep any inconvenienced patients happy. (More on this subject in Chapter 13 of this section.)

A good waiting room has comfortable seating, proper lighting, and interesting, professionally-relevant reading material for a start. Whatever else you add to enhance it–artwork, plants, toys for children, music, attractive product displays, a tea service or water dispenser–makes the space that much better. No matter the size of your waiting area, comfortable chairs that are easy for older patients to get out of are a good choice. If you cannot yet afford the chairs you would prefer, make this a priority purchase for the not-too-distant future. You'll also need a small table or two for magazines, educational materials, and signage. You may also want a sideboard or wall shelving for more educational information, product displays, or a lending library, and perhaps a toy box in one corner.

You also need to have lighting appropriate for reading but not so bright as to hurt patients' eyes as they emerge from a slightly darker treatment room. If you have good natural light it's a wonderful asset, but for cloudy days and evening hours you'll want a table or floor lamp (or maybe two).

Reading material in your waiting area can be for a general audience (think large coffee-table books, *National Geographic,* or *People*), for your specific niche market (think *Parents Magazine* or *Outside*), or TCM educational (*Acupuncture Today* or *Acufinder Newsletter*). If you do provide magazines, make sure they are current. Get a subscription or two (you can write off this expense) and once a month or so donate older issues to a low-income medical facility, a homeless shelter, or recycle them.

When patients arrive early or you are running behind, some will sit and surf, read their email, or text on their phones. Still, something to read is, at the least, courteous and, better yet, may be educational or good marketing. If you don't have much reading material, we hope your space is "friendly" for smart phones and wifi.

Consider a wall rack or shelf with books about Chinese medicine for sale (or lending), brochures about your services, and flyers about lectures, classes, or special events. This increases patient awareness about Chinese medicine and can produce extra income. A small bulletin board showing your community involvement or volunteer work, especially if patients can get involved, is excellent.

165

SECTION TWO: WORKING ON YOUR OWN

> **PRACTITIONER POINTER**
>
> "I operate both a private and a community acupuncture practice out of a large old home. The waiting area enjoys filtered natural light from four tall windows. Seating is arranged in comfortable groupings with big, plush pillows that invite people to relax. There's a basket with various herbal teas and the teapot is always on. Soft music comes in from the other room. Natural health magazines and my quarterly newsletter share the coffee table with big art books for those who want to browse.
>
> The unusal thing is a 9-foot Christmas tree that stands in the corner, fully decorated, all year 'round. At first I was afraid people might think it was too hokey, but the twinkling glow of the tiny lights in the evening somehow lifts your spirits and seems comforting in a familiar way. I not-so-jokingly tell my patients that every day is Christmas here, because we share in the gift of health and healing. They seem to like that."
>
> —C. Karen Stopford
> Norwich Community Acupuncture, Norwich, CT

▶ Treatment rooms

Treatment rooms should be havens of relaxation where patients feel safe, warm, and cared for. In addition to good tables and necessary supplies, adding a few special niceties can make visiting your clinic into an experience, not just a treatment.

Music

If you often leave patients to rest on the table for awhile, soft music helps cut down on background noise or overhearing private conversations in the next room. Clinic-appropriate music should be relaxing and acceptable to a wide audience. We all have different musical tastes, but a selection of Sirius® or Pandora®

stations allows great variety and without the hassle of a separate player in each room. Either way, the volume should be low enough that you can easily speak over it. If you choose to have a music system such as Sonos® installed and wired into each treatment room, make sure that:

1. **Each room has a volume and on/off switch.** While some patients will enjoy the soft sounds of smooth jazz, others will not want music at all.

2. **Some selections are music-or-sound without words.** Sometimes song lyrics are distracting. Ask for a few channels with natural sounds such as birdsong, rainfall, or ocean waves, which is totally relaxing for many people.

The nose knows
If you use it, the smell of moxa smoke can be controlled to some extent by air filtration units and opened windows. Other, less controllable smells that can permeate Chinese medicine clinics include often-used ointments and liniments for musculo-skeletal patients. If you have a bulk herb pharmacy, other aromas will also be in the air. Some patients will like these smells, but some may find one or another of them troubling, at least until they are used to them. Allergy patients (and you yourself with long exposure) may have a real problem with moxa smoke or bulk herb dust. If you decide on air filtration (either portable or attached to your furnace or A/C unit), check ratings online. A good one will cost between $300-$1,000 but can keep your air healthier and more patient-friendly if you are making either dust or smoke. Also consider aromatherapy in your waiting area. A wide variety of oils, candles, or plug-ins are available to offer subtle fragrance for your patients' olfactory pleasure.

Use your walls wisely
Acupuncture charts are educational and appropriate to hang in treatment rooms, but don't get stuck there. Other types of art

are also appropriate. If you specialize in pediatrics, consider bright posters with kid-centered themes. If you treat athletes, framed, autographed posters of the latest Olympic or professional stars could give the right feel. Inspirational poetry and quotations are another option. If you have the creative energy, it could be fun to have a different theme in each room. Nature, travel, medical, philosophical, or kid themes are all possibilities. I've seen one clinic that had five treatment rooms, each one decorated based on one of the five "elements." (Cheesy but fun.)

I also recommend lots of signage in your treatment rooms, bathrooms, hallways, waiting area, and where people check in and out, for example "did you know" signs with tidbits of information about Chinese medicine. More about that subject is discussed in Chapter 13 of this section.

Lighting

It is difficult to diagnose accurately without good lighting. Natural light is ideal, but in some treatment spaces it does not exist. Whether taking a history or doing a treatment, full-spectrum lights give you the best view of tongue and skin-tone, and help you with point location, exact bleeding of spider veins, or placement of small moxa threads.

Treatment room lights are best if adjustable. If not fluorescent, ceiling lights can be put on a dimmer switch. If you have to go with fluorescent lights, however, get the full-spectrum ones so the light is as true as possible. In that case, add an adjustable pedestal lamp in a corner to use when lights need to be dimmed during treatments.

Seating in your treatment rooms

Each treatment room needs at least two chairs. Three is better. It's best if you have a room with a desk and chairs for taking an initial patient history. At least in the early days of a clinical relationship, a patient may feel more comfortable sitting in a chair than on your treatment table to discuss their condition. An extra chair also allows a patient to bring a friend or relative if they wish and, in the case of treating a new patient of the opposite sex, an assistant or family member in the room avoids issues of sexual misconduct. Finally, with young patients, a place for a family member to sit is necessary.

Writing surfaces and storage areas
If you don't have a separate space for taking the initial history, you'll need a desk in at least one treatment room. Also, a cupboard for keeping treatment supplies, sheets or table paper rolls, towels, and treatment gowns dust-free and out of sight is preferable to having these items stored under the table or in a corner. You might instead use a rolling cart with two or more shelves or drawers. Either way, keep at least a day's worth of treatment items in each room so that you don't run out of anything you need in the middle of a treatment.

If you have smaller treatment rooms with no space for a desk, consider installing a corner shelf on which to write in paper charts or place your laptop if you are keeping electronic records. Another option that adds a touch of professionalism to a small treatment room is a drop-down desktop from a medical supply company; it looks just like a hospital room.

Flooring
If you have a choice, use carpet. Hardwood floors are lovely, but require daily dusting, are not warm for bare feet getting up from the treatment table, and add to the noise level. Carpet is quiet, cheaper, and warmer on bare tootsies! If you prefer hardwood or laminate flooring, use area rugs under the treatment tables for warmth (and decoration) and hallway runners for quiet.
If you're buying, get commercial grade carpet, like what is used

in an airport concourse! It will hold up better with the amount of foot traffic you hope to generate, and spending a little extra now will get you several more years out of the carpet. If you are a DIY person, download instructions on carpet installation and save on that cost, or request new carpet as part of your lease contract!

➤ Feng shui

Before your decor is set in stone (so to speak), consider hiring a feng shui specialist to give their opinion about the flow of qi in your space. You need not believe in the more esoteric, religious, or culturally-specific aspects of feng shui for this to be useful. Often the suggestions made will be very practical and not at all woo-woo. Just moving a lamp or a table, adding a plant or a mirror, or changing a wall color can have an impact on the feel and success of your clinic, and the cost may be much less than you expected. Want DIY feng shui? Pick up a copy of the user-freindly *Feng Shui Your Life* by Jayme Barrett.

➤ A final note

More important than your clinic decor or feng shui, however, are the human interactions that happen there. This will have the biggest influence on how it feels to people. How each patient is greeted, the tone of voice, dress, and demeanor of your front desk person, and what words they hear when leaving your clinic, either enhance or reduce the placebo effect of your treatments. This aspect of your clinic operations needs to be both sincere and systematic, based on real feeling but to some extent scripted. This is discussed in great detail in Chapter 13 of this section.

In terms of creating your interior decor, this work should be fun! Remember that you can easily change most of what you do if necessary, so don't get stressed about this. Any mistakes can be corrected or motifs updated with little effort. Paint is not expensive; furniture can be returned to stores; posters and signs can be replaced. So be creative! Try new things, fix them if they don't work out, and enjoy yourself.

Finally, whether your decor is designed or haphazard, your colors coordinated or not, the most important thing is to keep your clinic spotlessly clean, especially the bathrooms! This point cannot be over-emphasized.

POINTS TO PONDER FROM CHAPTER 6

- The impact of your treatments can be improved or diminished by the look, feel, and smell of your clinic.
- Make sure the outside of your clinic is as clean as the inside. Bathrooms must be spotless every day.
- Pick a complementary color scheme for your clinic rooms.
- Your waiting room needs comfortable chairs, pleasant reading light, and fun or interesting things for people to read, buy, or sample.
- Your treatment rooms need carpeting or area rugs to keep people's feet warm!
- You can get advice on color schemes and almost anything else to do with decorating from home improvement and paint stores.
- Consider a feng shui consultation to make sure the qi of your clinic space flows optimally.
- Remember that your clinic staff and what they say and how they say it is part of your overall clinic "feel."
- Be creative, have fun, make it beautiful.

Outside the Doc-in-a-Box | 7

Each of us has a different idea about how we define our "dream clinic." The purpose of this chapter is not to limit your ideas or push in any specific direction but to help you determine if either of the two out-of-the-box options might work for you. Both home-based clinics and mobile practices are possible options, each with their own positive and negative aspects (like most things in life). Before you decide on either of these, do your homework and stay within legal guidelines.

▶ Homework

Working out of your home can be workable. Low overhead, zero travel time, and less gasoline are tempting advantages for anyone first starting their own business. However, there are also reasons not to practice from home, such as business liability insurance issues, separation of work and social/personal life, zoning/parking conflicts, and the possible effect on your neighborhood. Just as everything has yin and yang sides, there are *pro's* and *con's* for every business decision.

The pro's

Working from home was once a common situation in many professions. When I was a child, our family doctor's office was a separate entrance in his home, which seemed very normal and quite welcoming. From bakers to storekeepers, people often lived upstairs from whatever business they owned.

> **PRACTITIONER POINTER**
>
> "It seems that many clinics are NOT places in which I feel relaxed enough to do healing work on myself. There are the phones, the noisy patients, the tired or impersonal acupuncturist, the music, the lighting, the colors, which combined, make for an experience that's too much like being in an allopath's office. So, having worked in other people's clinics and having had to tolerate the environment, I decided to create my healing space in a clinic that's in the first floor of my house and has its own entrance.
>
> "I have created a place that soothes the person the moment he walks in. At least, this has been the feedback I've received from many people."
>
> —Maria MacKnight
> Arlington, VA

If your space and location are workable, setting up a home clinic means your rent overhead is zero (depending upon how you do it). There are also tax deductions on heat and light as well as per square foot for a home office. Since your mortgage will not go up one dollar just because you are practicing out of your house, it can sound like an ideal setup for a beginning practice. The lower your overhead, the more profits there are for you.

Other advantages with a home-practice are that you won't be late getting to work (unless you oversleep!), you may get a break on your car insurance because you have no commute, you save on gasoline and wear-and-tear on your vehicle as well, you will be around while your children grow up, the bills for your clinic almost disappear when you leave on vacation, and you can write off a portion of your mortgage or rent payment to lower your tax bill.

The con's

Working out of your house means that you are never truly able to separate your business from everything else in your life. Some people thrive with this style of work-and-the-rest-of-life integration, which is great. But if not, your office is still just downstairs or down the hall. If you walk through it several times a day, patients or not, you may be tempted to flip on the computer, pay some bills, write a blog or create a Facebook post, do some research, or whatever, no matter the time of day or what else is going on.

Patients in your house is another consideration. If you cannot create a separate entrance into the clinic itself, patients will be walking through your "life" to reach the treatment area. Many of us have had this experience with various alternative therapists and issues like cleanliness, pets, children, noise, and even the color of your decor can make an impression. No matter how clean and pleasant your office/treatment room and waiting areas are, your personal space will become a part of a patient's opinion of you and your clinic in this circumstance.

With all your patients knowing where you live, you are also more open to the possibility of harassment. You don't have to be in practice for very long to know that there will be an occasional patient who is "peculiar" or even possibly scary. Having such people in your clinic a few miles away from your home is much more comfortable than having them in your living room!

The possible informality of a home clinic may also give patients "permission" to request late or early appointments. This may not be an issue for you, but how do you say no if this is not something you want to do more than on the *very* odd occasion? Setting clear hours of operation is extremely important in a home practice so that you get the rest and down time you need to be at your best when you are with patients.

Last there is the issue of liability. Treating patients in your home will usually increase the amount of home owner's liability insurance you must carry. You also will be wise to have the maximum ($1 million/$3 million) malpractice insurance coverage in addition, whether it is required in your state or not. One could "what if" these issues all day and it's not our intention to scare anyone; I [HW] had a practice in my home for several years with no particular problems. Still, while chances may be highly unlikely, if you were involved in a liability lawsuit and your clinic *is* your house, you could lose both unless your business legal model is set up carefully (Section 1, Chapter 6) and your insurance coverage more than just adequate.

Is it legal?
Once you've decided that a home office would work for you, the next step is determining if it is legal to do it. Unlike many European countries and small-town U.S. in the early 20th century where people often lived and worked in the same building, most towns now have zoning laws to determine what types of buildings, services, and production can happen in any given area. This is what keeps a factory or drilling rig from setting up shop right next door to your vacation beach condo.

Even if it is only one room, you must check the zoning of your house and neighborhood. To do this, call your city or county planning department and request your zoning by address (a zoning map for your city may also be available online). Then ask about rules for home businesses. (If you can get this information online, don't talk to anyone..yet.) If you do have a conversation, they will want to know that your business requires people to come to your location (*i.e.*, you are not planning a mail-order business with no other cars involved)—and that it is to be a health facility. Once you know the zoning, your options become clearer, although possibly fewer.

If you reside in either a commercial or mixed residential/commercial area or on a country road outside of town, you will run into few, if any, legal obstacles to setting up a small clinic in your house. If, however, you are in a residential-only zone, you have three choices: 1) forget the home-office option and set up your clinic elsewhere (maybe somewhere with great visibility and foot-traffic), 2) try to get a zoning variance from the city, or 3) decide you are small enough to fly under the radar for awhile.

Considering option #3 first, you could simply open your clinic without anyone's permission despite the zoning laws. I [HW] had a home office like this when my son was very young and I was only seeing a few clients a day. In my case I had a separate entrance, only one of my neighbors (who also had a home business) was the wiser because most were not home, traffic was minimal, and I was done each day before school let out. Still, you run the risk of unhappy neighbors (unless you've already convinced them to become your patients and they like the home clinic idea). If someone rats on you because of traffic or parking issues, you may only get your wrist slapped (a cease-and-desist order), or you may get a fine. At worst (if less likely), you could lose several potential referring neighbors and city employees and get some unfortunate newspaper publicity in the bargain!

A zoning variance or special use permit
A conditional land-use permit or zoning variance is what you need if you plan to set up a busy clinic (more than just one or two people per day) in a residential zone. These may not be easy to come by since your business will create at least some traffic and congestion. Rules for obtaining such a variance or permit vary slightly from city to city, but here's the basic procedure:

- Call the city planning department and tell them that you would like to set up an acupuncture clinic in your house. When they tell you your house is not zoned for that, tell them you wish to apply for a zoning variance. They will mail you the application or tell you where to find it online. Fill out and return the form, and then be prepared to wait.

- The planning department will send someone to investigate the feasibility of your proposal. If the city is not opposed to your clinic, they will place a sign in your yard inviting everyone in the area to comment on the proposed business for a specified period of time (60–90 days) followed by a public hearing. Given no neighborhood or city opposition, you can be given a conditional land-use permit or zoning variance.

> If you want to work from home, look into buying in the many new "mixed-use" projects that are springing up all over the U.S. This may improve your odds of practicing from home legally.

To make this go more smoothly, be a good neighbor. Mow an older person's lawn or dog-sit for someone going on vacation; it's great to be a good neighbor in any case, without any particular motive! While there's no guarantee this changes the minds of the toddler's parents two houses down, it may sway public opinion in your favor with some folks! Also be sure you have worked out a realistic estimate of increased car traffic per hour or day through the neighborhood. This is especially important to people with children and will likely be asked on the special use permit application in any case. If your high traffic times are not when most children are around, make sure your neighbors know that.

Except in very small towns, it can be difficult to obtain a permit to set up a business that requires people to come to you. If you wanted to manufacture items in your basement and mail them off to website customers, that is fine in most places. But if you are zoned residential, chances are not high that the city will allow a restaurant in your neighbor's house or a clinic in yours. So be prepared for this outcome.

Another fact regarding zoning variances—this permit stays with the property for which it was granted. It does not move with you or stay in effect at the property for which it was given once you have relocated. In other words, if you operate a business under a conditional land-use permit or variance, that permit expires the moment you move out unless you sell your house to another acupuncturist and therefore the new business will be exactly the same as the previous one.

The best scenario for establishing a home-based clinic is to purchase a property out in the country or in an area already zoned for a commercial business, which is not what most practitioners who want a home office have in mind.

I [HW] have seen many nice, professionally-operated home offices. Most had separate entrances, receptionists, and were professionaly run, irrespective of whether they had zoning variances. Depending on your situation, it could be a perfect option for you, but do be clear on the pros, cons, risks, and rewards if you choose this option for your clinic.

Accessibility

No matter where your clinic is created, people will need access to you. This means that not only will your patients need a place to park their cars or lock their bicycles, they will need clear, unobstructed access to your treatment rooms and an available restroom. Although your operation is small, check to find out if you need to be in compliance with the Americans with Disabilities Act. For more information about ADA law and how or whether it applies to you, see the link on the website. ●

Parking requirements vary widely by city and information about this will be part of your process if you are applying for a variance as described above. The number of parking spaces required often depends on the square footage of the clinic space, not the number of treatment rooms, which is something to consider when designing your clinic. If you've applied for your zoning variance and are going forward with creating this great clinic in your home, make sure to ask about everything you may need to know from the planning department or other relevant authorities in your city or county. You don't want to do anything you don't have to and you don't want to leave anything out that can come back to bite you later on.

Running a "Clinic-Mobile"

While there is a potential market for practitioners who are willing and able to travel to homes of those who are housebound, there are some obvious, and possibly difficult, obstacles to overcome. While many Boomers will remember the doctor coming to see them for measles or chicken pox when they were young children, the practice of home visitation has been largely abandoned by the Western medical community in the last 50 years. The main type of in-home therapeutic care available today is provided by home-care nurses. Thus, if you are thinking of creating a mobile acupuncture clinic, there are a number of real pro's and con's to consider and issues you must solve before you begin.

The pro's

Low overhead is a major advantage for a any small business owner. The lower your expenses, obviously the higher your profits. If your only real expenses are practice supplies, a reliable cell phone, brochures and cards, malpractice insurance, computer software, and your car expenses, then your overhead is pretty low. Assuming that you are able to charge what you need to for your work to be profitable, you could be very successful in this niche. Also, while a traveling business already has many possible built-in tax write-offs, the purchase of a new vehicle to start your practice could be a major tax write-off for your business. Whether your car is new or old, there are two options for declaring auto expenses: 1) Consider the vehicle a business expense, which allows you to deduct the entire price of the vehicle divided up over a certain number of years (consult with your tax advisor), as well as the cost of maintenance, fuel, insurance, everything. 2) Use your personal vehicle, keeping track of all business miles. This allows you to write off a specific amount per mile for all miles you drive *for the purposes of your work.*

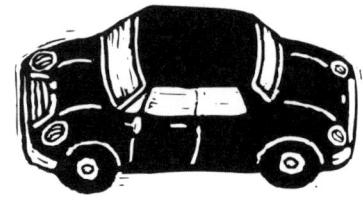

Either of these options requires that you keep precise records of the miles you drive. If the vehicle is owned by the business (possible if you set up as an LLC or an S-Corp), you have to log all miles for personal use, which reduces your deduction by the current allowable amount per mile. If the vehicle is your personal car, it is the other way around and you keep track of business mileage. The total business miles at the specified amount per mile will be taken as a tax deduction, in which case your type of business model does not matter.

Another benefit is that your vehicle can be excellent traveling advertising. A nice-sized magnetic car sign with your clinic name, phone number, and web address could be seen by hundreds of people every time you drive the car. You should consider doing this in any case, even if your clinic is not mobile!

The con's
Treatment price
When doing in-home patient care, you do not have the advantage of multiple treatment rooms and more than one patient per hour. Your treatment price will need to reflect this limitation. Additionally, your treatment price must include your travel time and expenses, plus a charge for the convenience

factor patients experience by not having to go anywhere to receive care. This will limit the size of your client base, but you can use the exclusivity factor as a marketing point.

Travel time and expenses
Time on the road is time that you are not seeing patients. Thus, you will need to be a precise planner, perhaps making appointment times and days for specific areas of town so as not to waste time and fuel, even if you bill for travel time. Also remember that, *unless reflected in your treatment costs*, all your travel expenses will come back to you only in the following tax year as a deduction, not as cash. All fuel, maintenance, and insurance costs will come out of your pocket now.

Liability
Treatments given under the roof of your patient may have a different liability cost than those given in your own stationary clinic. When considering a mobile practice, make sure your malpractice insurance includes a clause that covers you for this style of work. See if you need some type of "rider" for your policy to protect your traveling clinic.

Advertising
As stated above, your mobile clinic can be a moving advertisement. However, you'll need to be a courteous driver! Your phone number could be easy to remember if you cut someone off in traffic because you haven't left enough time to get to your next appointment! Also, be sure you know state and local rules for phone use while driving. You know you'll do this, so at least go hands–free. Also know that research shows even hands-free calls or texts increase your likelihood of an accident by a factor of two or three times.

In terms of other advertising and your website, the marketing advantage of an in-home visitation service is exclusivity and ultimate convenience. You could well be the only one in your area doing this. A Bluetooth enabled car could be a great advantage, and remember to keep your cell phone charged and set on vibrate when treating patients. Another option is to refer calls to an answering service and check in after each appointment. If fast response time will be an important part of your marketing, you'll need to figure out how to be available as close to instantly as possible.

➤ A last caveat

If you treat patients in their own homes or offices, especially those of the opposite sex, there are some precautions you may want to take to protect yourself. Since you cannot have an extra person present at each appointment to be a witness during each treatment, you are more easily open to claims of impropriety.

Make certain to *always* gown and drape properly, covering all body parts not being needled. Ask the patient to have a friend or family member in the room for all treatments and physical exams. If you are feeling uncomfortable about a treatment situation, consider using distal acupuncture for his sciatica or her pelvic pain—nothing local at all. Make sure that you are always dressed appropriately. Your white clinic coat may be even more important as a mobile clinician than for those working in a clinic or a hospital setting.

Especially for women practitioners but true for men as well, if you feel that a call from a potential new client is questionable or makes you uncomfortable in any way, you are better off to tell the person that your practice is full and refer them to a stationary clinic in their area. Don't put yourself or your practice into jeopardy from people who are sociopathic, weird, or mentally confused.

Every style of practice has both opportunities and limitations. If a home clinic or mobile clinic sounds like a the niche for you, we wish you great success. Either can be a workable and profitable business idea. We always love to hear from readers to find out how your practice is working, especially outside-the-box ideas!

> **POINTS TO PONDER FROM CHAPTER 7**
>
> - Working from home may be a good solution for you if you have a separate entrance, an easy-to-find location, and a flexible zoning situation.
>
> - If you live in a residential-only area, you may need a zoning variance or special use permit allowing you to practice at home. These may not be easy to acquire.
>
> - Don't make people walk through your "life" to get to your clinic. It is very unprofessional.
>
> - People may think you should be able to treat them just any time at all because you are at home anyway.
>
> - There may be patients whom you would prefer not to know where you live.
>
> - If you decide to have a traveling practice, remember that you must charge extra for your travel time and expenses.
>
> - Make sure there are no possible implications of sexual impropriety if you are practicing in your patients' homes.

Files and Recordkeeping | 8

Every medical facility in the U.S. is required to maintain accurate records about their patients. This includes us. Also, with implementation of the Health Insurance Portability and Accountability Act (HIPAA) in 2003, some forms are not optional. In this chapter and the next, we discuss records that you must maintain and others that you may wish to keep on every patient you treat. Samples of most of these forms are on the companion website. If you plan to keep your patient records on paper for the present, feel free to download these and "tweak" them for your own use. If you are planning to maintain electronic medical records (EMR), the software should include most or all of these. More on EMR below.

➤ Common, useful forms

Basic intake/medical history form

On this form a patient explains their current symptoms as well as their medical history. You can use this form as the basis for the questioning part of the Chinese four examinations. A good history form can help you save time, looks professional, and can protect you from certain legal liabilities. For instance, it can help prove that you did or did not know about certain signs, symptoms, pre- or coexisting conditions, or medications. You can have new patients fill out this and all your forms on their first visit, make forms available to be downloaded from your website, and/or email forms if necessary in advance of an initial visit. If you use email or patients can download, you can at the same time send directions to your clinic, an FAQ about acupuncture care, or any other appropriate educational materials you have in digital form.

184

Mandatory professional disclosure form

Required in some states, this form tells the patient what your educational background is, who licenses you to practice, what examinations you have passed, etc. It allows the patient to decide if your education and professional history are adequate for the treatment they seek. You may also be required to include your fee schedule and cancellation policy on this form.

Informed consent/permission to treat form

This required form is how each patient gives you specific, written permission to treat. It is a short statement of the risks involved with acupuncture and has a statement declaring that the patient understands those risks and is requesting treatment.

Patient confidential information form

A useful form if you will be billing any type of medical insurance and if you do mailings or other marketing directly to your patients. It gives you information about your patient, their family, their insurance coverage, their contact information, social security number, etc.

SOAP notes form (optional)

Used to record subjective, objective, assessment, and treatment plan information, you are likely to have learned to use this form in school. Subjective means the patient's report of what they feel, *i.e.*, their symptoms. Objective means the signs you observe in your examination, such as tongue and pulse signs, colors, smells, sounds, heat or cold, tightness of muscle tissue, etc. Assessment means what you believe is happening based on the combination of the subjective and objective information. Plan is what you decide to do to treat the patient. This information can be helpful if you ever need to give a deposition, support your treatment plan in a lawsuit, or for recalling your process when a patient stops care for several months and then returns.

Report of findings form (optional)

This can also be a PARQ form, which is short for procedure, alternatives, risks, and questions. This form can help you explain to patients what you plan to do for them and why, alternative therapies they might investigate, possible risks of the procedures, and then give the patient a chance to ask any questions. Give this form to the patient and keep a copy in their file.

Assignment of benefits for insurance form (optional)

Used only for insurance patients, this form tells the insurance company that your clinic is to be reimbursed directly for medical services provided instead of reimbursements going to the patient or some other third party. The patient-signed copy of this form goes to the insurance company being billed and a copy remains in the patient's file.

Financial policy form

This form discloses to the patient how your clinic operates financially. It tells them your fees for various services, your cancellation policy, whether and how you bill for insurance, what happens if the insurance does not pay, and, in general, what will be expected of them financially.

Follow-up care form (optional)

A short version of a SOAP form, on this form you write down what was done during each treatment and why. It can be used either for required insurance reporting or patient education.

Request for release of patient records form

For some patients, you need to have access to their current or past healthcare records from other practitioners. To get these, you need a release form that is sent to the practitioner in question with the patient's signature and information about where the information is to be sent.

Consent to the use & disclosure of health information for treatment, payment, or healthcare operations form

This is a HIPAA-required form that explains to the patient that their personal healthcare information may be used to plan their care, for financial and billing purposes, and other routine operations and information processing within your clinic. It also explains to the patient that they have the right to object to their private information being used in any published directory, to your sharing any information about HIV/AIDS, drug or alcohol abuse, or mental health conditions, and that they may give you permission now but later revoke it, which revocation must be done in writing.

Below is a checklist to help you be certain that you are keeping records in accordance with good risk management procedures. Remember, if a patient sues you for any reason, your chart notes are your only defense and will be the first thing your malpractice insurance agent or the lawyers on either side of any case will subpoena. If you are doing all the things on this list, your charts will be relatively unimpeachable, unless you are simply doing things that are outside your scope of practice or are, for some other reason, illegal or indefensible.

▶ Clinic Recordkeeping Checklist for Each Patient

- ❐ The patient name must be on all pages in your files.
- ❐ All pages should be secured into the treatment folder.
- ❐ Organize all notes chronologically (most recent date on top).
- ❐ Always write legibly, be consistent, clear and concise.
- ❐ Maintain records in ink, use the same pen for each entry on the same day.
- ❐ Do not alter the records after the fact, do not erase or use correction fluid. If an entry needs to be corrected, add a line referencing the entry and adding a correction and date.

SECTION TWO: WORKING ON YOUR OWN

- ☐ Fill in all blanks, do not skip lines or leave spaces, or line through large blocks of empty space.
- ☐ Do not "squeeze in" notes at a later date and do not indent on any line.
- ☐ Make additions and changes appropriately on a different line. You may reference the line on any specific page that you need to change and give a reason for that change.
- ☐ Record all patient contact!
  a. Missed appointments documented
  b. Telephone messages documented
  c. Entries dated, timed, and initialed
  d. Patient noncompliance documented
- ☐ Initial all reports from an external source (X-ray, lab, diagnostic, consultant) before filing them.
- ☐ Dictation, correspondence, and reports to insurance companies or other practitioners should be proofread and initialed before filing.
- ☐ Maintain a legend for any abbreviations used if needed for later reference.
- ☐ Document the reason for the visit and any unusual events; avoid or explain contradictions.
- ☐ All clinical findings (positive or negative) should be documented and the problem or complaint list kept current.
- ☐ Treatment plan documented and updated with each visit.
- ☐ Entries are objective and do not criticize other providers or their treatment methods.
- ☐ Properly identify the record, the record keeper, the technique employed, the table and/or room used, and the details of each treatment.
- ☐ Document any instructions given to patients.
- ☐ Informed consent is in the chart.

- ❏ Be certain that the "Release of Records Authorization" form in the chart is correct and valid.
- ❏ Referral letters or prescriptions are in the chart.
- ❏ Herb list is current, specifies when to refill, and any reactions or allergies.
- ❏ Document any educational materials given to patient.
- ❏ Customize the forms you use.
- ❏ Keep financial and clinical information separate.
- ❏ Retain the records forever because of the statute of limitations on malpractice cases.
- ❏ Signature of the provider of services.

Your malpractice carrier will suggest that you keep your patient records forever. A patient has up to two years from the discovery of a problem to sue you. While it is unlikely that a problem arising 10 years from your treatment could be traceable to you and a specific clinical event, it is not impossible. Basically, that means that you keep all paper files in storage, or scanned on a back-up drive, forever. See Section 1, Chapter 5 for more on this.

➤ Electronic Medical/Health Records (EMR)/(EHR)

Most important data in our world is now electronic or digital and less and less will be available on paper in the future. At the time of this writing, EMR is a possible freight train bearing down on U.S. practitioners of acupuncture, whether they know it or not. For those of us who practice in hospitals or in states that have already adopted acupuncture as an "essential health benefit" (see the next page), the necessity to convert to EMR will arrive soon if it has not already. Many acupuncture schools and colleges are moving away from paper records and toward EMR systems of one type or another. It's my guess that within several more years, and definitely as acupuncture becomes

ated into more standard medical settings, all of us will be expected to be comfortable with maintaining (or at least transmitting) patient records this way and billing insurance electronically as well.

One implication of the move to EMR is that acupuncture practice software needs to get and stay up to date in the areas of electronic transferring of records and electronic insurance billing. When doing research on software for your patient records, be sure you ask questions about these features and that you understand the answers you get.

POWER POINT

States that have accepted acupuncture as an essential health benefit as of 2013 (This info could change at any time!)

This will change and more states will be added over time. Right now this means that acupuncture is included as a preventive treatment covered by insurance companies in these states: CA, MD, WA, NM, NV, AK, and in CT as at least a "rider" to policies sold in that state. These policies usually allow 12 paid visits per year.

The implication here is that people will want to use their coverage and acupuncturists will need to learn to to play the game of insurance billing efficiently and effectively in order to be reimbursed at fair rates. The other implication is that acupuncturists will either need to use a service such as OfficeAlly.com or use electronic medical records and billing software to keep patient records. For more on insurance billing, see Section 3, Chapter 3 and, better yet, *Playing the Game: A Step-by-Step Approach to Accepting Insurance as an Acupuncturist* by Dr. Greg Sperber and Tiffany Andersen-Hefner.

CHAPTER 8 | Files and Recordkeeping

POINTS TO PONDER FROM CHAPTER 8

- There are many forms that are required by law in your patient interactions.

- There are other forms that are optional but can streamline patient care and make your clinic feel professional, caring, and organized.

- If you take nothing else from this chapter, read and follow the recordkeeping checklist.

- Electronic Medical/Health Records is coming our way. For practitioners who are willing and able to participate, it will mean leaving paper recordkeeping behind and learning to use medical records software to maintain patient records and bill insurance.

The Wonderful World of HIPAA Compliance | 9

> **The Health Insurance Portability & Accountability Act**

Also known as the Kennedy-Kassebaum bill, this act was passed in 1996 and became law in April 2003. Originally designed to help workers take their health insurance from one employer to another without a gap in coverage and for employees leaving the workforce who want to maintain their health insurance, it was expanded significantly into other areas of compliance to insure that clinics keep all patient records private. The act also limits the ways in which this private information may be communicated to anyone else. With regard to that, there are a few pieces of paperwork that you must present to your patient or that you must maintain in case of legal auditing. There are also rules about how you keep your patients' records private as well as codes that you use for insurance billing.

POWER POINT

Interesting facts about healthcare information

1. Twenty percent of the consumers in the U.S. believe that their health information has been used or disclosed inappropriately.
2. Seventeen percent of Americans report that they have taken action to avoid the inappropriate use of their information, including providing inaccurate information to healthcare providers, changing physicians, or avoiding health care altogether.
3. The Association of American Physicians and Surgeons report that 78% of its members have withheld information from a patient's record due to privacy concerns and 87% of its members have had a patient request that information be withheld.

CHAPTER 9 | **The Wonderful World of HIPAA Compliance**

In HIPAA's early days, there were rumors that you only had to comply with this law if you were doing electronic insurance billing. This was and is incorrect and almost everyone knows that now. Even if you don't currently bill electronically for insurance patients, all insurance billing must follow the Transaction Code Set section of HIPAA, which is easy to do (see page 198 below). And speaking of electronic billing, though not yet required by law, it is certainly the preferred method of insurance companies and both easier and faster to do. Furthermore, the privacy regulations and security standards of HIPAA apply to any clinic that gathers personally identifiable health information from any patient, whether you ever bill insurance or not. All patients have the right to privacy and security of their information. Details about these compliance requirements are discussed below.

> **POWER POINT**
>
> **Are You a Covered Entity Under HIPAA?**
> Covered Entities are defined as any healthcare provider who:
> - Transmits any patient information electronically, whether by fax, electronic transmission, or by email.
> - Has oral communication with a patient.
> - Gathers health information and writes it in a chart.
>
> Any health information that is gathered, whether stored on paper or in a computer, or is orally transmitted is Protected Health Information. Acupuncture clinics are covered entities by virtue of the above definitions.

What do you need to do to comply?

The several things you must do for your clinic to be in full HIPAA compliance are not complex for most small clinics, but you could get into trouble if you do not understand and implement these few simple requirements. You need not make these a big deal. Keep it simple and just do it.

1. **Appoint a Privacy Officer (PO)**
   You may be the clinic's PO or appoint someone on your staff if you are in a larger or multi-person clinic. Simply create a "To Whom It May Concern" letter for your Compliance Manual (discussed below) with the name of your PO.

   What does a PO have to do?
   - A PO must understand the privacy and security requirements under HIPAA as well as the related use of technology (hardware/software) in your practice.

   - A PO can appoint others to assist in compliance with privacy policies and procedures if need be. In that case, each person must have written instructions about all policies and procedures.

   - The PO trains newly-hired personnel, within 30 days of their hire date, about privacy and security standards.

   - The PO keeps a policies and procedures Compliance Manual. This can be as simple as a three-ring binder or digital folder in which you keep all required HIPAA forms.

   - The PO revises all forms in use in the clinic as needed. Updated forms should be kept in the Compliance Manual.

   - The PO monitors who has keys to entrance and exit doors. A list of who has keys and when they received them or returned them must be kept in your manual.

2. **Maintain a fax/email log**
   HIPAA rules allow for fax, email, and written communication about your patients to be used as needed in the normal course of their care. If you don't keep a fax/email log because your practice is very small with minimal in-or-outbound communications, a copy of any and all communication *that includes any private patient information* needs to be kept in the patient file and include the date and time of the incoming and outgoing fax or email.

An actual log that includes who sent and received the email or fax matters more if your practice includes many worker's compensation or personal injury patients, thus requiring regular reports to MD offices, lawyers, and insurance authorization offices. The same may be true if you bill a lot of insurance and have similar communications with many insurance companies. In these cases, a log can be helpful when the claims department states that "you did not send us the claim, the tracer letter, the requested form," and the like. Your fax and email log becomes your back-up that you did, in fact, send the required or requested paperwork.

3. **Create Business Associate Agreements**
   You may or may not need these, but it includes any legal firm, accountant, consultant, any group for which the acupuncturist is a provider, any billing service, interns or volunteers, or even janitorial services—anyone who has access to patient information. You need a short, simple agreement that assures the privacy of patient information with each business associate. These signed agreements go in your compliance manual (scanned digital or on paper).

4. **Make sure all patients have signed any form required by HIPAA in conjunction with their private healthcare information. Keep these forms in each patient's file.**
   What forms will you need to be compliant?
   - **Consent form.** Each patient (or legal guardian for minors) must sign a form showing that they understand that their Protected Health Information can be used for treatment, payment, and healthcare operations in your clinic.

   - **Privacy notice.** Each patient must be informed of your privacy policies and must sign a form stating that they have read and discussed the policies with someone in your clinic. This form is kept in each patient's chart. These first two forms could be combined.

- **Authorization form for release of protected health information.** The patient has to sign this form for the release of any and all health information. This form is limited to use for a specific period of time or a specific incident (such as a car accident). The patient has the right to tell you that they do *not* give you authorization to release any information regarding HIV/AIDS, substance abuse including drug or alcohol abuse, or mental health information.

5. Create a Compliance Manual
   What items need to be in your manual for compliance?
   - **Privacy Regulations Checklist.** This shows all HIPAA requirements and when you began implementing them.

   - **Requests for Restriction of PHI** (protected health information) from any patient who wants records or certain records not to be released.

   - **Patient communication list.** Any patient who has asked you to limit your communication to them or about them in any way should be on a list in your compliance manual. Before any communications are sent from your office or any protected health information is sent to another party (lawyer, insurance company, medical doctor, other), this list must be checked.

   - A description of your office security measures with regards to computers, faxes, email and paper files needs to be in your compliance manual.

   - Trading partners and vendors list

   - Fax/email log

   - Computer log of who uses/used any computer where you maintain your patient information, with date and time. This is most important in clinics with many users. If you are the only user, this may be a simple letter with a statement to that effect in your compliance manual.

- Business Associates Agreements

- Complaint log: A record of complaints from any patient with dates, main substance of the complaint, and who spoke to the patient.

- Access Codes for your computer

This manual can be paper or digital. If digital, you will need that scanner we talked about back in Chapter 1 of this section.

Review of the Areas of HIPAA Compliance

1. Are you keeping your patients' private healthcare information private and secure? This is the HIPAA baseline or starting point. If you are not keeping this information **private** and **secure**, make corrections and implement compliance.

2. **Privacy** means limiting the availability and use of *individual patient identifiable health information* within and from your office. This describes the "what" that is to be kept private.

3. **Security** is the "how," or the system you use to maintain that privacy. Whether on-paper charts or electronically maintained information, your method of limiting access to individual patient identifiable health information is what this means. For example, it can be as simple as stating that you keep all file cabinets locked or you maintain password-protected computer files, etc.

4. **Transaction Code Sets and Unique National Health Identifiers** means the codes used for transmission of information between two parties to carry out the financial or administrative activities related to health care. Codes now in use for these purposes are the International Classification of Diagnosis (ICD-9 or ICD-10) codes and Current Procedural Terminology (CPT) codes commonly used on the standard Health Care Financing Administration (HCFA or CMS) form. Secondly, each healthcare provider is now issued a

unique National Provider Identifier number to be used in all billing. See Appendix A on how to get your NPI (it's easy and free).

As you can see, there are a few things your office needs to keep track of for basic HIPAA compliance. Once you have the necessary compliance forms and notebook created, this is not difficult and will become just another aspect of normal office procedures. Privacy of communications and records is really the important thing to consider and control. There are samples of many of these forms on the companion website and several websites listed in the Resources section if you need further detail about HIPAA and its impact on practitioners. You need not make this harder than it is. If you are keeping your patient information private and secure and you have a system to prove that you do, you're unlikely to get in any trouble.

POINTS TO PONDER FROM CHAPTER 9

- If you collect personal information from your patients, you must comply with the privacy compliance sections of HIPAA.

- We give you lists of the minimal things your clinic must do to comply.

- If you bill insurance companies for your patients, you need to use ICD-9/10 codes and CPT codes for your billings. Eventually, you or your clinic will have a unique identifier number . . . but not yet.

- HIPAA is a minor pain in the ***. However, don't lose sleep about this stuff. Just do these few things and you are protected.

Hiring and Keeping Good Employees | 10

As we have said in other chapters, we believe that making the commitment to hire front desk help is essential to your overall business success. This can feel scary at first, but is absolutely necessary for your practice to grow and be successful. Without adequate help, you are always being pulled in too many different directions. This means you are not practicing the best medicine you can or providing your patients with the best customer service. In an age where good customer service is a huge part of everyone's marketing, this one change in your business can have more impact than almost anything else you could do for your professional life.

What should you look for in an employee to work the front desk? How much should you pay them? Can you hire someone as contract labor? What are the rules for being able to fire someone? This is pretty important stuff with many potential pitfalls. While there are no magic bullets here, we will give you the best guidelines we can.

Having had many, many employees myself [HW], I can absolutely promise you that this is and always will be one of the most difficult and mysterious parts of running a business. When you hire someone into a very small business, they become a part of your extended family very quickly. That means you get all of the craziness of anyone's life along with whatever wonderful things they may bring to your business. The problem is that, as a prospective employer, you are not allowed to ask questions like, "Do you have a girlfriend or boyfriend that drinks too much?" "Does your husband beat you?" or, "Has your teenage son ever been in jail?" Other than the general impression you get when you interview prospective employees, it can be difficult to ferret out the details of someone's life that will become a problem for them and, by extension, for you later on. That being said, there are great employees to be had, and we are convinced that you can make a better living and help more people with front desk help than without it.

> **POWER POINT**
>
> **Before starting to look, do your homework!**
>
> Start by making a list of what you are looking for in an employee.
>
> For example:
> - How many hours per week do you want someone?
> - How much can you afford to pay per hour?
> - Can you offer any benefits besides an hourly wage?
> - How long do you want them to commit to working for you?
> - Do you want someone in a certain age range? (You cannot advertise this, but you can make a decision in your mind about what you want.)
> - If your clinic grows and they don't want more hours or more responsibility, how will you handle that?
>
> There are many other questions you (and any clinic partners) may want to ask yourselves. The point is that the clearer you are about what you are looking for, the easier it will be to recognize the person who fits the bill when you meet them.

➤ How to find potential candidates

1. Consider looking within your circle of acquaintances or your client base. If you know lots of people in the town where you practice, you might consider putting out the word that you are looking for an employee. This has both advantages and disadvantages. It may save you money on advertising and time doing interviews, which are a huge drain on your time and

energy at best, and confusing and frustrating at worst. The major disadvantage is that you may damage a friendship because you don't want to hire someone's favorite niece who is looking for a job but doesn't fit your description of the perfect employee.

2. Write a specific job description. Once you have decided what your new employee will be responsible for, put it on paper—the more detailed the better. This document will become the basis for your advertisement and for your interviews. When well written, this tells everybody what is expected. An effective job description should include:
   a. the job title
   b. the job summary
   c. the job qualifications
   d. the job duties and responsibilities

3. If you only want part-time help and live in a city with an acupuncture college, consider hiring an acupuncture student. Now that there are close to 50 acupuncture schools around the U.S., you might find the perfect candidate within the student body of the local school. Especially if the school has mostly evening or weekend classes, a 24-hour per week job in your clinic could give the student valuable experience and solve your receptionist problem for a couple of years. Given the fact that few people in such jobs last longer than 2-3 years, this may not be a bad solution, especially if you are still in the early phase of growing your practice.

4. Consider retiree organizations. Older workers are mature, reliable, and have no child care issues. If you only want part-time help, they often have very flexible schedules.

5. If you do have to put an ad in the paper or on CraigsList, make your description of what you are looking for as clear as possible. Don't scrimp on words in your ad to save money. A clear description of the person you want to hire and what you want to hire them for can weed out lots of job seekers who

aren't right for you and will save you time in the interview process. Something like, "Alternative health clinic with two acupuncture practitioners seeks full time, reliable, mature front desk receptionist. Basic computer and good people skills a must. Medical office experience helpful. Position starts immediately. Fax resume to 333-3333."

It is illegal to put age or sex preferences in a job ad. However, if you put only a fax number or a P.O. box number, you can weed out many of the people who are not going to be appropriate candidates for whatever reason. You are not required to contact anyone with whom you are not requesting an interview.

If you get 25 faxes, you may only want interviews with 5-6 of the candidates. Some will be overqualified, some have the wrong background, and some will be too young. Call the ones that seem to fit and pay attention to their phone voice and language skills. Would you want this person answering your phone? Have a script for yourself with one or two questions about something specific from their resume. Tell each person that you are doing a short phone interview with many applicants before scheduling anything in person. If you can immediately tell that they are not right for the job, thank them for the resume and say you'll get back in touch with them by the end of that day if you want to schedule an interview. That way you don't string them along for more than a few hours and you don't have to take time to call them back. When you speak with someone who sounds great on the phone, schedule the in-person interview immediately.

This phone process will whittle down your list by one or two more, at least. You can manage 4-5 interviews in one afternoon or evening, if you are efficient. Don't schedule an initial interview for longer than ½ hour. Make a list of specific questions and try not to ramble. A possible list is included below.

CHAPTER 10 | Hiring and Keeping Good Employees

▶ What to look for during an interview

In a way, interviewing a potential employee is similar to doing a patient interview. You want to know what this person's "diagnosis" is, because that is who they are. Their TCM patterns could have a tremendous impact on your business! While you cannot ask to take their pulse or look at their tongue, you can get lots of information about them by the other types of examination in our medicine: looking, listening, and questioning. Here are some things to think about during an interview and some questions to ask:

1. Reference one or two items of interest on their resume. Ask them to describe the job, educational experience, or volunteer position that you are referencing and what they liked or did not like about it.

2. Find out why they left their last job.

3. Perhaps give them a short tour of your clinic and tell them in a few sentences about you and your services, but let them do most of the talking.

4. Notice if their nails are clean and shoes are polished.

5. Do a visual pattern discrimination from their face, skin, body type, carriage, and body language. For example, if they have serious liver lines between their brows, they might be very efficient but could they also be irritable with your patients? Do they have a reasonable amount of qi? If they are excessively overweight, will the phlegm and dampness affect their memory? What types of diseases do you think they might manifest and how might that impact their work? This may not be fair, but it is a reality, and it's also your money and reputation they will be managing.

6. Did they show up on time? If they will be unlocking for you in the morning, you cannot have someone who is chronically late working for you.

7. Look at their clothing, purse, or backpack. Do they seem organized or scattered?

8. Ask about long-term goals and aspirations. What do they want to be doing in five years, for example. You may not expect to keep them for 10 years, but you don't want someone who will disappear in six months.

9. Find out what they think is a lot of money. If they think $100 is a lot, for example, they may have a difficult time asking patients to pay what you ask. However, this issue may not be relevant for community acupuncture clinics.

10. Ask if they have had experience with difficult customers (sick people can be difficult) and what they do or say in such situations.

11. If they are clearly not a people person, end the interview as quickly as you politely can because they are not what you need.

12. Give them a timeline of when you will make this decision. It's unkind to keep people hanging on for days.

Once you have narrowed it down to two candidates, schedule a second interview with more pointed questions about compensation, working conditions, and your needs and expectations. You may want to do an online background check for police records and, since they will be handling your money, their personal financial history. You have to get permission from them in writing to do these checks. Costs vary but will be $35-$75 depending on how much information you want to find out.

You should have decided in advance how much you can afford per hour, what other perks you may be able to offer, a schedule for raises, a dress code, what types of behaviors are grounds for dismissal, acceptable personal telephone usage, vacation policy, holiday policies, whether you will use mediation for disputes, or anything else that needs to be discussed. For all office policies concerning the above subjects, it is absolutely essential to have it all written out as an "employee manual" which can be given to the employee for reading and signing. That way, there are no "he said, she said" issues to come up later because policies are in writing.

Contact everyone you interviewed, out of courtesy, within the next 24 hours. You can say something very simple, such as, "Thank you so much for coming in. We had many fine candidates for this job and we chose someone else at this time. We wish you the best of luck in finding a position soon."

If this is your first real employee, check state and federal labor laws online. Labor law compliance requires a few posters from the government concerning workers' comp rules that must be posted somewhere visible. You can find these online. Read them before you post them so you know what promises the government has made to employees on your behalf!

If you decide to have a payroll company handle your payroll, which I [HW] encourage you to consider, you may want to have this set up before your new employee starts working. See the following chapter for a discussion of taxes and payroll in general and Section 1, Chapter 6 for more information on the tax structures of various business models.

▶ Managing employees

This is a huge subject. There are entire books and weekend seminars that you can take on employee management, motivation, and reward structures. None of us is a human resources or employee management expert (even after many, many years in business), but we can give you a few general guidelines.

To begin with, arrange to spend an hour or so each day for the first several days training your new employee. You both need to feel comfortable that all the tasks involved in the job are

205

> **POWER POINT**
>
> **Things Your Employee Can Do When the Phone is Not Ringing**
>
> - Inventory your needles and herbal medicinals
> - Sort and prioritize the mail that is still sitting on your desk
> - Call insurance companies to check on patient benefits
> - Clean the bathrooms
> - Vacuum and dust all the treatment rooms
> - Call patients to reschedule missed appointments
> - Do outbound calls to patients who have not been in for several months
> - Do appointment reminder calls
> - Make copies of forms that are running low
> - Pull all the files (if they are paper) for tomorrow's patients and organize them by time
> - Write checks for bills to be paid and for you to sign; enter the data into QuickBooks
> - Dust the herb shelves and product display shelves
> - Fill out CMS 1500 forms and address envelopes to mail them or enter OfficeAlly data for insurance claims
> - Order needles and herbals
> - Fill brochure holders; put different ones in different rooms
> - Update your waiting area scrapbook
> - Clean and maintain water/tea/coffee service for patients

understood. Keep training sessions to no more than one hour of new material. Most people cannot manage more than that in their brain at one time. Perhaps they will only work half days for the first week and only on tasks for which you have trained them. The exception to this will be people with a great deal of medical office, computer, or phone experience.

Make sure your new employee has read, understood, and signed their employee manual *the very first day.* If you have a contract of any kind, that should be signed as well. If you do use a contract, make sure it is read over by an employment law attorney if not written by one in the first place.

I [HW] suggest you use a simple form stating that there is a 90-day probation period with two reviews of the employee's performance during that time. The first will be after 30 days to discuss the employee's progress and answer questions. The second will be after the 90-day probation period to determine if they move to regular employment (non-probationary) status. This gives you the chance to fire the person within that period without being liable for unemployment compensation, for which your state and federal accounts would be assessed. If you make the mistake of keeping the wrong person because you don't have the courage to fire them when the first signs of trouble occur, you can end up paying a lot of unemployment for someone who only caused you trouble when they were on your staff.

My belief, learned the hard way, is that if something does not feel right with an employee, you are better off to cut your losses and let them go as soon as possible. The longer you maintain a dysfunctional relationship with an employee out of fear, misplaced compassion, or simple laziness, the worse off you will be both emotionally and financially in the end. Believe me, you will end up firing them sooner or later, and sooner means less complexity, less unemployment compensation liability, and less potential issues for a lawsuit. The more grown-up you can be about this the better.

If the employee will be collecting money, make certain they understand your fees for various services. Better yet, fill out the "charges" part of the chart and hand it to them as the person is leaving so there is no guesswork. There should be a daily income sheet or computer "form" on which the name of the patient and what was collected from them is entered. At the end of each day, check receipts against this form. This must balance against bank deposit slips, credit card machine tallies, etc. At least for the first several months of any new employee's tenure, you probably want to do all the bank deposits yourself.

POWER POINT

What to Do When You Are Having Trouble with an Employee

- Give them a first warning that the behavior is not acceptable. Give them a specific demand about what needs to change, with a deadline if appropriate. Put a note in their employee file with the date, the infraction, the conversation, and your specific request/demand. Tell them that this note has been made.

- If there is a repeat of the infraction, give them a final warning. Document this conversation similarly to the first one. This documentation gives you what is called "cause" or grounds for dismissal. It is this "cause" that keeps you from having to pay unemployment if you do have to fire them.

- If the specific behavior does not improve, fire them after the final warning. If the very first infraction is totally unacceptable (theft, showing up drunk, absence with no phone call, abusive behavior to your patients, etc.), you can fire them on the spot. Make sure you have a list in your employee manual of unacceptable behaviors for which people will be dismissed immediately.

- Remember that good documentation of all these situations is your legal protection against lawsuits or unfair unemployment compensation requests.

▶ **Long-term employee maintenance**

Treat good employees as well as you can afford. It is my experience that if you take care of your employees, they will take care of you and your patients. Remember that your staff is a huge part of your customer service and can be either a wonderful asset or a terrible liability. Small gifts to recognize jobs well done, a paid day off here and there, birthday remembrances, and a simple "thank you" when called for, are all important in the long-term health of your employee/employer relationship.

By the way, before we get to the end of this chapter, the answer to the question about hiring front desk staff as contract laborers is *no.* The IRS has very specific rules about the definition of contract labor and there is no way that your front desk person can fit within that definition. If you get caught doing this, you will owe huge amounts in back taxes! There are websites where you can look at the rules to confirm this for yourself, including www.IRS.gov, but I promise you we are telling you the truth.

Every practitioner we have spoken to about the advantages of having the right someone to take care of their front desk has stated, *unequivocally*, that this person makes their life easier and allows them to make more money with less stress. So take the time to find the right person with the right fit for your clinic. Train them well and treat them well, and this could be "the beginning of a beautiful relationship."

POINTS TO PONDER FROM CHAPTER 10

- A good employee is one of your clinic's most valuable assets. Take time to find the right person.
- Write a very specific job description including the job title, description, qualifications, and a list of specific duties and responsibilities.

"Points to Ponder" continue on the next page

- Consider alternative methods of finding an employee such as canvassing your patients, notices at the local acupuncture college, retiree organizations.

- If you put an ad on Craigslist, don't scrimp on text. A clear, well-written ad can save you a great deal of time. Put a P.O. box or fax number only and collect resumes. Do not put a phone or address on the ad!

- Our guidelines for the interviewing process can save you lots of time. During the interviews, remember what you know about diagnosis. Think twice before you hire someone whom you suspect to have serious health issues.

- Write a short, clear employee manual with your policies for vacations, holidays, personal phone use, grounds for dismissal, and anything else of importance to you. Your new staff person must read and sign that they understand this information on the very first day of working for you.

- Train your new hire carefully; give them a 30-day review and a 90-day "you-are-now-really-an-employee" review. If you think it's not a good fit or are at all uncomfortable, fire them sooner rather than later.

- Document any conversation about a problem or infraction of employee rules. Good documentation with employee issues, just like good documentation with your patients, is your best protection if a legal situation arises.

- With the right person answering your phone, you can make more money, have less stress, and run a more successful and professional clinic.

The Tax Man Cometh: Here's How to Be Ready | 11

One common reason for new business failures is that people forget or don't know to pay their taxes. None of us like to pay them, of course, but they are a part of business life for everyone, regardless of how anyone feels about it. Even if you are lucky enough to live in a state that does not assess income tax or sales tax, you still have to pay federal payroll taxes plus Medicare and Social Security. In this chapter, I'll discuss all the types of taxes that you may incur, with information on how to pay them. Still, please know that while every state and municipality may be a little different, the appropriate office will be more than happy to help you pay what you owe!

Helpful links: We have listed some very useful links for helping you determine your tax situation. For state tax information for all 50 states, you can go to http://www.statelocalgov.net/index.cfm, a portal site to hundreds of agencies. From there you will be able to find out about your business tax requirements and know who/where to call for help if you need it. The people who work in these departments want you to call if you need them. Their job is to help you succeed. Otherwise how do they collect taxes?

For soup-to-nuts information about mall businesses and taxes, visit http://www.irs.gov/Businesses/Small-Businesses-&-Self-Employed. For information on IRS rules and regulations, use the link to the main IRS website, http://www.irs.gov/. At this site you can find the most recent tax laws, publications, withholding requirements, and listings of federal schedules and payment guidelines.

▶ Self-employment taxes

Business owners operating as a sole proprietor, a partnership, or an LLC-paying-yourself-as-a-partnership must pay quarterly state and/or federal self-employment taxes (Social Security and Medicare, or FICA for short) as well as estimated income tax. If your state has a similar requirement and you need help to determine your state's quarterly tax requirements, follow the link listed above or contact your state tax department by phone. The percentage you need to pay the feds depends on the amount of income you took out of your business. The same may be true in your state. However, in some states the income tax is flat, which actually makes life easier. For example, Colorado has a 4.8% income tax for everyone with nothing further to figure out.

1. **Who needs to pay self-employment taxes?** According to IRS rules, a self-employed person not paid by salary, who makes over $400 per calendar year must pay these taxes.

2. **What are self-employment taxes?** These taxes, a combined 15.3% of your income up to $113,700 at the time of this writing, are the result of Social Security and Medicare benefits (12.4% and 2.9% respectively). Self-employed people have to pay this, the same as if we worked for any employer. This money is deducted from the paycheck of every employee in the U.S., no matter where you work. When you work for someone else, only half of this money is deducted from your pay and the other 7.65% is paid by the company you work for. Being self-employed means you are both the employee and company at the same time and, therefore, pay both halves. (Sorry.)

3. **What are estimated taxes?** These are an estimate of what you would have been paying to Uncle Sam in income tax if you had been receiving a paycheck from an employer.

4. **When are these payments due?** All federal self-employment tax and estimated tax are due quarterly on April 15, June 15,

September 15, and January 15, paid on your income for the previous quarter of the year. You can download the appropriate forms for payment from the IRS website. Look for form 1040 ES. Once you start paying these taxes, the IRS will send you (or your accountand will give you) a forms packet with instructions and payment coupons each year.

As stated above, you are liable for the 12.4% Social Security tax only on the first $113,700 of your income. Above that amount, you will still owe income taxes and 2.9% for Medicare no matter how much you make, but not the 12.4%. To review these federal taxes, there are two types that need to be paid. The 15.3%, which accounts for your self-employment tax (FICA), and your estimated income tax payment, which is what you believe you will owe in federal income tax at the end of the year divided up on a quarterly payment system.

Your quarterly self-employment taxes (Social Security and Medicare [FICA]) are paid using a Schedule SE (Form 1040). Your estimated taxes are filed with a 1040 ES (Estimated Tax Payments for Individuals) form. Instructions for both these forms are easy to find at the www.irs.gov website. There are tons of websites with help for first timers.

▶ Keeping track of what you owe

Once you've done some basic research to figure out how much you owe, create a system for setting aside the money for these quarterly payments. Here's how I did it for years when I operated a sole proprietor business. I had a special savings account to set aside money either weekly or monthly. I saved 15.3% plus whatever I figured I'd owe in estimated tax. For this example, let's say my combined FICA plus state and federal estimated tax is 30% of my total take home pay of $6,000 per month, I would put $1,800 into that account every month. The money was still in an account collecting interest and looking good on my credit report, but I had removed it from the business checkbook bottom line and from the temptation to spend money that really was not mine. When the time came to pay the IRS, the money was there and I've stayed out of trouble.

The other way to handle this is to create a corporation or an LLC (see Section 1, Chapter 6) and pay yourself a combination of salary (on which all your taxes will already be paid and you will receive a regular W-2 form at the end of the year) and cash dispersals (on which you will not owe Social Security taxes but you will owe estimated income tax!). Again, it is a good idea to discuss the advantages of various business models with a tax accountant to make certain you are keeping track of everything correctly and that you create the business model that works best for you. If you choose to be paid a regular paycheck, we suggest you consider working with a payroll company, which, for a very small fee, will handle your paychecks, payroll and all related taxes, and take this entire issue off your plate, while at the same time making sure your taxes are all paid on time in full.

▸ Ways to cut down your tax liability

One of the great things about being in business in the U.S. is that there are many things you can legitimately pay for from your clinic bank account instead of paying yourself and then buying from your personal bank account. Learning to do this legally and skillfully lowers what you need to pay yourself which in turn lowers your tax liability. We suggest you discuss all this with a tax accountant, but everything from clinic clothing, magazine subscriptions, many travel expenses, certain types of entertainment expenses, computers and electronics, even a car including its insurance and repair costs, can be purchased by your business. If you create a corporation, the list of what you can buy through your business is even longer and more beneficial. There are a couple of book resources that we have included in the Resources for Going Further section in the back, which will give you more information about the size of this envelope and how far you can push it and still be within the law.

▶ Other types of taxes that vary by state and city

Unfortunately, this is not the end of the chapter on taxes! There are a few other types of taxes that may or may not affect you. Don't worry too much about these, as they are either very minimal amounts or are deductible expenses that lower your federal tax liability.

Sales tax

If you live in Alaska, Delaware, Montana, New Hampshire, or Oregon, you can skip this section, because you have no sales tax! For the rest of us, we must collect and pay sales tax for any sales in our clinic of herbs, supplements, books, or other retail products. Sometimes people ask if we can avoid sales tax on herbs because prescription pharmaceuticals are not taxable. Unfortunately, the answer is no. Chinese herbal products are classified by the federal government the same way nutraceuticals such as vitamins and minerals are classified. This classification gives us a great deal of freedom, but we cannot have things both ways, which means we must collect sales tax on these product sales, the same as any other retailer. If you have either state and/or local sales tax, look up online which office(s) to contact for the appropriate forms and payment schedules.

Use tax

A use tax is considered a compensating tax or complementary tax. Use tax is assessed and due on property or taxable services when sales tax has not been paid because you purchased it in another state. At the time of this writing, the U.S. Congress is trying to find a way to assess sales tax for online purchases, which may make the concept of use tax go the way of the dodo bird. If this act does/did not pass, we can continue to buy things from mail order companies in other states and not pay tax on these items. Few of us bother to assess and pay the use tax due on these purchases in any case. However, if you buy an item and did not pay sales tax to the seller, but you used or consumed that item in your own state, technically you owe use tax on it. My advice is not to worry about this tax unless someone sends you an assessment request; you've enough on your plate in your first years of practice! Again, if the federal law covering this goes into effect, then use tax may become a thing of the past.

Property tax
If you purchase a building this is automatic, so be sure to consider this expense as part of your rates for renting space to other practitioners.

Unemployment tax
For all your employees, you will be assessed both state and federal unemployment tax. Most states have a very low rate (Colorado is .0203 of wages). Federal unemployment is 6.2% *but* you get a tax credit of 5.4%, making the actual rate .8%. One thing to realize, however, is that if you hire and fire employees frequently, your state rates can be increased! In the chapter on hiring good employees, I have discussed how to avoid frequent firings!

> **POWER POINT**
>
> If you use the services of a payroll company, unemployment tax will be included in their monthly assessment and you need not think about this tax or your Self-Employment tax any further.
>
> Payroll companies are inexpensive and take a complex job off your plate for very little money. They are highly recommended!

Business property tax
This is an extremely low tax that is assessed by some states or cities on business property that has a life of more than three years, such as furniture and equipment. The rates you pay will decrease as the property decreases in value year to year, and many states have an exemption on the first $2,500 of things you

buy. Once on the radar for this tax, the authority in question will send you a form on which you are expected to add new purchases and cross off discarded items. The annual amount you pay is quite minimal, if your state assesses it at all.

POINTS TO PONDER FROM CHAPTER 11

- There are several taxes that all of us must pay to participate in business in our country.

- You can find out online for what state taxes you will be accountable (sales, income, use, property).

- If you are operating as a sole proprietor, LLC, S-Corp, or otherwise not taking *all* your income through payroll, learn how to determine how much estimated tax you need to pay and create a system for setting that money aside for your quarterly payments. If you tend to be forgetful, create a way to "ping" yourself so you make your payments on time.

- Do the same as above for your employment tax (Social Security and Medicare, also called FICA) unless you are taking a salary, in which case these are taken out of your pay automatically.

- If you sell products, find out how to pay your state/city sales tax and do it on time to avoid penalties.

- Depending on your state and situation, you may owe other types of taxes discussed in this chapter. Create systems that are as stress free as possible for these to be paid on time and in full.

- If you have salaries for yourself or employees, using a payroll company to handle this for you is inexpensive and highly recommended.

Managing a Successful Herbal Dispensary | 12

A good herbal dispensary can be a great asset both to your patients and your income. In most towns and cities in the U.S., there is not a "Chinatown" where you could send patients to another pharmacy even if you wanted to. That means your dispensary is also a convenience for patients. You can choose to carry only ready-made formulas in capsules or tablets, granule extracts for writing your own formulas, a complete traditional bulk herb pharmacy, or all of the above. How to manage this income source effectively and without stress for your clinic is the subject of this chapter.

➤ **Having a bulk herb pharmacy**

If you choose to create a bulk herb pharmacy, you may be the only clinic in town with this service, which could be a serious marketing advantage. The downside includes the initial cash outlay for storage jars and shelving, determining how to price your formulas, and the fact that you will sometimes need a medicinal you don't have but would be great for this patient right now. That said, this is the standard of care in China and is an effective and reliable delivery method for herbal medicine. My experience is that patients are far more accepting of cooking and drinking nasty-tasting herbs than you think they will be.

Begin by planning carefully what medicinals will be included in your initial setup, but don't purchase any herbs (bulk or otherwise) until you are ready to begin dispensing them to patients. You can be ready by doing some research during your last year in school, checking out several suppliers' prices and shipping policies, sourcing jars, and considering shelving systems. Once you have a real clinic, it will be easier to finalize your storage decisions. Then make a one-time large herb order as close to your opening day as you can. You can often get a nice discount as a first-time buyer if the order is large enough, and free shipping as well (be sure to ask if they don't offer). There are now distributors all over the U.S., so you can usually find a source with very short shipping times.

A bulk pharmacy, if you are well trained and legally allowed to dispense herbs, can start out reasonably small and grow with your clinic. My husband and I had a bulk dispensary selection of close to 400 ingredients after several years in practice. While that is perhaps ideal, it is not necessary to start out with so many ingredients. You can get off to a very nice start with 100-150; just because you know how to use it does not mean you are likely to need *wu gong* (centipede) on your first day of practice unless you are specializing in migraines!

While doing your last few clinic shifts at school, keep notes on the formulas you write and dispense to your patients. See if you can whittle your selection of herbs down to fewer than 150. The list you create will be the items included in your initial order.

Another option is to order the ingredients of 10-15 base formulas and a few others with which to modify those formulas. Example base formulas might include the most important one or two from each category in the formulas book, or the most important ones used in your chosen specialty. To find more specific advice on choosing base formulas or the most useful 100 single medicinals, see Bob Flaws' and my [HW] book, *The Successful Chinese Herbalist*. Chapter 11 gives "starter" lists of the singles and formulas you will likely need to start. You might also look at Bob Flaws' *Seventy Essential TCM Formulas,* which gives the 70 formulas taught at the Shanghai College of TCM.

Next, and you can do this while you are still in school, create a database of the cost-per-gram of each herb so that determining what to charge for your formulas is easy (you will also need to do this if you create a granule extract pharmacy). There are 453 grams in one pound, so if a pound of *dang gui* is $15, your cost is about 3¢ per gram and you will need to charge 5¢-6¢ per gram to patients when that medicinal is included in their formulas. Be sure to take into account the costs for paper bags, plastic baggies, labels, and labor as well when determining your cost per packet of herbs. These and many other details about creating and managing a pharmacy are also discussed in *The Successful Chinese Herbalist*.

Bulk herbs can be kept nicely in glass or plastic jars, either one gallon or half-gallon depending upon the shape and bulkiness of the specific medicinal. However, purchasing enough jars can be a sizable expense and needs to be planned for in your start-up budget. Price these locally and save on shipping.

➤ A granule extract pharmacy

There are many options available in North America and Europe for good quality extract granules. While more expensive than bulk herbs both for your initial purchase and for your patients, the convenience factor may be worth it to everyone involved. Granules also require less shelf space, which can be important in small clinic spaces. Figuring out costs to your patients, which formulas and singles to carry, and managing inventory is exactly the same as for a bulk herb pharmacy. For everything you could ever need to know and understand about maintaining a top-quality granule pharmacy, see Eric Brand's excellent book, *A Clinician's Guide to Using Granule Extracts*.

➤ Prepared or ready-made formulas

If you use only prepared herbal medicines (capsules, tablets, or tinctures), base formulas are a little more difficult to modify, although there are ways. You can use granules to modify these formulas and have the patient swallow their pills or capsules with the modifying "tea." You can also use simple add-on tablet formulas such as *Si Wu Tang* and *Er Chen Tang* to modify your main formula. While not a perfect system, it is a common method of prescribing in Taiwan, and has a good track record (See Eric Brand's granule book for more details on this method of prescribing.) Also, if you are specializing in gynecology, for example, you will require a different group of formulas than a sports medicine or dermatology clinic, so you need not carry every formula in the book. However, if you create a list of the 50+ formulas you know you want to start with, you can get quotes on those from several companies to help you plan your start-up budget. Also find out if these companies give case purchase discounts, first-time buyer discounts, or offer free shipping for purchases over a certain quantity or dollar amount.

▶ Good Manufacturing Practices (GMP) compliance

GMP compliance is a large topic, with all-day classes and many articles available on the subject at the time of this writing. All I will say about this subject here is that you should ask herb companies if their invoices include batch numbers and if Certificates of Analysis and product testing results are available at their websites if there were ever a problem with any of their products. For a more in-depth discussion of GMP, see Eric Brand's book or the revised (2013) edition of *The Successful Chinese Herbalist,* which includes a chapter on this subject.

▶ Managing dispensary inventory

Keeping an herbal dispensary inventory is similar to keeping an acupuncture supply inventory, but for a larger number of items. You begin by counting the herbs/products in your initial order (or what is on hand if you've been maintaining a dispensary but not keeping inventory!!) and then compare that to the number of pounds/ bottles of that medicinal or formula you need to keep on hand. The difference between these numbers is the number of bottles or pounds you will order. This is one of the jobs that a good front desk person can be taught to do.

If, however, your clinic has more than one practitioner, you may need to do something a little more complex to be sure that all products are being sold, not given away. To really work in this situation, all herbal products need to be accounted for as they are sold and as replacements are ordered. If you are using a software program that keeps track of sales and inventory, this is easier. It is also easier if you have a full-time front desk person who is actually selling the products and ordering the replacements! If not using a computer, however, you must create a paper inventory tracking system where someone writes down each time a product is sold or when the last pound of any bulk or granule herb is opened. All incoming inventory must be accounted for in the same way.

Each month, inventory must be done and each herb or formula compared to its own numbers. If you started off on March 1 with six bottles of *Cold Quell*® and if four were sold and six were purchased by April 1, you should have eight on the shelf (6 – 4 + 6 = 8). If you ended up with fewer than eight, it's time to either have a group office meeting or to reconsider your method of doing product displays in your waiting area.

This chapter on operating a dispensary is only an introduction compared to what might be said on this subject. A more thorough exposition about starting and operating a successful pharmacy is the subject of *The Successful Chinese Herbalist: How to Prescribe Correctly, Gain Patient Compliance, and Operate a Profitable Dispensary, Revised 2013 Edition*.

CHAPTER 12 | Managing a Successful Herbal Dispensary

POINTS TO PONDER FROM CHAPTER 12

- Your pharmacy can be a major source of healing for your patients and profit for you.

- You can do well with any type of dispensary: bulk, granules, or ready-made tablets and capsules.

- While you are still in school, do research about pricing and policies from a variety of companies. Ask about discounts for new grads, initial orders, or case purchases for ready-made tablets and capsules. Find out order requirements to get free shipping on an ongoing basis.

- Determine a list of the first 50+ formulas and/or the first 100+ single medicinals that you want to start with. Get quotes on these from several companies.

- Create a simple inventory system to keep track of your herbals. This is even more important if you have multiple practitioners using the dispensary. Most good clinic management software programs include an inventory module. This function should be part of your front desk person's job description.

- Ask your suppliers about their GMP compliance and whether their GMP systems will aid you with your compliance as well. At the very least, product testing reports should be available for each batch and batch numbers should be printed on your invoices.

Patient Management, or How Do You Keep Them Coming Back Happy?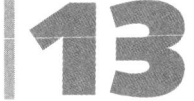

This aspect of clinical practice is vital for your long-term success. Finding new patients is an effort, but may actually be easier than keeping each one as an active patient for years to come, which is the subject of this chapter. Doing this well is, like most things in life, a confluence of many factors. The goal is to both help patients be successful in using our medicine to get well and keep their perceptions about interactions with your clinic positive. In Chapter 6 of this section, we discussed the importance of the look and feel of your clinic. In addition to these more subconscious responses, however, there are many aspects of patient interaction where you, your staff, and your clinic systems have the opportunity to shine, or not.

▶ Initial impressions

Patient communication begins well before a new patient arrives at your clinic. Your tone of voice answering their questions on the phone could form a first impression. Their response to your website, which they are likely to have perused before calling, can have a major influence on today's healthcare consumer. If you do a good job with all these preliminary points of contact, your next opportunities for patient approval (or not) include the atmosphere of your waiting area, the professionalism of your front desk staff, and the quality of your bedside manner. All

> **POWER POINT**
>
> **People search for health care online**
>
> - 85% percent of smart phone users like to read website content about products and services before they buy.
>
> - 35% of U.S. adults have gone online to figure out a medical condition; of these, half followed up with a visit to a medical professional.
>
> - 20% of internet users have consulted online reviews of healthcare service providers and treatments.

these factors could have a potential patient thinking either that you may be a good addition to their healthcare team or that you are a quack. Since keeping patients is essential to professional survival, your attention to these initial interactions is vital.

▶ Close encounters of the telephone kind

Second only to your website as an *initial* influence, early contact with your clinic may well be by telephone. Whether you are handling calls or you have front desk staff, phone contact needs to be scripted, at least to some extent. Start by writing down several ways that your phone may be answered and allow your front desk person(s) to choose the option they like best. Whatever you have them say, it is most important that:

- They (or you) don't mumble or speak too quickly. Remember that the caller cannot see you, making relatively slow speech and clear enunciation very important. You don't want the person to hang up because they could not understand what was said by the person who picked up the phone!

- They sound upbeat and helpful, not bored, preoccupied, or surly. Prospective patients should know the person who answers the phone is happy they called and happy to help them.

- There is actually someone to answer the phone during normal clinic hours, such as 8-to-4 or 9-to-5! Would you expect any doctor's office to have only an answering machine with music in the background that says, "I'll get back in touch with you within one working day"? If we wish to be perceived as professional medical providers, we have to act like other care providers in our culture. That means having normal business phone hours during which people can reach a real person, even if that person is not you.

- They have some scripted answers to commonly asked questions so that they sound competent and professional.

- They have some idea what to do with people calling about a problem or complaint.

- They know approximately how much time various proce-dures require, what initial paperwork needs to be completed (and how to email it or tell people where it is on your website), and if there is any other information you need from a new patient prior to their first visit.

> **POWER POINT**
>
> **What are the most commonly asked questions at an Asian medical clinic?**
>
> Here are some common questions from prospective patients. Write some scripted answers for yourself and especially for any front desk person working for you.
>
> - How long do your appointments last?
> - What do treatments cost?
> - What kinds of things can your clinic treat besides pain?
> - Does acupuncture hurt?
> - How many treatments will I need?

When writing short scripts to answer these and other questions, remember that you want each answer given by your front desk person speaking to a prospective patient to lead to something like: "We could see you at 2 PM on Friday or at 10 AM on Monday. Would either of those work for you?"

▶ Forms and paperwork

Whether available for download from your website, sent by mail or email, or patients fill them out in your office, there are many required forms you'll use to gather information from your patients (covered in Chapters 8 and 9 of this section). In addition to fulfilling HIPAA and other requirements, your forms communicate a lot about you as well as how you do business and give other information that you feel is necessary or helpful to new patients. Remember that an informed patient is a happier and more compliant one; none of us likes to feel confused. These have been covered before so we won't belabor each one here. Just make sure your forms are neat, easy to read and understand, that they communicate professionalism, and that you or someone is available to answer any questions that a patient may have.

Forms you need for an initial exam and visit:

- Personal patient information—Name, phone, email, address, emergency contact, etc. How do they prefer to be contacted? Who referred them? Are they under the care of an MD or other provider?

- Health history—Chief complaint, secondary and other more minor complaints, medical history, prescription drug and supplement use, last medical exam and reason for it, recent surgeries. This form is designed to flesh out why the person is there, what they have done about it in the past, give you a social and family history, and point to any communicable or life-threatening disease or disorder they may suffer concomitantly.

- Financial policies—How much your services cost, accepted forms of payment, if you have a sliding scale. Describe how it works here. If you bill insurance but want patients to know they are responsible for any unpaid balance, tell them here. If you offer a payment at time of services discount, describe it in detail here. It is very important that people sign this page to show they understand your policies. Some clinics take an imprint of a credit card to use in the case of nonpayment; if this is your policy, describe it here. The more you tell people on this form, the less difficulty you will have in getting paid later.

> **PRACTITIONER POINTER**
>
> "If an initial appointment has been made at least a few days ahead, I like to mail people's paperwork to be filled out in advance so that I can include a small packet of information and directions to my clinic. I do this both because it looks professional and gives the person confidence in my services before they even get inside the door, and because it gives us time to get patient records from other providers if necessary."
>
> —Gary Klepper, DC
> Paonia, CO

- Office policies—Do you have observers or interns from the local acupuncture college? Do you have a required cancellation window of 24 hours or more?

- Privacy policy—HIPAA rules require you to tell patients how you will protect and use their personal health information. Please see Section 2, Chapter 9 for more details on this.

- Insurance forms—If you accept insurance, make a copy of both sides of their card and then have the patient complete a form giving you all the necessary information for insurance billing. Be sure this includes the insured's name, date of birth, address, and Social Security number. This form also needs a release of information statement and a signature block so there is no misunderstanding that you will share information with the insurance company. If you accept assignment of benefits, you'll need them to sign an assignment of benefits agreement as well.

- Consent to treatment—If your malpractice insurance does not require the use of a specific form, create one. This form tells people what the risks associated with your services are: acupuncture, herbs, tuina, cupping, guasha, moxibustion, and the like. This is not meant to scare people. However, if you say that a possible side effect of acupuncture is bruising and they have read and signed the form telling them this, they will be less likely to be upset about getting a bruise.

- Arbitration agreement—Although a touchy subject, some malpractice insurance companies give you a price break if you have patients sign an arbitration agreement. This form waives the patient's right to a jury trial, saying that they *can* sue you if they want, but they will arbitrate instead of going to trial. More and more professionals of all kinds are using this type of form, including medical practitioners and real estate brokers.

The more information you give to your patients, the more professional you appear and the less likely there is to be a misunderstanding between you. When you do this effectively, you are telling them that they and their information is safe with you. Without saying it, you demonstrate that you are a medical professional they can trust.

▶ An initial exam that WOWs

This book is not about teaching medical exam-taking. However, the fact that we often spend more time face-to-face with one patient than many physicians spend in a day with *all* of their patients combined is definitely in our favor, so make the most of that time. Remember that an initial exam is like a first date or a job interview; it is an opportunity to really shine. The person may never have seen an acupuncturist, but it's likely they've seen a doctor before. For this reason, doing a history and exam that is thorough, smooth, gentle, and caring makes a real difference for their first acupuncture experience. How about a lovely silk brocade cushion to take patients' pulses? (Remember your fascination the first time a good practitioner took your pulses?) Make this a memorable experience for each new patient!

Take your patient's blood pressure (in some states this is a requirement before every treatment. Even in states where that is not the case, for certain conditions like headaches or dizziness, you should take it every visit). No matter what, always take it on the first visit. Patients are used to this from Western medical providers. It conveys professionalism and shows that our process is still grounded in a reality they are familiar with. You may also do a simple urinalysis to check for sugar content if it seems relevant to their case.

When taking their first history, let your patient talk but control the flow of conversation. Start with some open-ended questions that give you more general information, some of which the patient is unaware they are giving (strength of their overall qi, emotional affect). As you move toward a clear-cut pattern discrimination, ask more "yes/no" questions that give you the specifics you need ("Is the cough wet and productive or dry?"). Listen to the patient's "story" as much as you are able, but keep them focused (gently) on the information you need so that you run on time, which is good for you and for all your patients.

As an active listener, we must avoid the tendency to simply stare at our computer and make notes as they talk. Make eye contact and really listen. Repeat some of their statements back to them for confirmation; patients appreciate knowing that you have heard them. "So, Mr. Jones, your pain is in the left lower side of your abdomen and eases once you have a bowel movement. You also have burping and discomfort after eating. Is that correct?" Make sure the patient knows you understand their complaints.

During your physical exam, explain your actions as much as you can. What are you doing and why? Why do you need to touch me there when my pain is over here? Why do you look at my tongue? What do you feel when you take my pulse? By telling a patient, in simple terms, what you are looking for during a physical exam or what you are trying to accomplish with your treatment, you give them more power over their own body. We want our patients to feel that they are participants, not passive receivers of care.

Allow a new patient to ask questions. While you must control the time, give patients an opportunity to learn about what you think is going on and what you think you can do about it. Answer the questions that you can and keep your metaphors as simple and straightforward as possible. It is easy for people to understand analogies from the natural world, but Chinese medical or quasi-spiritual jargon may turn them off or scare them away.

If you do a PARQ or report of findings form, that helps you to inform your patient about any possible side effects (usually minimal) they may expect from your treatment. You might also give them some treatment options from which to choose (different modalities and/or different durations of care). With some patients, you may simply need to tell them to come back X number of times over the next X number of weeks. With most, however, it works better to give them a couple of treatment plans to choose from. Everyone likes to feel that they have choices and the judgment to make a choice on their own.

▶ Communicators win

The common thread here is clear, compassionate, professional communication. Talk to your patients about your diagnostic and treatment processes as much as you can. Answer their questions and let them know where you think you can make a difference. Also let them know when you've made a mistake and take care of any patient miscommunication or errors in your treatments promptly, seeing any problem through to a satisfactory resolution. Don't let someone walk out your door angry, upset, or frustrated if you can help it.

> **POWER POINT**
>
> **The bonding call**
> We suggest that you *always* call every patient within 24 hours after the first treatment. This is called a *bonding call* and it tells the patient that you really care about what happens to them and how they are doing. Make sure you have their chart in front of you when you make the call and can ask one or two specific questions about their response to treatment. If they have not made a second appointment already, this is your opportunity to suggest it.

▶ Getting the second appointment

We all know most patients need several appointments to get well. When you read Chinese medical journal articles, you never see a protocol that was successful in only one visit! Most of the time, a treatment plan will include 6-8 visits for an initial course of treatment, with 2-3 courses of therapy for full resolution if only using acupuncture. It is up to us to help patients understand how our medicine works. Tell the patient you believe you can help them (unless you don't believe you can) to restore balance in their body, decrease pain, improve the function of bodily systems, and that to do so will require a course of therapy that is sensible and manageable for them.

Explain to each patient that they can expect improvement in their problem only with a series of treatments, and as close together as possible. We know this is how acupuncture works best. For herbs, let the patient know how long you believe the course of treatment needs to be and what they can do in their lifestyle to improve their odds of being able to lower the dose or get off the herbs completely. Otherwise, you are shortchanging your medicine and not giving your patients the best care. Remember, patients will subconsciously pick up on any lack of confidence you inadvertently display, in which case you probably won't see them again. If confidence in the medicine or your skills is a problem for you, either take courses to improve your clinical skills (and thereby your confidence in yourself) or write yourself an affirmation to help you manage your demons until real experience takes care of them for good.

Also make sure patients know that they can get their preferred appointment times if they make them enough in advance. If it is legal in your state to sell treatment packages at slightly reduced prices, this may help motivate patients to come in for more treatments. I have also seen clinics that charge a small membership fee ($10) with which you get a certain number of

CHAPTER 13 | Patient Management, or How Do You Keep Them Coming Back Happy?

treatments over a specified period of time for a reduced rate. Let patients know if you have these options, but don't push people who aren't interested. Check with your state association or regulatory board about these types of offers before offering patients something that may be illegal.

As a patient's course of treatment is coming to an end, schedule a short consultation to decide if treatment is complete or in what way it might continue. It is does not serve your long-term success to string people along, but neither does it serve a patient to cut treatment off if you believe more is warranted. Be honest with your patients and with yourself. If you have done 10 or more acupuncture treatments or weeks of herbal medicine and the patient's condition has reached a plateau, it may be time to make a referral to a senior practitioner in your area, or to a different type of care altogether. Also be sure to give patients a rest between courses of treatment to account for the tendency of the body to habituate to any therapy.

If you are largely an herbal practitioner, you can do very well starting off each patient with a 4-5 day supply of medicine, after which time they come in for a short appointment for you to evaluate progress and adjust their formula. Once their results are somewhat stabilized, they may be able to call in for refills for several weeks without a visit unless there is some problem or change in their situation (the exception being female patients who require a different formula each week of their menstrual cycle). An herbal practice like this could allow you to manage many, many patients with a good portion of your income coming from filling your patients' herbal prescriptions.

Another pointer for herbal practitioners is the issue of dose. I can't tell you how often I've seen patients who were properly diagnosed and the proper formula prescribed but given such low doses that they came to believe, "Chinese herbs don't work." So,

233

think carefully about how much medicine a patient would be getting with a standard decocted formula in China. If you are not doing bulk herb decoctions, take a look at the concentration ratio of the medicine you are giving your patient (pills, powders, tinctures). If you don't know the concentration ratio from the bottle, call your supplier and find out. Pills may get good compliance, but make sure your dosing would come close to the standard of care in China. Otherwise, patients may be wasting their money and, worse, not getting better. This will do nothing for your reputation or the reputation of our medicine. This is especially true in the case of acute or serious disorders. So remember, good patient management with Chinese herbs means giving the right dose.

▶ What to do about the disappearing patient

It happens to all of us. A patient comes in once or twice and never makes another appointment or doesn't show up for one already scheduled. Maybe you "cured" them in one or two sessions, but it is more likely that something in your new-patient procedure needs improvement. Try to reach that patient and learn what you could be doing better. Of course they may be embarrassed to tell you what was wrong with their experience or they may not even be able to articulate it. They may not return your messages or, if they do, you may not get honest answers to your questions. Still, if you can get them on the phone, we suggest the following approach. It may disarm them enough to actually try and tell you about their experience of your clinic and care. If you already did a standard bonding call with the patient, then you know how they *seem* to have responded to their first visit. If not, this may be the first thing you need to add to your procedures.

First ask how they are doing. Ask if they would like to reschedule or if they have any questions about your exam or treatment. Tell them you are sorry if their experience was not

CHAPTER 13 | Patient Management, or How Do You Keep Them Coming Back Happy?

everything they expected it to be and that you'd be happy to assist them in finding another practitioner or another type of service to solve their health problem. That alone should disarm any "armor" to some extent. Explain that, as a healthcare practitioner, it is your responsibility to close their file with some "release from care" and you need to know that they are better or have determined another way to manage their problem.

Depending upon how they respond to this, ask if they have any advice about what you or your staff could have done better or differently that might have changed their decision to discontinue care. Thank them for trying acupuncture and assure them that, should they have further problems or questions about their health, you would be most happy to help them if you can. This is a class act, and anyone that you'd really want to associate with will recognize it. Some may even reschedule on the spot. If not, tell them that you will put them in your inactive files and consider their record closed for the present time but that any other practitioner of any discipline is welcome to request a copy of their files if it would be helpful in their future care.

If you get advice or a complaint, don't be defensive. Listen carefully, take notes, and decide if their statement is valid and if

> **PRACTITIONER POINTER**
>
> "I have noticed an interesting phenomenon when a patient is getting ready to leave the office. I have found it makes a difference whether I say, 'Do you want to call, or do you want to schedule now?' versus, 'Do you want to schedule, or do you want to call?' They have a greater tendency to pick whatever I say second."
>
> —*Valerie DeLaune, L.Ac.*
> *Juneau, Alaska*

there is anything you can do to improve in whatever area(s) they bring up. Discuss what they tell you with your staff or partners and try to find a way to respond that is workable for you. If you do this phone call *with every dropped patient* and listen to any advice you receive, the numbers of "disappearers" will decrease with time.

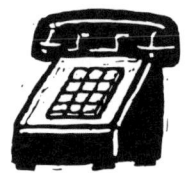

▶ Staying in touch with patients

When a patient terminates care, even for the right reasons, you want to stay in touch with them from time to time. In the marketing chapters, we discuss at great length various ways to keep in touch with your patients. See Section 4, Chapters 2, 4, and 7 for lots of ideas.

▶ Developing confidence

As stated above, if you are unsure of your diagnostic or clinical skills, patients will know it. So, even if you are method acting, conveying a sense of confidence in the treatment room puts the patient at ease that they are in good hands. Choose a treatment and do it. Write a treatment plan and follow it. If, today, you can only think to needle St 36, do it with presence and a confident heart! Your patients *want* to trust in your judgment and experience. Don't try pulling the wool over their eyes, but know that you have learned and can do this work, so do it!

At the same time, while patients want to feel at ease, they also want to feel in control of their lives, which brings us back to skillful communication. Give a patient knowledge about her body and an understanding of how you and Chinese medicine are going to help her and you are empowering her toward better health. Do this with confidence and you will have an educated patient who cares about her health and who will, in turn, have the confidence to send you her friends and family members. That is how you grow your practice.

POINTS TO PONDER FROM CHAPTER 13

- Good communication and self-confidence are two important attributes for managing patients to everyone's advantage.

- Take a look at the recommendations in Section 2, Chapter 6 because patient management includes a lot more than paperwork and phone calls.

- Consider writing standard "scripts" to answer basic phone questions. These scripts should always lead to the appointment-making phase of the initial phone conversation.

- In order to serve your patients well, you need to help them follow through with the treatment plan you create. Make sure they know that, in order to work with you, a certain number of treatments or a certain amount of herbal medicine will simply be what happens in your clinic.

- Don't under-dose with Chinese herbal medicine; not giving enough medicine for the person to experience relief from their symptoms is a waste of that patient's money.

- Your clinic forms should be thorough, clean, not a Xerox-of-a-Xerox, typo free, and easy to understand.

- Use a bonding call within the first 24 hours of a first treatment to find out how a patient responded and to answer their questions.

- If you lose a patient before the treatment plan is complete, find out why and how you could change your clinic procedures, phone practices, décor, or whatever is necessary so that you will not lose another patient for those same reasons.

- If you don't have enough confidence in your skills as a practitioner, decide what you need to do to change that feeling and go do it. When you have confidence as a clinician, it is contagious and growing your practice is much easier.

Using the Services of Other Professionals 14

Sometimes we all need help. A misconception among many small business owners is that doing everything yourself will make you more profitable. This is not true in many cases. In fact, using other professionals not only frees up your valuable time, but also can end up saving you money.

Some services described in this chapter you may not need right away and can do yourself until you get busier with patients (yard work, cleaning service). Others it may be better to start with from the beginning (bookkeeping). Because many of you already know about these services, I've listed them below but discussed only some of them in any detail in this chapter. My only other advice is to barter where you can, at least until you have a full practice, but get help when you need it. Don't let a gap in service, cleanliness, or operations keep you from operating the best clinic you can.

> **Who ya gonna call?**

Here's a list of some service providers you may need as you start-up and grow your practice:

- Bookkeeper
- Tax accountant
- Attorney
- Paralegal
- Building contractor
- Electrician or plumber
- HVAC expert
- Answering service
- Janitorial
- Yard maintenance
- Snow removal
- Laundry service
- Medical transcription
- Insurance billing service
- Computer geek
- Web designer
- Marketing specialist
- Graphic designer
- Printer
- Bank
- Herb preparation service
- Insurance broker

▶ Bookkeeper

A bookkeeper records business transactions that occur during any given accounting cycle such as checkbook reconciliation and bank transactions, ensures that these are recorded properly, and keeps copies of all supporting documents. Bookkeeping services are not hugely expensive so, if you are really bad at this type of work, we suggest you find one with whom you are comfortable working.

▶ Tax preparation service

As a long-time business owner, I suggest you have your taxes prepared and filed by a professional. Just as you have invested thousands of hours in education for your profession, tax preparers are trained in the labyrinth of tax law and can save you both money and headaches. Unless you were a tax preparer in your pre-acupuncture life, doing your tax return is best left to a professional. You may also find it useful to have this person look over the books in October and give end-of-year advice for things to do before 12/31 to lower your tax bill.

▶ Lawyer

While many forms and waivers used in our profession are standard, it is not a bad idea to have a lawyer verify their legality, especially if they are going to be signed by patients or sent to insurance companies. For those of you creating a corporation, partnership, or LLC, having a lawyer draft or review your articles of incorporation and by-laws and advise you about your structure gives you peace of mind. Also, before signing a lease or purchasing a piece of property, running your contracts or agreements by an attorney can protect you from making any really expensive mistakes.

If the cost of an attorney scares you off, find a government-supported legal aid office or a low cost walk-in legal office that hires young lawyers to read documents and make suggestions on how to protect yourself legally. Many towns and cities have such services. Alternatively, contact the local Small Business Administration or SCORE office and ask if they have an on-staff legal advisor who could read the document in question. If you live in a university town with a law school, try contacting them to see if they have a low cost legal clinic. For simple document checks and other minor legal questions, you may also try the services of a paralegal.

If you cannot find inexpensive legal help, try barter. If a lawyer likes your work he or she may refer their clients or law partners, so a barter arrangement may have some marketing value as well.

The times that you *really* want help from an attorney are when you hire anyone for whom you want to create a contract or operating agreement, when you are creating a corporation or LLC, when you have questions about firing employees, when you have serious trouble with anyone with whom you have already entered into a contract, when you are offered a contract by another employer (hospital, MD, DC, school, publishing company), or when you create any legal document or possibly-could-be-legal document.

▶ **Paralegal**
Unlike a lawyer, a paralegal cannot give legal advice. They can, however, draft articles of incorporation or other business or personal legal paperwork. For the price, a paralegal is a good choice for some of this work in the early days of your practice. If you do need a lawyer, a good paralegal will tell you.

▶ **Building contractor**
A good contractor is a valuable asset if you need one, but check them out carefully. You can ask for references, but Angie's List or Yelp may be more reliable before you hire. Even though contractors must be licensed in most states, shoddy

workmanship is not a punishable offense! On the other hand, if the contractor is good, there will be no shortage of people online raving about their services. Also, verify the contractor is licensed, bonded, and insured. **NOTE:** If you plan to hire a contractor, I strongly suggest you get a personal referral, check out Angie's List, Yelp, and any other local business review sites! Do your homework before you hire.

▶ Answering service

On the whole, telephone service is not a strength in our profession. I believe poor phone service is one of the fastest ways to fail. If you cannot hire help from the get-go, consider an answering service. People want to talk to a real person. Let's say someone is in intense pain or has the urge to quit smoking NOW and decides to pick up the phone and ask for your help. If no one answers, they may lose the impetus to pursue care.

You also must faithfully check messages on an hourly basis when you are in the office and on a daily basis when you are not.

▶ Receptionist or office manager

This is not really an outside service, but I'll reiterate anyway. A receptionist or office manager is vital if you are a serious practitioner. I guarantee that you will love having this employee! The phone is answered, patients are greeted and checked out, forms are filled out, and inventory managed. If you find someone good and you can pay a decent salary, they will do your insurance billing, keep your patient files organized, clean restrooms, and tidy treatment rooms between patients as well! Nothing says "professional medical practitioner"

> **POWER POINT**
>
> Remember that HIPAA law requires you to have a business associate agreement form on file for any service provider who is in your space on a regular basis and may have required or inadvertent access to your patients' medical records.

SECTION TWO: WORKING ON YOUR OWN

like a skilled receptionist. When did the MD herself ever pick up the phone when you call for an appointment? This person is not a luxury but a requirement if you want to dedicate yourself to the work you were trained to do for the welfare of your patients. Not convinced? Read Chapter 10 of this section again.

▶ Janitorial service

A medical office of any type needs to be really, really clean. Many companies offer reasonable rates for once-a-week cleaning. Professional companies are bonded and insured.

▶ Yard maintenance

For clinics with a lease agreement, this has already been discussed. If you own the building yourself, then at least basic yard upkeep is necessary. If you like mowing and yard work, that's great, but don't neglect this chore because you have no time. Pull those weeds if you want to pull in new business from anyone walking or driving by!

▶ Laundry service

If you have towels, sheets, and gowns for your patients, a laundry service can save you time, energy, and hassle. Do the math on the amount of laundry if you are seeing 8-10 patients a day, four days per week. A laundry service will pick up and deliver, and everything will be clean, folded neatly, and ready for use. Prices vary and there are usually minimums, so shop around.

▶ Medical transcription

This kind of service may be less important as we all move to digital recordkeeping, but may appeal to busy clinicians and illegible writers. This person or company will take your recorded medical notes (you may need a special type of recorder) and transcribe them into written form for your patient charts (paper or digital). If you have an interest in this, look online for pricing for these services.

CHAPTER 14 | Using the Services of Other Professionals

➤ Insurance billing service

Insurance billing services are more widely used now by many medical professionals, though MD offices have been using these services for years. When you bill electronically, it's convenient to use such a company, the most famous one being OfficeAlly, which at the time of this writing is free to practitioners, fairly easy to use, and makes you HIPAA compliant with regard to this aspect of your practice. See more details on our website under Important Web Tools, Miscellaneous Web Resources.

➤ Computer geek

A good computer tech is a well-loved asset for almost every business and could save your bacon time and again. One hard-drive crash is all it takes to prove it. This person is able to help with major and minor computer disasters. They should also help keep your systems secure, up-to-date, protected from viruses, and help with computer-related problems or questions that arise. Find a good techie before you need one.

➤ Web designer

Websites are either a powerful tool for marketing success or a serious waste of time and money. For more on website marketing, see Section 4, Chapter 7. Here I want to say only that if you have a site and it is not well-designed and well-optimized, you will not capture the interest of potential patients. You will have to write the copy and find the photos for all the parts of your site, but making sure that people will see it could require professional assistance.

➤ Marketing firm or specialist

In Section 4 on marketing I have not suggested anywhere the use of marketing services, which are expensive and may not really do exactly what you need. Even with the help of a good one, you cannot avoid the need to create a wonderful clinic, keep your skills sharp, and network within your community.

▶ Graphic designer and artist

A graphic designer specializes in creating logos and effective text and visual effects for printed or online marketing pieces. Having all this work in digital files on your computer allows you access to it for everyday publishing needs of all types. If you have no visual arts skills, you need this type of service now and again.

As for artists, everyone likes seeing original artwork, especially by someone local. Why not offer local artists a "gallery space" that you rotate quarterly or semiannually? If you live in an art-friendly community, this is one more way to become known as a community team player as well as a supporter of the arts.

▶ Printer

Except for your business cards, in the early days of your practice you may be able to do most of your printing in-house if you purchased that good printer we talked about earlier. However, as your practice grows it will become more cost and time efficient not to be doing most printed materials yourself.

NOTE: As publishers who have printed more typographical errors than we would care to remember, we can only say proofread, proofread, proofread. It is extremely disheartening to have 1,000 copies of something that looks really beautiful only to find a nasty typo that no one noticed. Hire a professional proofer if you can, or have 2-3 people read your printed pieces backwards and forwards (we mean that literally) before you send them to the printer!!!

▶ Bank

You will need a place to put your money and get credit card draft capture. Check out local banks first; it's great to do business with local people when you can. Compare costs of a business account as well as the benefits at several institutions. There is a lot more to say about banks. See the website for a longer discussion.

CHAPTER 14 | Using the Services of Other Professionals

> **Herb preparation service (bulk or granule)**
> If you live in a large city, especially one with a decent-sized Chinatown or lots of OM clinics, you may want to farm out an occasional bulk herb prescription to one of them if you don't have that type of dispensary. At least check out who's out there and their prices, timing, and delivery services. In addition to whatever is local, more than one major U.S. distributor and several of the granule herb companies will do custom prescriptions and drop-ship them directly to your patient.

> **Insurance broker**
> We've already discussed the two types of insurance that you want to carry as a medical business: medical malpractice and general liability. Discussing insurance can feel uncomfortable for some because, when you need it, usually something unfortunate has happened. Looked at another way, however, insurance is a safety net for your practice and for all the patients you are able to help. If an accident or inadvertent mistake forced you out of business, many people would lose your services and your family would lose your income.

POWER POINT

Another service you need is a professional acupuncturist! It is important when you go on vacation to have another practitioner to whom you can refer your patients if they need care. This practitioner's contact information should be left with your answering service and/or on your phone message machine. This relationship should, of course, be mutual and is very valuable. Leaving town without coverage for your active patients is, in some states, legally actionable as patient abandonment. Furthermore, shouldn't we all have someone with whom we regularly trade acupuncture and Chinese herbal care for ourselves?

POWER POINT

Checklist for choosing a business bank

1. Can you get a personal banker to call when you have a question or problem? This is very helpful in many ways.
2. Do they offer free online banking for businesses?
3. Do they charge per check that you write? Under what circumstances will they waive that fee?
4. Do they charge per check deposited? Under what circumstances will they waive that fee?
5. Can you use any credit card processing service you like (Costco for example)?
6. Are there minimum balance requirements?
7. Are there new customer perks and how long do they last?
8. What are the ATM card charges?
9. Are there any perks for small businesses such as yours that will save you time or money?
10. Is the bank friendly and do they seem enthusiastic about having your business?
11. Do they offer reasonably priced lines of credit to help you manage cash flow? What else will they do to help you grow your business?

Concerning malpractice insurance, it's alarming how many practitioners don't feel it is necessary. Arguments usually center on a state's not requiring it or that "no one ever gets hurt with acupuncture." Not true: there are over 500 legal actions against acupuncturists every year. Even if you believe you practice safely and within your scope, it does not mean that no one will ever sue you, justly or not. Also, remember that malpractice insurance covers more than just the cost of redressing any injury to the patient, it also covers the cost of your defense.

Lastly, if you want to work in an integrated setting such as a hospital, if you want to get paneled by any major insurance companies, or if you want to volunteer for any of the many acupuncture-NGO organizations, malpractice insurance will not be optional.

POINTS TO PONDER FROM CHAPTER 14

- There are many professionals in a variety of fields whose services will benefit you, save you time, and lower your stress level. This chapter gives you a long, if not comprehensive, list to consider.

- The belief that you have to be able to do everything in and for your clinic in order to save money is not true.

- If you don't have enough money right away, work out a barter system with some of these much-needed pros.

- Remember that in order to be paneled by any major insurance carrier or to work in an integrated setting such as a hospital, you must have malpractice insurance.

SECTION THREE

GETTING PAID

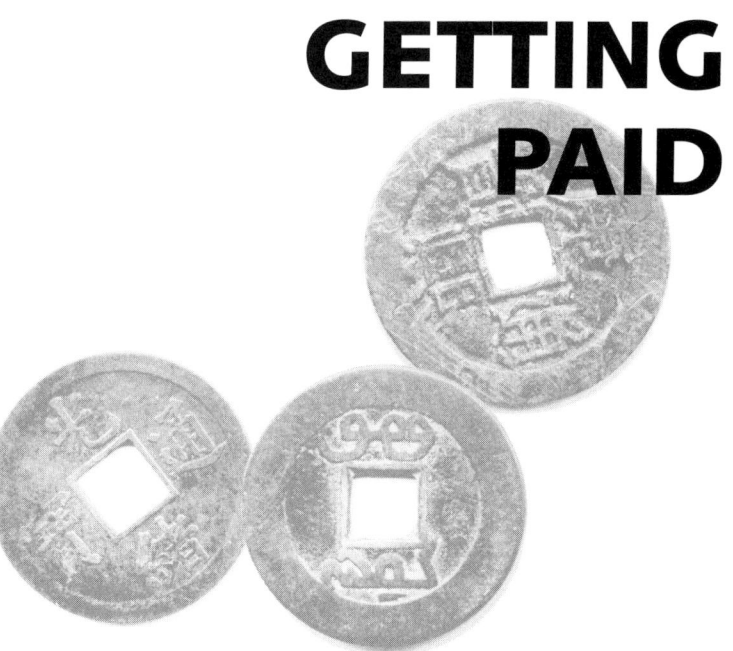

Attitudes About Money | 1

Few of us grow up without some issues where money is concerned. Add to that the fears that a new practitioner may have about the level of their skills compared to someone down the street who's been in practice for years, and you have a perfect recipe for new practitioners of our medicine not being emotionally capable of charging and being paid what they could be and probably should be for their services.

In the case of the typical acupuncturist or other alternative healthcare practitioner, we must also acknowledge the common psychological stumbling block that some people encounter about charging people money when they are already sick or in pain. In this chapter, we'd like to try to help address some of these gut level issues that many people may have.

Money is such a fundamental and wholly integrated part of modern life that it touches every part of everything we do. In our culture, money can mean many things: survival, comfort, success, prestige, love, power, and access. Many books have been written on the subject and, if you believe that severe "money neuroses" are negatively affecting your personal or professional life, we encourage you to explore the resources listed in our bibliography. (See the Resources for Going Further section.)

> "Though mothers and fathers give us life, it is money alone which preserves it."
> —Ihara Saikaku

Within the scope of this book, however, we want to suggest several things with relationship to money. The first is that, as a businessperson, you need to understand your own money issues and figure out ways to work with them so that you don't sabotage yourself where making a living is concerned. We do have some suggestions with regard to this to share in this and other chapters.

Second, with regard to "taking money" from sick people, we strongly suggest you remember that you are offering them services to help end or mitigate their suffering. If there is no appropriate exchange of energy for those services, it is commonly acknowledged among practitioners around the country that people are far less likely to actually get results from your treatments.

Third, and even more important and fundamental, we want to suggest to you that, *while greed or the love of money may be the root of all evil,* money itself is not. In fact, I'd [HW] like to suggest that very few, if any, good things come from poverty. If you truly consider all the worst ills in this world, many of them have a very direct relationship with poverty and its alter ego, greed. The desperation that leads people to become terrorists, to kill endangered species, to tear down the rainforests, or to murder or maim or sell others into slavery—these are most often due to poverty.

> **PRACTITIONER POINTER**
>
> "The most important thing for me to become successful was to overcome my poverty consciousness and believe that I could make it work and that I was worth the price of my care. We need to believe that we are worth it. Then my business changed completely and I am much happier in my work."
>
> —Nancy Bilello
> Denver, CO

As you read this book, I encourage you to think about the good you can and will do with the prosperity that we want to help you create. What would it be like if you could give away vast (or even modest) sums of money? Why do other types of health practitioners or other acupuncturists deserve more than you? Why can't you get to a place of financial comfort and prosperity similar to others? If you really don't like money and are uncomfortable with charging patients, can you come up with a practice that allows you to give it away for free and be supported in the world by some other method? However, if money and any discussion about it is *really that uncomfortable* for you, perhaps you need to find new ways to think about and relate to money in your life or get some help from a psychologist-money counselor. (Yes, these problems are common enough that such people do exist.)

Since we don't live in a fairy-tale world where no one needs to create a source of income, try for a moment to think of money in all its forms as a method of energy exchange, a form of qi, if you will. We all simply exchange our time and energy in lesser or greater amounts to get what we want or need to survive in the world. Our car requires so much energy per week to buy and maintain and no one expects to own a car and maintain it for nothing. Similarly, our house, food, utilities, and clothes all require some exchange of energy. No one should expect to get your services for free either (unless that is your choice). You should not feel that you are doing your patients a disservice by charging what you need to make a decent living. If you don't, you will burn out and not be able to help anyone. Remember that 30-50% of acupuncture graduates are not in practice within five years of graduating, whether they have paid back their school loans or not! If you get your head and heart right with money, you are far less likely to be on the wrong side of these statistics.

> "Money is the seed of money, and the first guinea is sometimes more difficult to acquire than the second million."
>
> —Jean Jacques Rousseau

▶ Family messages

Everyone "downloads" the family line (or lines) about money. Our deepest true beliefs about this mysterious stuff are probably pretty hardwired before we are five or six years old. So think back and look at what the cliches were that you heard in your household. Things like, "money doesn't grow on trees," "do you think I'm made of money?," "a penny saved is a penny earned," or "money is the root of all evil." (That is not, by the way, what it actually says in the Bible. It is the *love* of money that is the root of all evil according to the Old Testament.) In any case, we all got these messages, and, as young children, we mostly believed what we heard.

The problem with all this is that whatever we learned about this most fundamental part of life can have a way of coming back to bite us if it does not mesh well with reality. For example, if we believe deep down that a camel has a better shot at getting through the eye of a needle than a rich man has of getting into heaven, this could make it difficult for us not to unconsciously sabotage our own efforts at financial success, even if practicing Chinese medicine is not really going to make us hugely rich (which it probably won't in any case). That is why it is important to really look at our personal money beliefs and become as conscious of them as we can. It is the "stuff" that is left unconscious that is most likely to stand in our way in life. When we know what our issues are, at least we can be more aware of and, hopefully, more in control of our responses.

Think about your parents and their money "styles."

- Was Mom a worrier and Dad a big spender?

- Was Mom always trying to get more money out of Dad, who tried to keep control of every last dime?

- Did you ever get into trouble as a child in relationship to money? What impact did these things have on your beliefs about money? What impact do you think this has or will have on your business life?

CHAPTER 1 | Attitudes About Money

- What one thing in your relationship with money would you like to change?

- Can you give yourself an assignment to become more conscious about how you work (or don't work) with money?

- What about keeping a journal about your responses to money: spending it, making it, accepting it, sharing it?

Almost everyone has some issues around money. It's pretty hard not to. However, if you think there are issues here that are beyond your ability to work with on your own, look for a counselor or psychologist to help you sort through this part of your life. For someone trying to operate a small business, it is more important than you might believe and can have an impact on your close relationships as well as your professional success.

One final note. If you have beliefs about money that are pretty negative and you don't want to change them for whatever reason but you still want to practice acupuncture, our suggestion is that you get a job. Find another practitioner, hospital, MD, or public clinic that will pay you a flat salary with no requirement for you to collect money, market your services to any extent, or have any money decision-making responsibilities. We have heard of such positions. Here's another possibility. You might try offering your services to an organization that will send you to somewhere in the Third World to do acupuncture in a free clinic. Such organizations do exist and can do wonderful work in the world. This allows you to leave the creation of money for your services and supplies completely to someone else. You will, in this case, probably not be paid at all, at least

> **PRACTITIONER POINTER**
>
> "I believe that people decide where to go for health care based on where they believe they can get the best care and not based on who has the lowest prices."
>
> —Jonathan B. Ammen
> Boston, MA

not in the form of money. But if you are not looking for money in exchange for your work, this style of practice is an option and not a bad one. However, even a life of voluntary simplicity that feeds your heart and not your pocketbook may take some work on your part to create. Either way, getting clear on your relationship to money and how you truly feel about it is fundamental to your success.

POINTS TO PONDER FROM CHAPTER 1

- Do you have a healthy relationship with money?

- What if you could give away millions, or even just hundreds, every year?

- Patients who don't exchange anything for health services often do not get well.

- What did you learn from your family about money and what is the impact of those messages on your business life? If the impact is negative, what could you do to change it?

- If you really have issues that are handicapping your life, get professional help.

- If you don't want money in exchange for your work, find a way to give it away that will allow you to live in harmony with your beliefs.

Methods of Payment for Your Patients | 2

As a healthcare practitioner and an acupuncturist or herbal medicine specialist, you are providing a valuable service. There are several different forms of payment that you may consider in exchange for your services. It is a good idea to have at least thought about each of these in advance. For each one described in this chapter, decide whether, when, and how you will accept these methods of exchange.

Some practice management gurus suggest that you should classify your patients by the way that they pay. Doing this keeps you abreast of your clinic's actual sources of income. Most professional software will have a report you can use to track this, or you may use different colors of file folders for each payment type if you maintain paper files. You may never want to have too many patients of any one payment type, except, of course, cash patients! If you keep things apportioned, rather like a stock portfolio, your income flows from more than one stream. For example, if all you see is insurance patients from the major employer in town and they change their plan to no longer cover acupuncture, you may then see a serious drop in patients!

If your practice is heavy on insurance and managed care patients, try to bring in some workers' comp or more cash patients. If you have plenty of cash patients, look for a few barter patients and get some things you want or need without

POWER POINT

Community acupuncture clinics are an exception to some parts of this discussion. As cash-only practices [some do barter or trades as well], they do not bill any insurance unless it is some type of hybrid clinic. People pay what they can within the clinic's range of charges, $19-20 being the average that clinics around the country seem to make per treatment.

> **PRACTITIONER POINTER**
>
> "Not having a diversified cash base can have its drawbacks. The month that the U.S. went to war in Iraq (February 2003), the cash base in our clinic went from 75% to 45%. People everywhere were spending less money. Although our acute patients remained steady, the chronic ones were more likely to drop off treatment plans or space their treatments farther apart. Our solution? We spent time with each of our patients talking to them about their insurance coverage. Some of them were self-insured, while others had company policies that they could chose from. We gave all of them information on insurance companies that we bill for acupuncture with great success. Within 45 days, we had recovered our total patient base by increasing our insurance billing."
>
> —Eric Strand
> Gresham, OR

using cash at all. Encouraging a variety of payment types keeps your practice better prepared to handle any economic challenge that may arise and affect one or another type of payer.

▶ Cash

Cash payers should make up the largest portion of your payment pie-chart, whether actual greenbacks, checks, or credit cards. These are all equal, which is one reason that you cannot offer patients a cash price lower than you give insurance companies: the check the insurance company sends you *is* cash. Checks and actual greenbacks are nice, but you will find that many patients will use debit or credit cards if they can, including Health Savings Account debit cards. Patients and even visitors to your clinic buy more of the products you have on display for sale if they can use a credit card for their purchase, which brings us to a discussion of credit card accounts.

> **POWER POINT**
>
> The clinic financial policies form that each patient must read and sign should state that, while you are willing to bill for insurance payments *if the patient's policy reimburses for acupuncture and the annual deductible has already been met*, the patient is, finally, responsible for the payment of all fees. You may also say that payment is expected at the time services are rendered "unless other arrangements have been made in advance of treatment." If unsure of the patient's insurance status at the first appointment but the patient says they want to bill insurance, tell them that until their insurance status can be verified you will give them a superbill so they can get reimbursement directly from their insurance company for all or any part of the fees they pay to you.

➤ Credit card machines

Credit card processing is no longer an option for businesses; even a hotdog stand at a street fair has at least a Square® these days. There are a number of sources for getting your equipment and processing services.

- When interviewing banks to establish a business account, talk to them about their merchant services department and charges for credit/debit card processing fees and equipment.

- Costco (or Sam's Club) is a good source for merchant services accounts if you are a member and the bank is more expensive.

- Some state and national acupuncture associations have merchant services agreements with very reasonable processing fees for their members.

- If you are renting space in someone else's clinic but keeping your money separate, Square® or a similar service is a very nice option. You will still need a merchant services deal with the bank where the money will be deposited.

Stay away from companies that send out postcards offering low processing fees. Many times such companies go out of business or stop providing customer service. Go with the larger companies that have been around for awhile.

When shopping for credit card service, know that there may be three different types of charges on your account: 1) the lease or monthly payment for the machine, 2) a monthly fee for using the merchant services (not all accounts have this fee!), and 3) a percentage and/or flat fee taken from each transaction.

If you purchase a machine, monthly charges will be less but your initial outlay could be $250-$900 depending on the speed and age of the equipment. Another option is to make monthly payments with interest, a better route if you want to own a machine but don't have cash up front. As with any product, however, if your machine breaks [they don't break easily] or becomes outdated [they stay usable for a long time], you have to fix it or buy a new one. You can buy used quite cheaply through Ebay, but check with your card services company to be sure the machine you want to bid on is still usable!

If you lease a machine, you can lease by the year. If the machine breaks, the company will fix or replace it at no charge. However, you are paying rent that never stops. In my experience, there is no right or wrong way to do this. I have both rented and purchased credit card machines. The equipment is usually reliable, rarely

POWER POINT

Several companies offer credit card swipers (GoPayment®, ROAMpay®, Cube®, Square®) that attach to a smart phone and deposit funds to your bank account. At the time of this writing, sketchy customer service seems to be the largest problem with these, so review them carefully at online forums, blogs, Yelp, etc. Convenience is good, especially if you do live events, but this market is still developing. Products will, no doubt, improve with time.

needs servicing, and will last several years before it is too outdated to use. If you can get used equipment for a good price, it's not bad to own it. We have two machines, one of which is many years old and still works fine.

The percentage you pay on each transaction varies depending on the company and volume of credit business you do. On-site sales where the credit card is present, get you a better rate than mail order sales. A good rate is anything less than 2.0%, especially if your business is brand new. You may not get the best rates until you've been taking credit cards for a year or more and companies see that you are reliable, so find the best rates you can with the shortest time requirements. After a year, look for a better deal. Tell banks you are shopping for a new merchant services provider. You do not usually have to change the lease or buy out of your equipment in order to change service providers.

➤ Time-of-service cash discounts

You may wish to discuss specific questions about this with the insurance commissioner in your specific state, but in most states it is not illegal to offer a payment-at-the-time-of-service discount. According to an article by John Frostad, L.Ac., in the Winter, 2002 issue of *Extraordinary Points,* this type of discount is legally defensible because it saves you time and postage, reduces risk of nonpayment for services already rendered, and means you don't have to wait for payment. While there don't seem to be any guidelines on minimum or maximum discounts in this case, to be legally defensible the discount should roughly equal the value of the time you would save if not having to bill for your services and wait for payment, say 10-15%. You do not have to offer such a discount to patients for whom you are billing their insurance, but you must offer the discount if they are paying you directly but billing their insurance themselves. You also do not offer this discount to a patient to whom you will be sending a bill after services are rendered, but very few practitioners in our field do this. Whatever you decide to do with this option, make sure your financial information forms for patients are clear.

> **Fee-for-services insurance**

Despite the obvious advantages, if you take only cash patients you lose out on several other types of paying patients, insurance patients being one of those types. Fee-for-service insurance is where you bill the insurance company every time you see the patient and they send you a check of some amount. The remaining balance, if any, is billed directly to the patient or to the patient's credit card that you have on file. This is likely to be the second largest group of patients you will have.

Acupuncture coverage is growing. These days more employees are requesting acupuncture and alternative care to go along with their major medical coverage, which means that more insurance companies are scrambling to add alternative care coverage so they don't lose their payers. Also, under the 2010 Affordable Care Act, six states have voted to add acupuncture as an essential health benefit, espcially for preventive care. So far, this coverage is for 12 visits per year, although exactly what that means in terms of coding and reimbursement is not yet clear. If you live in CA, CT, MD, WA, NM, or AK, however, you need to find out what this coverage means for your patients and how to participate to everyone's advantage.

People with insurance want to use their benefits. If their policy covers your services, getting them to reschedule for more than one appointment is not difficult. Therefore, insurance patients will typically follow through with the course of treatment you suggest and often take more treatments than a cash patient, as long as your treatment plan shows that the care is *medically necessary,* a favorite phrase in the world of insurance companies. What this phrase means in practical terms for us is that things

CHAPTER 2 | **Methods of Payment for Your Patients**

like "stress reduction" or "zang-fu balancing" have no billing code, are not medically necessary, and will be denied. That said, all insurance plans recognize pain as a medically necessary treatment issue and will cover it if they cover acupuncture at all. All of the ICD-9/10 codes related specifically to pain are in the 7xx.xx series: low back pain is 724.2; shoulder pain 719.41; ankle pain 719.47. Therefore, your best option with insurance billing (if you are *not* in the state of California and if the patient is *not* coming in with a diagnosis from an MD) is to bill for pain. If the patient complains of RA or OA, bill for the areas of the body where the pain is and you are far less likely to have difficulty getting reimbursement. For more on insurance billing, see Chapter 3 in this section.

POWER POINT

Find out what insurance programs the largest companies in your area offer their employees and if your services are covered by the policies they use. By establishing a relationship with the human resources (HR) director at each company, you can find out this information. If you find local companies with coverage for acupuncture, send the HR director information on acupuncture and what it can do for people: treatment or prevention of colds and flu, quick pain management and resolution resulting in decreased down time and increased productivity, or whatever you specialize in. Ask if you can send enough flyers to put something in each employee's pay envelope and on the bulletin board in the employee break room, and offer to give a free lecture about acupuncture care as part of the company's lecture series. Just letting people know that acupuncture is a covered benefit may be enough to spur an initial few patients. Once word gets around about the great results you provide, you have yourself a nice patient population to draw from.

SECTION THREE: GETTING PAID

> **Managed-care organizations**

Not the friendliest method of payment available to us, but it is one of the ways that patients will want to pay. Like insurance (but worse for practitioners), managed-care networks function as a middleman between the practitioner and the insurance company. A managed-care network is an organization that offers to collect a panel of providers for insurance companies for some set rate per insured each month. This does two things. One, it gives the insurance company a quick way to ensure that their clients are getting quality care from trained, licensed, and insured providers. Two, it controls costs by limiting the amount the company pays for any given treatment to any given provider.

In order to participate in a managed-care network, you have to be accepted onto their panel. To do this, contact the provider relations department of that network, submit an application, and occasionally an application fee. If accepted, the network will send you a copy of your contract and a fee schedule with acceptable billing codes. This means that you are limited not only in how much you can collect from the insurance company, but also in what CPT codes you can bill for. Also, being a provider for a managed-care network means you cannot collect any other money from the patient beyond a predetermined co-pay.

Think about this for a moment. If you typically charge $75 for an acupuncture visit but the managed-care network only pays $50 ($40 plus a $10 co-pay you collect from the patient at the time of the visit), you have essentially cut your rates by a third. The rest of that $75 is ungettable. So, should you do this or not?

If you have done the budget exercises and have a clear idea of what your clinic needs to make per hour, you will already know the answer to this question. For example, if you have the ability to see only one patient per hour and your clinic needs to generate $65+ per hour, then accepting a patient through this network means you are operating at a loss. On the other hand, if you can see more than one patient per hour (by having more rooms or shortening the treatment time) and you keep your billing time efficient, then you are still operating in the black.

Another way to think about managed-care patients is to think of what that patient means to you over the course of a year or the potential life of that patient's need for your care, which could be several years. Chances are they can get X number of visits per year under the limitations of their policy. Say 12. Okay, that represents $600 to your bottom line. If you are not completely booked every day, it may be foolish to throw away $600, especially if you could schedule these patients on your least busy days or times to keep your appointment book full all week. Also, consider that this patient might send you referrals who may not be managed-care patients.

Whether you decide to accept managed-care patients or not will vary depending on many factors, as you can see. Do some careful math so that you have real numbers to back up your decision. For considerable detail on this and all insurance subjects, see *Playing the Game: A Step-by-Step Approach to Accepting Insurance as an Acupuncturist* by Sperber and Hefner-Andersen.

▶ Medicaid

This is a state insurance program for low-income people. The payment rate for these programs is extremely low (in California around $16-$17 per visit) and patients are allowed only two visits per month. Despite this, to have a state-controlled insurance program paying for acupuncture services at all is a governmental acknowledgment that acupuncture works, though not all states offer this coverage. Medi-Cal, the name of the program in California, pays at the above rates. The Oregon Health Plan used to cover acupuncture but stopped in recent years due to budget woes. If you are interested in working with low-income patients, contact your state's insurance commission and find out if acupuncture is covered, at what rate it is reimbursed, how many visits per month patients are allowed, and how complicated the paperwork is (this could be the deal-breaker). If it is covered in your state, you believe in offering services to the economically disadvantaged, you have a clinic with multiple treatment spaces, and you can work on several patients at the same time with simple protocols, you might be able to make this work at least a day or two per week. If the

> **PRACTITIONER POINTER**
>
> "At Alternative Healing Network, we use music and free events to get people in the door of our wellness centers and to grow our mailing list. As a non-profit, we've also gotten a few grants to expand the types of services we can offer to local underserved populations, but we mostly generate our own funding from our sliding-scale wellness centers. Our free clinics are supervised off-site clinics for students from the local acupuncture college, which is great experience for them. In this way we've been able to give thousands of free treatments at the same time as we've built a real presence in our community and a solid demand for our paid services. No one is getting rich, but paid staff members make a living. Everyone is an employee with guaranteed minimums and bonuses above a certain threshold and all full time staff are eligible for Federal Student Loan forgiveness. It's been really hard work, but really rewarding.
>
> The secret to making this type of clinic work is finding the right people who want to give back to their community. We also started small and things grew organically."
>
> —Ryan Altman
> *Adams Ave. Integrative Health, La Mesa Integrative Health*
> *AltHealnet.org*
> *San Diego, CA*

paperwork is too complicated, consider ways to give free treatments one or more times per month or to donate proceeds of one day per month to a cause in your area.

There are many underserved in our nation and it's great to help them. However, before you consider taking on this type of patient, make sure you are still able to operate your clinic at a profit. Your landlord won't take pity on you if your rent is late because you are treating people out of the goodness of your heart. As the Practitioner Pointer on the previous page describes, you must balance pro bono work with treatments that bring in income. Again, the more you diversify, the more you are able to do things like treat people for free or for very small payments.

➤ Medicare

Medicare (federal health insurance for seniors and the disabled) does not yet cover acupuncture. However, the fact that we are not covered does not exempt us from association with this department or government. Many seniors will come to your office with dual coverage, *i.e.*, Medicare plus a supplemental insurance program. In this case, Medicare is the patient's primary insurance and, before you can send a bill to the secondary insurance, you need to get it denied by the primary provider.

Here's where the system has a "catch-22" and one option for how to get around it. Even though everyone in the insurance world knows that Medicare does not cover acupuncture services, you still have to get a denial of benefits. However, when you send your claim form to Medicare to get your required letter of denial, they may take 2-3 months to get back to you and then return your claim form with a letter telling you that since they don't cover acupuncture, they cannot even deny your claim!

To get off this merry-go-round, you need just one generic "we do not cover acupuncture" letter to use for all future billings to each senior patient's secondary insurance carrier! If you look on the website that comes with this book in the Insurance Forms section, there is a letter of denial in the insurance forms section, which you can download and try to use. ● We hope it will work in at least some cases. That being said, this type of patient should comprise only a very small proportion of your payment pie because of the time and paper-work involved.

> **Workers' compensation (WorkComp)**

Workers' compensation is an insurance program for employees who are injured on the job. Not all states' WorkComp programs pay for acupuncture, but many do. Colorado's law is quite forward-thinking when it comes to this type of insurance. The acupuncturists there are not considered primary care physicians and are not allowed to evaluate and diagnose WorkComp cases, but they can be selected as the individual's choice of care once the patient has been seen by their primary care physician.

WorkComp pays quite well in some states. However, plans and coverage vary widely from state to state and plan to plan. Rehab from various types of pain conditions are the most commonly covered events, and there may also be state-specific CPT codes.

PRACTITIONER POINTER

"In 2012, I averaged $71 gross per patient visit, with 30% of that being cash, the rest from insurance or workers' compensation. WorkComp patients average the most return on a patient visit.

I have one full-time employee for the phone, help with records, insurance billing, inventory maintenance, all the office jobs.
I see 60+ patients per week and need 20 per week to break even."

—*Bertram Furman*
San Diego, CA
http://www.acupunctureandyou.com

Call your state's Insurance Council and ask about coverage for acupuncture, rates of reimbursement, and the following items:

- Are there any special forms or reports?
- What CPT codes are acceptable and payable by Workers' Comp?
- How many treatments can a patient receive?
- And, most importantly, do you need a referral from an MD before treatments can be billed?

Some practitioners have a very large proportion of this type of patient. If you have lots of medium to large manufacturing companies in your area, your clinic has multiple rooms, and you can stay focused enough to do a patient every 30 minutes for a few days per week, you could even specialize in this type of patient. See Chapter 5 in this Section for more specific information on working with WorkComp patients.

POWER POINT

A few words of caution on billing auto insurance companies:

- They have lawyers—lots of them. Make sure the services you provide are indeed medically necessary and that you have very good, clear chart notes. Do not try to string out a patient's treatment plan so you can make your overhead for the month; company auditors will catch you, and rightly so.

- Make sure the patient signs in for each and every treatment. It is not uncommon that a patient will seek legal assistance to deal with their insurance company. Your records may be subpoenaed regarding any case. If the patient didn't sign in on the date you say they received acupuncture, the only proof is in your word and

"Power Point" continues on the next page

SECTION THREE: GETTING PAID

> the patient's—and that may not be enough to hold up under legal scrutiny. Paying bills and taxes is hard enough. Don't be forced to send money back to the insurance company that you actually earned!
>
> - Send in your claims in a timely manner. If the patient is getting other medical care at the same time, remember that the insurance company pays bills in the order received, and you could get th short end of that stick!

▶ Personal Injury (PI)

As long as acupuncture is licensed in your state, auto-accident insurance probably pays for it. Still, this is another call-and-check situation. If you can bill auto insurance for personal injury, it is worth considering taking this type of patient. Unlike other forms of insurance coverage, unless there is complex litigation going on with your patient's case, they pay what you bill (within reason), there is no co-pay, and there is no deductible. In most states, personal injury insurance will cover all *medically necessary* treatments or modalities up to the full medical coverage amount in the patient's policy. This could cover a lot of acupuncture, enough to really help your patient's chances of returning to full and pain-free health. The patient does not have to worry about amassing large medical bills that need to be paid out of pocket. See Chapter 4 of this Section for more detail on dealing with PI cases.

▶ Trade or barter

I have always liked trades and barters as a form of payment; these are a good way to acquire services you want or need while staying outside the cash economy. Straight trades are just that. "I do this for you and you do this for me." Bartering means, "I'll do this for you at no cost and you give me X number of

CHAPTER 2 | **Methods of Payment for Your Patients**

dollars off your product or service" or the other way around. This can be advantageous for you some of the time, but make sure the terms are clear in advance. Even and email exchange can be your evidence of what was agreed to on both sides.

I have done straight trades for massage, haircuts, and barters for lots of things over the years. For trades, if you want a particular service, do a straight time-for-time or service for service. For barters, negotiate based on what feels fair. Please note that,

POWER POINT

Hardship Waiver Forms and Sliding Scales

It is not illegal to have a sliding scale or to discount your services based on financial need. Many medical clinics, Planned Parenthood for example, have such discount programs, usually based on federal poverty guidelines. We have a link to the most recently published federal guidelines on the website (Patient Management Section) along with a Financial Hardship form to have people fill out if requesting a discount based on financial need. ● Unless you have a community acupuncture style clinic, you may wish to ask patients requesting a discount for proof of their assertions (most recent bank statements or last year's tax return).

You do not need to offer these discounts to patients for whom you are billing insurance. You also need not advertise that your clinic has discounted services but only provide information if they inquire about such a discount program or if you think it is appropriate for a specific patient. There are no minimum or maximum discount amounts mandated by law. In deciding what your discounts should be, remember that people will benefit more from your services if they exchange something fair for them in return.

271

according to the IRS, you are supposed to report the fair-market-value of these services on your return. I'm not sure how they would know, but I have to give you this information for the sake of full disclosure.

➤ Free

Free is an option for every practitioner and sometimes you will want to do it. There are a variety of reasons for this and all of them seem correct at the time. I like free consults and fundraising events where I am giving away my time and work, in moderation. You might consider giving regular patients a free treatment on their birthday or treating low-income people free on the last Wednesday of each month as a community service. Just remember that free treatments must not compromise your ability to support yourself. And, statistically, patients who don't pay anything for treatment don't get well as fast as those who pay something. It seems that there needs to be at least some kind of energy exchanged in order for patients to get the results they are seeking from your care.

> **PRACTITIONER POINTER**
>
> "I pay myself first. Not the rent, electricity, herb company, or phone company. I am the most important bill in my business. I include my bill as part of the overhead and, as always, I 'goal' for the result and it always comes to fruition. When there are moments in the month that I think it might not happen, I think in my mind that I can cut back on my bill to myself. Then I call my mentor. She tells me that if I were electric or water, I would be turned off. So focus on your purpose and the practice will provide. Sounds like religion but, damn, it works month after month."
>
> —*Susan Schiff*
> *Delray Beach, FL*

➤ A final note about freebies and payments

We don't suggest that you give away "an introductory treatment" as a promo. Yes, you will get calls and people coming in for those free treatments, but 90% of them are "tourists" who will not come back when you discuss your fees for further care. They got it free the first time, so why should they consider paying you? This does nothing for your long-term growth and even less for your sense of value. If you want to give away something, offer free 15-minute new patient consultations. This is a good idea and you can state this offer on your after hours phone message, on a little sign in your office, the back of your business card or brochure, and on your website or Facebook page. When you do these, have a form with 3-4 questions that you ask. See the Patient Managment & Record-keeping section on the website. 🎧 Listen to the person attentively for a few minutes. Then give a fairly standard response, including a closing statement something like:

"I have experience helping people in your situation, but I'll need to do a complete exam and history to know everything about your specific case. I'm happy to help you with your health issues and I think Chinese medicine/acupuncture may be a wonderful resource for you. We take new patients on Mondays and Wednesdays. If you like, I can have our front desk person schedule an appointment for you at a convenient time."

Give the person some literature and your card. This is where your eye contact and general demeanor sell you to that potential patient. So don't give away treatments except in rare situations, as part of the resolution of a problem with a patient or as a demo at speeches and live events. Remember that in life, time is the one thing that you cannot ever get back.

POINTS TO PONDER FROM CHAPTER 2

- In order for your income to be balanced, it's a good idea for your clinic to accept more than one type of patient based on the various ways patients can pay.

- Cash patients are great. However, you may find that insurance, PI, Workers' Comp, and managed care patients are more reliable sources of income during tough economic times. So don't count them out unless you are a community acupuncture clinic.

- If you don't have a credit card machine, get one. You will find that patients are happier to pay you that way than to write a check. They may be more willing to take their herbs or buy other products you sell in your clinic if they can pay with a credit card. There are many companies who sell credit card machines and card services accounts. Try Ebay for used equipment. Shop around for a reliable, well-priced service.

- Regular health insurance, Workers' Compensation insurance, personal injury, and managed care patients can all be a part of your practice mix. If you have adequate clinic space, are well organized, and have a good front desk person, you can probably figure out a way to make each of these types of patients add to your bottom line.

- Trade or barter only for things you really want, not just to do someone a favor. You won't give them a good treatment if you don't really want what they are trading for in the first place.

- Be careful about free treatments. Patients who don't give back any kind of energy in exchange are less likely to get better than patients who do.

The Ins and Outs of Billing Insurance | 3

The status of insurance coverage for acupuncture in the U.S. has changed from a decade ago, due to changes in various states' laws in response to the 2014 implementation of the Affordable Care Act and due to the fact that we've been in the insurance marketplace that much longer. I have met many acupuncturists who bill their patients' insurance companies with great success.

The purpose of this chapter is to help you decide whether to do insurance-billing and to explain a few basics of how to work with insurance companies to have the smoothest possible relationship. Although paper forms are becoming a thing of the past, this chapter also includes information on the forms you will need, how to complete them, and, hopefully, how to get paid promptly. If you are serious about becoming proficient at billing insurance, however, you will need to take a course or two and to find other books that are specific to this subject. There are many such resources available, some of which are listed in the Resouces section at the back of this book.

This chapter is only an overview and cannot easily be kept up to date with ongoing changes in laws or the vagaries of policies of various insurance companies. Some of the issues that could be discussed here have been presented in other chapters. That said, here we go.

> ## The insurance learning curve
For anyone not specifically trained to do it, insurance billing can be, at first, confusing and stressful. Still, once you conquer the learning curve, insurance opens the door to a new patient population and the financial growth that implies. It's also worth

pointing out that patients with insurance for acupuncture care are often willing to get more, and more regular, treatment. Still, the operations of and communication with insurance companies can feel both opaque and inconsistent. Each company may pay a different rate for the same service, whatever *their* definition is for "usual, reasonable, and customary" amounts, of which you may then only receive a percentage. Some companies allow (or even require) you to collect a co-pay, others do not.

POWER POINT

Basics to remember when accepting patients who want to use their insurance benefits

- An insurance policy is a contract between the patient and the insurance company. Fundamentally, it has little to do with the practitioner. The benefits are available to the patient, not to you specifically.

- The patient controls the monies paid out from the insurance policy. They can choose to pay or to stop payments to any and all providers.

- If benefits have been assigned to you, as treating practitioner, then your office procedure should without question have a procedure to verify the insurance benefits *before you accept the assignment.*

- Before any payment is made, you must decide how much credit you are willing to extend to a patient, and how much time you are willing to extend that credit: 30, 60, 90 days or more.

- If you accept assignment of benefits, be sure the signature is on file for both:
  a. release of information form
  b. assignment of benefits form

"Power Point" continues on the next page

- Do your insurance billing on a regular 30-day basis. If the patient is not notified of a balance due for a service you rendered, then the patient does not have to pay unless you have an agreement based on the time limit you are willing to extend credit. (See the fourth bullet point above.) It is good business practice to bill every 30 days for any unpaid balance, even if the insurance was supposed to reimburse for those treatments.

- Always remember that the insurance company will pay their percentage of what they deem is allowable based on the patient's policy. They may not pay the expected 80% of the total charges. They might pay only the amount that they (the insurance adjusters) deem "medically necessary." In most cases this is far less than the 80-100% you might be expecting.

While some insurance companies pay whatever you bill (*e.g.*, personal injury insurance), others may only pay 50%. Whether you can retrieve the balance from the patient is established by the type of insurance coverage as well as any contractual agreement you may or may not have with that company.

Types of insurance

In order to figure out whether and how various types of insurance will pay for your services, it helps to understand how each type works with their clients. This was all discussed briefly in the previous chapter.

Fee-for-services insurance: This type of insurance coverage reimburses to the provider directly as long as that provider (in this case, you) accepts an assignment of benefits from the insured person. The amount reimbursed for your services is usually some percentage of what is called in the insurance world "usual, customary, and reasonable" charges. Each company has what they call a *relative value scale* (RVS) for all types of medical services, including acupuncture, by which they determine reimbursement for the different services covered by their range of policies. Based upon the company's usual, customary, and reasonable RVS listing for acupuncture, they may pay for all, a portion, or none of your services. Based upon each patient's specific coverage, he or she may or may not be required to pay you an additional portion of the bill, called a co-pay. We discuss below how to find out if and how much a company pays and whether the patient is responsible for any co-pay.

Managed care: Managed-care organizations are brokers between insurance companies and healthcare professionals, credentialing practitioners in each of the professions they cover and placing them on a "panel." Patients with managed-care coverage have the option to select practitioners only from among those on the panel, and services from all paneled practitioners are reimbursed at a predetermined rate based on the contract. Some companies require a patient co-pay ($10-$30 for example). Practitioners apply to be included on panels; there may or may not be an application fee. Some companies take a portion of the amount paid to you each time services are billed. Patients who choose a credentialed practitioner on their plan save money.

Medicaid: This state-administered health care for low income Americans is discussed in Chapter 2 of this section, p. 265.

Medicare: This federal insurance plan for seniors and disabled persons is administered under the Social Security Act. At the time of the printing of this book, there is still no coverage for acupuncture under Medicare. There was a bill before Congress to amend both the Social Security Act and Title 5 of the U.S. Code so that qualified acupuncturists' services will be reimbursable under Medicare Part B and also under the Federal Employees

Health Benefits Program. However, its main sponsor has now retired and, because of the 2013 budget cuts under sequestration, it is unlikely that any new services will be added for Medicare coverage any time soon.

Workers' compensation: This subject is large enough that we have given it its own chapter. Coverage for acupuncture varies from state to state but can be a good way to expand your income. The most important caveat for practitioners who want to bill this type of insurance is to learn the rules regarding billing and paperwork and follow them to the letter. See Chapter 5 of this section for more details.

Personal injury (PI): PI insurance covers people involved in auto or other types of accidents. Payment for acupuncture varies from company to company and state to state, but can be very good. Some PI cases allow you to get paid as you treat, and you do not need an MD referral to treat the patient as you do in many WorkComp cases. PI cases do, however, require meticulous recordkeeping, and there can be an element of risk to consider. For example, in PI cases where there is an unresolved lawsuit against the allegedly responsible party, you may have to wait some time for reimbursement, and, if the patient loses their case, and you may not get paid at all! If you choose to take such lawsuit cases for the potential long-term payoff, it is important to have a good working relationship with the attorneys involved, maintain all paperwork to document what you are doing, and be in touch with all parties involved regularly. (See the "skunk test" below to help you determine if an attorney is someone you do or do not want to work with.) It is also wise to have a clear assignment of

> **PRACTITIONER POINTER**
>
> "It is wise to have a clear understanding with each patient that they are ultimately responsible for payment of all services rendered through your clinic."
>
> —Anonymous

> ## POWER POINT
>
> **"Skunk Test" for attorneys**
>
> 1. Will the attorney sign your lien *and* return it to you?
> 2. Will the attorney send you a copy of the settlement statement?
> 3. Will the attorney provide complete insurance information?
> 4. Will the attorney give you all information on the defendant?
> 5. Will the attorney provide you with all of the information about the plaintiff's medical payment from the automobile insurance?
> 6. Will the attorney give you the information about the claims adjuster? This should include the address and phone number as well as the claim number.
> 7. Will the attorney help you collect on the medical payment part of the auto insurance?
> 8. Who is the attorney's acupuncturist?
> 9. The attorney in PI cases often does the billing for all medical services to the insurance company(s) involved. This often means that the payments for these services are being sent to the office of the attorney. Does the attorney deduct a fee (can be up to 30%!) of the checks before sending on the payment to the practitioner?

benefits contract ● with the patient and with the law firm working on their behalf. Most PI billing requires regular accompanying chart notes and reports, so don't take on a lot of this type of patient if record-keeping is challenging for you.

▶ Finding out who pays what

To determine which insurance companies reimburse for acupuncture and related services, you must first find out the *state laws* about insurance coverage for acupuncture. In some states, there is no requirement for insurance companies to cover acupuncture at all, though in a few states it has now been designated as an essential health benefit under the terms of the Patient Protection and Affordable Care Act (PPACA) going into effect in 2014 (although how this will be interpreted by each state remains to be seen). Another provision of PPACA is "Non-discrimination in Health Care" language, which prohibits health plans from discriminating against providers whose services are within their state-defined scope of practice. In other words, plans can no longer require acupuncture services to be rendered only by an MD if acupuncture is a separate, licensed profession in your state. Contact your state government insurance authority to find out the position of your state with regard to coverage for acupuncture.

If your state allows or requires insurance reimbursement for acupuncture, one effective way to make local connections is to call the human resources department of major companies within 20 miles of your clinic. You want to know specifically what insurance carrier each company uses for its health care plans and whether employees have policy options that include acupuncture. If any plans do, ask about the extent and type of that coverage. For instance, is there a deductible on their policies, a limit to the number of visits per year, is coverage only for certain types of problems, and is there a co-pay? There is a form on the website with a list of questions you should ask.

When you have made all of these phone calls (and kept good notes!), go online to find the 800 number for each insurance company mentioned. It may require persistence to get a real customer service rep on the phone, but when you do there are several things you want to find out from them.

1. For a patient with such-and-such policy number or type is there coverage for acupuncture treatment?

2. Is there a deductible on this type of policy and how much is it? Is there a co-pay?
3. Is there a yearly maximum dollar amount for acupuncture benefits?
4. Do they honor an assignment of benefits from the insured?
5. May acupuncture treatments be administered by licensed acupuncturists (or only MDs or DCs)?
6. Do they only cover certain CPT (Current Procedural Terminology) or RSV codes?
7. Do they require reports and at what intervals?
8. Do they require a medical referral from an MD?
9. Are there any other forms or paperwork specific to their company that they need to send you?
10. Do they prefer that you bill electronically? (Yes, this is upon us now. Eventually *all* billing will be electronic. There is more on this subject in Section 2, Chapter 8)

It is also true with more companies all the time that you can view specific policies and coverages at insurance company websites, which may not answer all your questions, but can save time and hassle. Practitioners wanting to bill insurance for their patients need to be comfortable with online research.

POWER POINT

We have included a Phone Verification of Insurance Coverage form on the website for you to use when you call. You may also want to write down the phone number for provider services right on the patient's form. Once completed, this form should be kept in the patient's administrative file with all other financial records. FYI, if you keep paper records, consider two separate files for each patient: one includes all examination and treatment records, the other all financial, billing, insurance, HIPAA, and other administrative forms and records. Electronic records already have such internal file management.

Many companies reimburse for all services at a different rate for "in-network" and "out-of-network" providers. If this is the case, you may wish to apply to get on their panel, though you can choose to be reimbursed as an out-of-network provider. If you want to get on the panel, ask to be transferred to the provider services department, where you can find out if they are accepting applications from acupuncturists in your area or if the panel is closed at the present time. Request an application regardless of the panel status, fill it out and mail it back (or complete it online). You never know when their situation may change.

Being able to say "yes" when a prospective patient asks if you are in-network for their policy is excellent if you need to grow a private practice. Still, since not all insurance policies have panels (though more probably do than don't in these days of cost cutting), you can simply wait until a prospective patient asks if you accept their company's insurance before deciding about this. Tell the patient that insurance plans vary and if they give you their name, birthday, policy number, and company contact phone on their insurance card, you will happily contact the company to find out if coverage is available (do this as promptly as you can). Don't let a patient convince you that they "are sure they have acupuncture coverage." Always determine available benefits and policy rules yourself. More time-consuming, yes, but we all know how confusing conversations with insurance companies can be. Don't assume that a patient understands her policy and don't assume that a patient will be completely honest with you! After you've done a few of these phone calls, you will know red flags or potential problems when you hear them.

▶ Verifying benefits

When a new insurance patient first comes for treatment, make a copy of both sides of their insurance card for their file. All cards have an 800 number for providers (that's you) to obtain policy coverage information. Tell the customer service person at that

SECTION THREE: GETTING PAID

> **POWER POINT**
>
> **Forms that you will need to use if you are going to accept insurance patients**
>
> 1. Assignment of Benefits form
> 2. Power of Attorney to cash checks written-to-the-patient-but-sent-to-your-office form
> 3. Superbill forms
> 4. CMS-1500 forms (or bill online)
> 5. Claim forms provided by the patient
> 6. Insurance tracer letter/form
> 7. Insurance company basic information form
> 8. Patient Confidential Information form
> 9. Notice of Doctor's Lien for PI cases
>   See the website for samples of all these forms.
>
> As of 2007, you also need a National Provider Identifier (NPI#) to bill insurance. See Appendix A for how to apply.

number that you are calling to *verify benefits*. They will ask you a number of questions about the patient and type of benefits requested. You may also be asked to provide your social security or tax ID number, clinic name, and phone number. Write down all information you receive or use the form on this book's website. Once you have a confirmation or denial of coverage, you can provisionally add that policy from that company to your list of those that do or do not cover acupuncture.

▶ **Getting on a panel**

As discussed above, a panel is a group of practitioners certified by a management agency or broker to make it easier and cheaper for insurance companies' clients to use their services. The certifying agency ensures that the insurance company's clients will be receiving services from practitioners with appropriate training and credentialing, in accessible and professional clinics that afford patient privacy, and who carry a specified level of malpractice insurance.

Getting on a panel can be as easy as calling the company and asking if they are accepting applicants for their acupuncture panel in your city or area. The application and certification packet, as well as a contract you must sign, will likely be on the company website. There may or may not be an application fee. The application will cover everything you would expect it to and then some.

Read through all the instructions prior to filling it out, especially if it is on paper. A messy application will not inspire confidence in the certifying agent(s). Use black ink if the application is on paper and make a copy of the form beforehand so that you can start over if you flub the first one. If your handwriting skills are poor, ask for help from a friend or find an old typewriter (libraries often have one of these).

POWER POINT

As a new practitioner learning to work with insurance billing, tell the representative on the phone just that. They will usually help you. Insurance companies (or at least many of the people who work for them) want you to succeed and want you to communicate with them effectively. The more successful we are as practitioners, the more companies will agree to cover our good work. Before you call, always have a pen in hand and write down the name of the person to whom you are speaking, call the person by name (Miss Jones, Mr. Smith), thank them sincerely for their patience and help, and see if you can get their extension number. If you can make a friend at every insurance company you bill, there may be someone to help you if things don't go smoothly later on.

A mailed application may include a contract. It will tell you how much and for which services/codes you can bill. It will also contain information about required malpractice insurance, filing grievances, how disputes will be handled, and whether you may bill patients for any difference in the billed and paid amounts. *Make sure you read thoroughly and understand clearly the entire contract before you sign.*

Upon receiving your application and signed contract, the company will verify educational and licensing claims, call references, and verify your malpractice and general liability insurance if required. They may or may not send an inspector to your clinic to ensure patient privacy and safety, acupuncture practices, and disposal of medical waste. Some companies may send you a list of things for you to photograph and send to them. The completed application and results of their investigation and inspection will be forwarded to a jury of people who vote on your candidacy. Once accepted to a panel, you receive notice from the company, a list of acceptable billing codes and fees, and a copy of the contract that you signed which now has a counter-signature from a representative of the company.

There is no limit to the number of panels you may join. Once on a panel, your name and clinic information will be added to the list of practitioners from whom members of that insurance group may receive treatment. Be sure to ask the company representative how long it will take for your name to appear on the listing at their website and keep following up until your information has been added.

Some managed-care panels are controversial within the profession because of low reimbursement rates and a tendency to slow payment and difficult communication. I suggest you contact colleagues in your in your state association about their experiences with the panels you are considering joining.

CHAPTER 3 | The Ins and Outs of Billing Insurance

▶ Know the insurance codes

There are two sets of codes to become familiar with in order to bill insurance companies and *get paid.*

ICD-9 or 10 (International Classification of Diseases, 9th or 10th edition) codes tell the company what condition you were treating. There are books available that list these codes in lengthy detail. The codes are important to you because, without both a thorough exam and history and a specific diagnosis for each patient who wants to use their insurance to reimburse for your services, you cannot establish *medical necessity.* Without adequate proof of medical necessity, an insurance adjuster is likely to deny coverage for your services.

Current Procedural Terminology (CPT) codes are five digit numbers used to bill for the procedures you administer. These procedures include, but are not limited to, intake and examination, follow-up evaluation, acupuncture and electro-acupuncture, moxibustion, cupping, and tuina or other bodywork and manipulation (if allowed in your state). Listed below are common CPT codes, their associated procedure, and when you can use them. Remember that the types of codes accepted can vary by company, so make sure to ask.

▶ New Patient Evaluation and Management [E&M] codes

These codes are only used for the first time you see a patient or if you are seeing a patient whom you have not seen for three years or more. In California and some other states' workers' compensation laws, you may use these codes for any *new* injury even if you have seen the patient within three years prior.

A new patient exam code is billed separately from any treatment you give and is followed by the number of minutes spent face-to-face with the patient or patient's family and the severity of the chief complaint.

99201 – 10 minutes; presenting problems are minor
99202 – 20 minutes; presenting problems are low to moderate
99203 – 30 minutes; presenting problems are moderate
99204 – 40-50 minutes; presenting problems are moderate to high severity
99205 – 50-60 minutes; presenting problems are high severity
97041 – Colorado and some other states' WorkComp New Patient E&M code (no matter the number of minutes)

All the above codes have three requirements for use:

1. You must take a medical history, the scope and comprehensiveness of which increases from: a focused history regarding the problem (99201), an expanded history regarding the problem (99202), a detailed patient history (99203), or a comprehensive patient history (99204-99205)

2. You must perform an examination, the scope and comprehensiveness increasing from: focused on the problem (99201), an expanded examination regarding the problem (99202), a detailed patient examination (99203), or a comprehensive patient examination (99204-99205)

3. You must make a medical decision of increasing complexity from: straightforward (99201-99202), low-complexity (99203), moderate complexity (99204), and high complexity (99205) *The last two codes will require an accompanying report proving necessity in most cases and should be used rarely.*

At the time of this writing, it is not clear if insurance companies will pay for E&M codes billed by acupuncturists. There have been reports that some companies have stopped paying for these codes if not billed by an MD office. Other practitioners say no, they get these codes reimbursed regularly. It may be worth a try to bill them, unless you are on a panel and are specifically told you cannot bill for them.

Established Patient Re-evaluation and Management codes

These are used for a follow-up examination, a re-evaluation, and for established patients who present with a new condition. In order to bill one of these codes, you must again take a history of the problem, perform another exam, and make a medical decision. As stated above, these codes are separate from any acupuncture or other service you provide. The codes below are followed by the number of minutes spent face-to-face with the patient or patient's family and the severity of the chief complaint.

99211 – 05 mins; presenting problems minimal
99212 – 10 mins; presenting problems minor
99213 – 15 mins; presenting problems low to moderate

> **POWER POINT**
>
> **Using Evaluation & Management Codes (E&M)**
>
> These codes are used instead of office visit codes. E&M codes include various components and the provider is paid one fee for all of these parts:
> 1. Medical history
> 2. Physical examination
> 3. Medical decision making (MDM includes diagnosis and creation of a treatment plan)
> 4. Counseling of the patient
> 5. Level of severity of the problem
> 6. Coordination of benefits (time for phone calls, report writing, etc.)
> 7. Time. This is the most important for acupuncture practitioners because we spend more time with a patient than most other types of medical providers.
>
> Find out what each insurance company will pay for specific codes. Contact the benefits department of any insurance company directly to get this information.

99214 – 25 mins; presenting problems moderate/high severity

99215 – 40 minutes; presenting problems moderate to high severity

97044 – Colorado and some states' WorkComp re-evaluation code (flat fee no matter how many minutes are spent).

Similarly to the two initial examination codes 99204 and 99205, the last two re-evaluation codes, 99214 and 99215, should be used rarely as they are likely to receive extra scrutiny and require extra paperwork to establish necessity.

▶ Acupuncture-specific CPT codes

These codes are used to bill for acupuncture services. Below we explain the use of these codes as well as we can, as it can be a little bit confusing. Here goes:

97810 – This is the basic acupuncture treatment code. It is a time-based code used to bill for the initial application of one or more needles and active one-on-one patient contact for 15 minutes. That means the time spent palpating and preparing points for treatment, positioning the patient, washing your hands, disinfecting points, inserting and manipulating needles, checking on the patient in the middle of the treatment, and taking needles out. It can include up to three minutes of what is called "pre-service" or "post-service" activities such as charting time. Neither this nor any other 15-minute increment includes time that patient spends lying on the table quietly.

97811 – This code is for a second (or third) increment of time (a minimum of 7.5 minutes up to 15 minutes) working one-on-one with patients, usually relating to insertion of a second group of needles, but not the same needles used for 97810. The first set of needles should be disposed of according to this billing model. This code is used for each subsequent application of needles (without electric stimulation) regardless of whether you reposition the patient. This code is used only when 97810 was used for the first 15-minute increment. You bill this in 15-minute increments of time or any portion thereof.

97813 – This is the primary electro-acupuncture code. It is used the same way as 97810 except that there was the application of electro-stimulation on one or more needles. This code should **not** be used with 97810 or 97811. For a second time-increment of electro-acupuncture, bill using the following code.

97814 – This is the second increment code for electro-acupuncture. To use this code, you must have first used 97813. Time requirements for this code are the same as 97811. Please also note that, in some cases, electro-acupuncture is reimbursed at a slightly higher rate than regular acupuncture, perhaps $1-$2 per increment.

97782 – Cupping. This code may not be billed concomitantly with either acupuncture code with some insurance companies. This code is not accepted for WorkComp billing in every state, or with every insurance company.

97802 – California WorkComp code for cupping. (We suggest that you take a state or insurance-company-sponsored course in how to bill WorkComp accurately for best reimbursement. See Chapter 5 in this section for more details.)

97783 – Moxibustion; may not be billed concomitantly with either acupuncture code with some insurance companies and is not accepted for WorkComp billing in many states.

97803 – California WorkComp code for moxibustion

97124 – Massage/tuina; billed in 15-minute increments. Time blocks are billed after 7.5 minutes up to 15 minutes. For example, 15 minutes of tuina is billed as one unit of 97124, while 22.5 to 30 minutes of tuina is billed as two units of 97124. This code is listed once on the CMS-1500 and then modified in the unit block for each 15-minute period. (Use the same code for each 15-minute increment. Some companies will not reimburse when billed with acupuncture codes.)

97250 – Myofascial release

97140 – WorkComp code for manual therapies in some states; *i.e.*, trigger point therapy. This code may not be reimbursed by some companies as it is considered to be a part of acupuncture.

If you provide services through managed-care or PPO plans where you are a paneled member, your level of reimbursement for any and all of these codes will be specified in advance. If a service you wish to bill for is not listed, call and find out from the provider services department any limitations or specifics about which codes will be reimbursed at what level and which ones may be used on the same billing form.

➤ Treatment procedure for the best billing outcome

So how do you put this together for good care of fee-for-service insurance patients and fair reimbursement for your time? Here's one suggestion.

When you see a new patient, you can bill one of the new patient EM codes (such as 99202 or 99203). After quickly writing up a preliminary treatment plan, start with the patient face up on the treatment table (gowned for treatment if needed). Use a first group of needles such as Liv 3-LI 4, perhaps adding one other point related to the patient's major complaint or main pattern discrimination, or a point to help the patient relax such as Yin Tang, as appropriate. This set of needles will be billed as 97810. Now allow the patient to rest while you complete your chart notes and consider options for the next part of the treatment.

After 7-10 minutes, remove the initial set of needles. A second set of needles, either on the front or back will be even more specific. After the second set (code 97811) of needles are inserted, the patient may rest again as appropriate. Depending on the time available and specific needs of the patient, you may add a third session of needles or do moxa, tuina, cupping, therapeutic exercise, or whatever is indicated. You will then bill for one 97810, at least one 97811 code, and any other codes based on the specific treatment. Remember, each 97811 code requires at least 7.5 minutes of hands-on time in addition to the 15 minutes of hands-on time for 97810. Hands-on time for any billed session may include the time you require for point location, sterilization, or other necessary point preparation as described above, but not resting quietly on the table.

This is one system or idea for making the system work for you and for the insurance company while giving your insurance patients the best possible care for their money. The key is to bill only one unit of 97810 or 97813, and then add units of 97811 or 97814 or other codes based on your actual treatment.

Be sure to document everything. Be clear about initial insertion and re-insertion sets of points. You might note them as Ac1, Ac2, etc. Accurate chart notes are required by law and can be reviewed by the insurance company at any time, so bill only for things you actually do, neither more nor less.

▶ International Classification of Disease (ICD-9) codes

Diagnosis codes that are universally accepted by the insurance industry are called ICD-9 (or ICD-10) codes. These consist of a three-digit number followed by a decimal, possibly followed by one or two more digits called modifiers. These numbers are written in block 21 on lines 1-4 of the CMS-1500 form in order of severity. Diagnosis codes are chosen based on the patient's chief complaint(s), but be careful what codes you choose as many insurance companies restrict the selection of diagnoses acceptable for acupuncture treatment. Some companies will tell you what types of disorders are covered under the patient's plan when you call to verify eligibility. Others will not, so it is best to be conservative when choosing them. For example, it is likely to be easier to get paid for treating shoulder pain than to get paid for fibromyalgia.

On the following pages you will see some of the more common ICD codes in use for acupuncture. We recommend you purchase a book of codes, available at most bookstores or online. If you purchase acupuncture patient management software, such as Client Tracker or AcuBase, there are some pre-loaded codes. Ask these companies when they last checked for code changes, since these codes are updated occasionally.

▶ Tips for getting your codes reimbursed

Insurance companies often reimburse for acupuncture only for specific ICD codes. When calling to verify benefits, ask if the diagnosis in your case is covered. They may be willing to tell you, especially if you have made a friend at the company. When unsure, use a symptomatic ICD code that is a part of the overall diagnosis and more likely to be accepted, such as pain in a specific area of the body. For example, if a patient presents with an MD diagnosis of **847.2** (Lumbar strain/sprain), this may not be covered for acupuncture treat-ment. However, a patient with lumbar strain/sprain is obviously suffering from **724.2** (Back Pain, Low), a more generic pain code that is likely to be on the list of acceptable codes. If you bill for a code not on their list, it will be sent back with a statement of non-coverage. So if you cannot get specific information about acceptable billing codes from the insurance company you are billing, use the most generic codes possible when you fill out your billing form for that patient.

▶ Filling out the CMS-1500

Insurance companies will pay for our services as long as we play the game by

> **PRACTITIONER POINTER**
>
> "I decided to really learn how to bill insurance effectively. I've worked with American Specialty Health, Kaiser Perma-nente, all the major companies. My billings get paid more than 90% of the time. One key is to always verify benefits in advance of treatment. Patients who have insur-ance want to use it. I help them to do so if I can."   —*Lori Gritz San Diego, CA*
> *www.gritzacupuncture.com*

POWER POINT

Sample of frequently used ICD-9 codes

Headaches:
- 784.0   Headache
- 951.9   Cranial nerve(s) injury
- 307.81   Tension headache
- 625.4   Premenstrual headache
- 627.2   Menopausal headache
- 346.1   Migraine, common
- 346.2   Migraine, variants of
- 346.8   Migraine, other forms of
- 346.9   Migraine, unspecified

Musculoskeletal pain:
- 789.0   Abdominal pain
- 781.2   Abnormality of gait
- 756.10   Abnormalities of m.s. system, unspecified
- 724.6   Arthritis, gouty
- 714.30   Arthritis, rheumatoid, juvenile
- 733.22   Bone cyst
- 848.42   Chrondosternal sprain or strain
- 737.4   Curvature of spine, unspecified
- 737.41   Curvature of spine, kyphosis
- 737.42   Curvature of spine, lordosis
- 737.43   Curvature of spine, scoliosis
- 719.7   Difficulty walking
- 839.61   Dislocation of sternum
- 737.1   Kyphosis, acquired, postural
- 905.6   Late effect of dislocation
- 907.9   Late effect of injury, unspecified nerve
- 905.7   Late effect of sprain/strain
- 905.8   Late effect of tendon injury
- 908.9   Late effect of unspecified injury
- 737.2   Lordosis, postural
- 354.8   Neuralgia, intercostal
- 729.2   Neuritis, neuralgia, radiculitis, unspecified

"Power Point" continues on the next page

SECTION THREE: GETTING PAID

715.9	Osteoarthritis, unspecified
712.0	Osteoarthritis of spine
268.2	Osteomalacia
306.0	Osteomyelitis, unspecified
733.02	Osteoporosis, idiopathic
733.01	Osteoporosis, senile
733.00	Osteoporosis, unspecified, wedging of vertebra
733.99	Other bone disorder
782.0	Paresthesia
720.0	Rheumatoid arthritis
848.3	Sprain/strain, rib
845.1	Sprain/strain, ankle, unspecified
719.59	Stiffness in joint, multiple sites

Please note that ICD-9/10 codes can change. You may need to replace your ICD-9/10 book every few years to stay up to date. You may also want to get a copy of the *AccuCodes Book* from the H.J. Ross & Co. by calling 1-800-562-3335. This book is easy to use, well organized, and covers all the major pain codes that acupuncturists commonly use.

their rules, one of which is to understand how to properly fill out their standard form, the CMS-1500. CMS stands for Center for Medicare/Medicaid Services. See the example on page 299 or print out the filled-in CMS from our website. Now let's go through the form block by block. (It's really not difficult after you have done it a few times!)

Starting at the very top of the CMS, there is a large margin with "PLEASE DO NOT STAPLE IN THIS AREA" in large letters in the left-hand corner. This space is for the name and address of the insurance company. This information should be placed directly above and to the left of

P O W E R   P O I N T

Using Modifier-25 for E&M Codes

If you perform acupuncture on the same day as you do an evaluation and will be billing an E&M code as well as one or more treatment CPT codes on the same form, always use Modifier-25 on your E&M codes or you will not be reimbursed. For example, 99202 becomes 99202-25.

the boldface words on the form "HEALTH INSURANCE CLAIM FORM" which is written towards the upper-right corner.

The numbers below correspond to the numbered items that must be filled out on the CMS form.

1. Make an "x" in the appropriate box related to the type of insurance policy you are billing. For patients with insurance through their employer, the Group Health Plan box is appropriate. For Workers' Comp or PI cases, use the box that says "other." For private health plans that are not purchased through an employer, you may also use the Group Health Plan box. Champus is a type of U.S. military coverage but is mostly not applicable to acupuncturists.

1a. Insert the insured's identification number. It is on their insurance card. It may or may not be their Social Security number. Some insurance companies assign their own number.

2. Insert patient's last name (ALL CAPS), first name, middle initial.

3. Insert the patient's date of birth using eight digits. (You must use four digits for the year.) Check box male or female.

4. Insert the insured's last name, first name. (This is not always the patient's name.)

5. Insert the patient's street address.

6. Insert the patient's relationship to the insured.

7. Insert the insured's address.

8. Insert patient's marital and employment or student status.

9. Leave blank.

10. Insert appropriate type of case (*e.g.,* Workers' Comp, PI.)

11. Insert insured's group number if there is one on their insurance card, date of birth, and sex (a), and employer (b). Don't worry about (c). For (d) check "no".

12. Insert "Signature on file" and date. (You must actually have a form on file signed by the patient, at least on the patient confidential information form in order to fill in #12 this way.)

13. Insert "Signature on file." (Same as #12 in parenthesis.)

14. Insert date of current illness or injury or the first day you saw the patient.

15. Leave blank.
16. Complete only if you took the patient off work.
17. Complete only if referred by an MD and the insurance only covers services referred by an MD.
17a. Leave blank.
17b. The referring physician's NPI number goes here.
18-20. Leave blank.
21. Insert appropriate ICD-9 diagnosis code, using up to four of these. If there is more than one, put them in order of severity, the most severe first. You may also list the codes in order of the level of specificity, the most specific diagnosis first. For instance, 737.4 is the code for general curvature of the spine, whereas 737.43 is the code for scoliosis specifically. List 737.43 first since both are applicable.
22. Only complete for Medicaid.
23. Only complete for MediCal in California.
24a. Insert date of service.
24b. Insert place of service. The number 11 means at an office. The number 12 means at the patient's home.
24c. Leave blank.
24d. Insert appropriate CPT code.
24e. Insert "1-2" if you used two diagnostic codes, 1-3 if three, etc.
24f. Insert fee for specific service.
24g-i. Leave blank.
24j. Your National Provider Identifier (NPI) number must go here and must go on each line where a CPT code is listed.
25. Insert your tax ID or Social Security number.
26. Insert patient's account number.
27. Mark "Yes," if you have sent an assignment of benefits and the checks are to be sent directly to you.
28. Insert total charges for the claim.
29. Always "zero."
30. Insert total charges for the claim.

CHAPTER 3 | The Ins and Outs of Billing Insurance

1500
HEALTH INSURANCE CLAIM FORM
APPROVED BY NATIONAL UNIFORM CLAIM COMMITTEE 08/05

Name and Address of the Insurance Company goes here.

1. MEDICARE / MEDICAID / TRICARE CHAMPUS / CHAMPVA / GROUP HEALTH PLAN / FECA BLK LUNG / OTHER	1a. INSURED'S I.D. NUMBER (For Program in Item 1)
	123-45-6789

2. PATIENT'S NAME (Last Name, First Name, Middle Initial): **DOE, JOHN A.**
3. PATIENT'S BIRTH DATE: **11 15 81** SEX: **M** ☒
4. INSURED'S NAME (Last Name, First Name, Middle Initial): **DOE, SALLY M.**

5. PATIENT'S ADDRESS (No., Street): **1234 Main Street**
6. PATIENT RELATIONSHIP TO INSURED: Child ☒
7. INSURED'S ADDRESS (No., Street): **1234 Main Street**

CITY: **Anywhere** STATE: **NY**
8. PATIENT STATUS: Married ☒
CITY: **Anywhere** STATE: **NY**

ZIP CODE: **11234** TELEPHONE: **(315) 222-3344**
Employed ☒ Full-Time Student
ZIP CODE: **11234** TELEPHONE: **(315) 222-3344**

9. OTHER INSURED'S NAME (Last Name, First Name, Middle Initial):
10. IS PATIENT'S CONDITION RELATED TO:
11. INSURED'S POLICY GROUP OR FECA NUMBER: **H8374521X**

a. OTHER INSURED'S POLICY OR GROUP NUMBER:
a. EMPLOYMENT? (Current or Previous) ☐ YES ☒ NO
a. INSURED'S DATE OF BIRTH: **05 10 82** SEX: **F** ☒

b. OTHER INSURED'S DATE OF BIRTH:
b. AUTO ACCIDENT? ☐ YES ☒ NO PLACE (State)
b. EMPLOYER'S NAME OR SCHOOL NAME: **Anywhere Printing Co.**

c. EMPLOYER'S NAME OR SCHOOL NAME:
c. OTHER ACCIDENT? ☒ YES ☐ NO
c. INSURANCE PLAN NAME OR PROGRAM NAME

d. INSURANCE PLAN NAME OR PROGRAM NAME
10d. RESERVED FOR LOCAL USE
d. IS THERE ANOTHER HEALTH BENEFIT PLAN? ☐ YES ☒ NO

READ BACK OF FORM BEFORE COMPLETING & SIGNING THIS FORM.
12. PATIENT'S OR AUTHORIZED PERSON'S SIGNATURE
SIGNED **SIGNATURE ON FILE** DATE **9/1/2014**
13. INSURED'S OR AUTHORIZED PERSON'S SIGNATURE
SIGNED **SIGNATURE ON FILE**

14. DATE OF CURRENT ILLNESS/INJURY/PREGNANCY: **09 01 2014**
15. IF PATIENT HAS HAD SAME OR SIMILAR ILLNESS, GIVE FIRST DATE
16. DATES PATIENT UNABLE TO WORK IN CURRENT OCCUPATION

17. NAME OF REFERRING PROVIDER OR OTHER SOURCE: **DR. MARK SMITH**
17b. NPI: **Dr. Smith's NPI #**
18. HOSPITALIZATION DATES RELATED TO CURRENT SERVICES

19. RESERVED FOR LOCAL USE
20. OUTSIDE LAB? ☐ YES ☐ NO $ CHARGES

21. DIAGNOSIS OR NATURE OF ILLNESS OR INJURY:
1. **848.3** 3. **719.5**
2. **354.9** 4.
22. MEDICAID RESUBMISSION CODE / ORIGINAL REF. NO.
23. PRIOR AUTHORIZATION NUMBER

24.	A. DATE(S) OF SERVICE From / To	B. PLACE OF SERVICE	C. EMG	D. PROCEDURES, SERVICES, OR SUPPLIES CPT/HCPCS / MODIFIER	E. DIAGNOSIS POINTER	F. $ CHARGES	G. DAYS OR UNITS	H. EPSDT Family Plan	I. ID QUAL	J. RENDERING PROVIDER ID. #
1	09 05 14 / 09 05 14	11		99202 / +25	1-3	75 00			NPI	Your NPI # GOES HERE
2	09 05 14 / 09 05 14	11		97810	1-3	55 00			NPI	NPI #
3	09 05 14 / 09 05 14	11		97811	1-3	45 00			NPI	NPI #
4	09 05 14 / 09 05 14	11		97124	1-3	25 00			NPI	NPI #
5									NPI	
6									NPI	

25. FEDERAL TAX I.D. NUMBER: **84-1234567** SSN ☐ EIN ☒
26. PATIENT'S ACCOUNT NO.
27. ACCEPT ASSIGNMENT? ☒ YES ☐ NO
28. TOTAL CHARGE: **$ 200 —**
29. AMOUNT PAID: **$ 0**
30. BALANCE DUE: **$ 200 —**

31. SIGNATURE OF PHYSICIAN OR SUPPLIER INCLUDING DEGREES OR CREDENTIALS
Sally Jones L.Ac.
32. SERVICE FACILITY LOCATION INFORMATION
ABC Acupuncture Clinic
1231 Broadway #2
Anywhere, NY 11235
33. BILLING PROVIDER INFO & PH # **(315) 211-1222**
SALLY JONES, L.Ac.
1231 Broadway #2
Anywhere, NY 11235

↑ YOUR NPI # GOES HERE ↑

OMB APPROVAL PENDING
NUCC Instruction Manual available at: www.nucc.org

If you want to get some of this paperwork off your plate, consider hiring Office Ally (www.officeally.com) to do your billing electronically.

31. Insert signature of practitioner and date.

32. List the address where the services were performed.

32a. Insert your clinic NPI number here. If your clinic NPI is the same as your personal one, list your personal one.

33. If billing from the same location as your clinic, list your name and phone# with the same address as in 32. This is where the check will be sent and how it will be made out.

33a. List your personal NPI number here again.

The original goes to the insurance company; keep a copy for your records. If you bill electronically, you still have to fill out the online version of the form, but our advice is to use OfficeAlly for this. They even screen your codes and other entries, improving chances for reimbursement.

▶ What to do when you don't receive timely payment

If you have created any friends at the company, contact them first and see if they can help you find out what happened to your bill. If you have no "insider" to contact directly, send the company a copy of the CMS form with an *insurance tracer letter*. Insurance companies are required to respond to tracer letters in writing with an explanation within 10 days of receipt. What may happen when you send an insurance tracer is that, instead of a letter of response from them, you will simply get the payment.

▶ Final thoughts

This chapter is only an introduction and by no means the final word! Also, this information may change at any time for many reasons. Serious insurance billers who really learn how to do this can make money and make it work! However, save yourself a lot of aggravation and take a good course or two, and purchase a book such as Sperber and Andersen-Hefner's *Playing the Game: Accepting Insurance as an Acupuncturist*. The more educated you are and updated you stay, the more likely you are to be successful, which is good for you and for your insurance patients.

POINTS TO PONDER FROM CHAPTER 3

1. If you're willing to do the paperwork to play the insurance game successfully, you can increase your income significantly by taking insurance reimbursement.

2. There are several types of insurance you could agree to accept. These include basic fee-for-service private or group plan insurance, personal injury, Workers' Compensation (see Chapter 5 in this section), managed care, or Medicaid.

3. Before agreeing to take an insurance patient, you must find out if their policy covers acupuncture, under what circumstances, for up to how many treatments, with what type of required reports, and with or without a co-pay.

4. It is usually easy to get on managed care insurance panels by calling for a copy of their application, but find out how much they reimburse and for which codes before you decide if you can afford this use of your time.

5. You must know how to use CPT codes and ICD-9/10 codes in order to prove medical necessity and get reimbursed for care.

6. Workers' Compensation CPT codes may be different from other insurance codes.

7. All insurance companies require the use of the CMS-1500 form. Instructions for filling out a CMS-1500 are listed in detail above.

8. If you don't get paid in a timely manner, file an insurance tracer letter; they must respond to you in writing within 10 days.

9. See Appendix A on applying for your National Provider Identification number.

Personal Injury Patients: Yes or No? | 4

Approximately 2.25 million people in the U.S. are injured in traffic accidents each year. These people are all potential personal injury (PI) cases that could end up in your clinic. Other incidents that may become PI cases include bicycle or sport event accidents or a fall in a commercial establishment or the parking lots adjacent to them.

Every state in the U.S. requires people to have their vehicles covered by insurance, and almost all of these policies have a provision for medical care. While whiplash of the neck and head is the most common injury in auto accidents, any body part may be affected. Headaches are the most common symptom and these may not even show up until several weeks after the actual accident.

If you are interested in PI cases, there are many things you need to know and questions to ask in each case. First, you should find out if your state auto insurance system is *no fault* or *tort liability* by law. In a no fault system, the injured person's insurance will usually be responsible for all medical treatment related to any vehicular accident. This situation is usually easier, since any litigation over who caused the accident will likely not affect reimbursement for medical care. If your state has a tort liability system, medical treatment coverage responsibility will depend upon which party was at fault.

If the injured person was at fault, usually they must use their regular health insurance or pay out-of-pocket. If the injured person was not at fault, they may be covered by the insurance of the at-fault party or under their own auto insurance in the bodily injury coverage and/or the uninsured motorist coverage. If their policy does not include this coverage, they may, again, be forced to use their regular health insurance. In such cases, the health insurance company may sue the at-fault person or that person's auto insurance company. This is called *subrogation*. If who was at fault is unclear, complex litigation or mediation between the insurance companies can take many months. Whether medical bills will be paid in advance of the completion of these legal proceedings is something you must find out for each specific case.

One place to start doing research is with your own auto insurance carrier. Your personal insurance agent will, at the very least, be able to explain the fault/no fault situation in your state. You may also be able to find out a great deal about how they handle PI cases, the extent of uninsured motorist coverage for injuries on your own policy and their most standard policies, and whether acupuncture care is a reimbursable service. If covered, under what circumstances? For example, does the patient need an MD prescription for acupuncture care, what types of progress reports are required, and how are funds disbursed? If you have a good relationship with your insurance agent, you may be able to get all sorts of information about the best way for you to be successful in caring for PI patients, or if you want to do it at all.

If you make the decision to treat auto (and other) accident injury patients, there will be more paperwork, and your chart notes must be written in detail. All this paperwork will be part of a medical-legal file in most cases. There must be comparative exams to document progress throughout the course of treatment, the possibility of the need for future medical treatment related to the injury, and the possibility of residual problems in spite of whatever treatment is given.

In states where we are not considered primary care providers (most of them), your patient may also need a referral or prescription for acupuncture from an MD. In such cases, you may have to prove medical necessity for more than a specified number of treatments with reports that show specific progress such as increases in range of motion or mobility, lower levels of pain, improved functioning of specific bodily systems, etc.

When any new patient calls your office to make an appointment, it is important to determine if they are seeking care because of injuries from a car or other type of accident. If it is not discussed in your initial phone conversation, then your patient confidential information form should have specific questions that reveal if any type of accident has played a part in their major complaint and if they expect their own (or any other person's) auto insurance to cover their treatment fees. If so, you will need to contact the insurance company(ies) involved to find out:
- if your services can and will be reimbursed and in what amount of time,
- if there are specific paperwork or reporting requirements,
- if you will be reimbursed for the time required to create these reports, and
- if there are any limitations on your regular fees or procedures for care.

If you need to contact the patient's or the at-fault party's legal counsel, you need to find that out as well, along with the lawyers' contact information before you begin treament with this patient.

Upon determining that a patient is a PI case and what the expected payment method and time frame is, there are other special forms that need to be completed by the patient with regard to the accident and the injuries sustained. Additional paperwork (See Insurance-Related Letters & Forms on the Website.) necessary for payment may include the following:

- **Auto Accident Information Form**
  This form provides information about the patient, attorney, insurance coverage, and basic information about the accident.

- **Phone Verification for Acupuncture Benefits**
  This form (discussed in the previous chapter) is used with all types of insurance patients. It is used to gather needed information regarding a patient's policy and benefits, in this case from their auto insurance company. Any other expected health insurance benefits also should be verified.

- **Assignment of Benefits to you or your clinic**
  This form is completed and signed by the patient and then is sent to an insurance company and any lawyers involved in the case to guarantee that the check will be sent to the provider (you) and not the patient.

- **Rescission of Attorney Assignment of Benefits**
  Some attorneys want to do the billing for all their client's medical services through their office. In such cases, the insurance company payments are sent directly to the attorney's office. Some attorneys then take a cut of up to 30% (!?!) of the reimbursement for medical services, sending the remainder to the healthcare provider. This is both illegal and unfair. If it happens to you, send a Rescission of Attorney Assignment of Benefits to the insurance carrier.

- **Power of Attorney** (limited to endorsement of checks)
  The patient signs this form so that if a check comes to your office made out to the patient, you can endorse and deposit it into your checking account.

SECTION THREE: GETTING PAID

- **Medical Lien** (agreement between medical provider and attorney). In a PI case, both the attorney and the practitioner have paperwork completed and signed by the patient. The medical lien is a legal agreement between the acupuncturist and the attorney that allows your office to get paid.

- **Copy of Accident Report** (this usually is obtained by the patient from the local law enforcement authorities)

- **Personal Injury Questionnaire**
  This form can replace the auto accident information form listed above. Completed by the patient, it provides demographic information about the patient, the attorney, insurance coverage, and other information about the accident.

Most of this paperwork is completed by the patient. The forms need to be in your files even if you don't use all of them right away. With any luck, you will never have to use some of them at all.

A key factor in most PI cases is the attorney or attorneys involved. They can either make your involvement easy or very difficult. Listed below are questions that should be asked and answered if there is legal representation and especially if you will be dependent upon their office in order to be paid.

- Who is the attorney?
- What is the address and telephone number?
- Who is the paralegal if there is one involved?
- Who is the secretary in the attorney's office that you will usually deal with?
- Will the lawyer sign the lien if there is one?
- Will the lawyer return said lien to your office promptly?
- Will the lawyer send you a copy of the settlement statement?
- Will the lawyer provide complete insurance information?
- Will the lawyer give you all information on the defendant?

- Will the lawyer provide you with all information about the plaintiff's medical payments from the auto insurance?
- Will the lawyer give you information about the claims adjuster? This should include the address and telephone number as well as the claim number.
- Will the lawyer help you collect on the medical payment part of the automobile insurance?
- Who is the lawyer's acupuncturist if he or she has one?
- Does the lawyer's office ask you to send all bills for your services to their office as intermediary to the insurance company? (This means that the lawyer's office will bill and collect payment from the insurance company for your services.) The practice of a lawyer's office taking a percentage of the check before paying the medical provider is illegal in most states.

If the answer is "no" to any or all of the above questions or "yes" to the very last one, there is the possibility that you may not get paid, that the attorney may ask you to cut your bill, or that the money will only be paid in the distant future. What you want and need in these cases is a PI attorney who will help both your patient to get the care they need and you to get the payment you deserve. If you have any suspicions about the lawyer, do some digging to check out their reputation (Yelp, Angie's List, Craigslist, Facebook, LinkedIn) and make sure the patient knows about your concerns. And remember, if this all seems like too much work and too many potential pitfalls, you do not have to accept the patient for care.

As stated in the beginning of this chapter, during the process of a PI lawsuit, an insurance company may ask for an independent medical examination of the injured patient. This is a normal request in a lawsuit, or under the policy conditions of the patient's insurance. As a care giver, it is professional to apprise the patient of their rights, which should include the following:

- You, the acupuncture patient, have the right not to be verbally abused.

- You, the acupuncture patient, have the right not to have to wait an unreasonable time for the scheduled examination.

- You, the acupuncture patient, should not be submitted to disrespect regarding your choice of medical providers for your injuries.

The insurance company's doctor may ask questions concerning the injuries your patient received as a result of the accident, for example, how your patient sustained the injuries. The insurance company's doctor may *not* ask about the following:

- Questions about the patient's personal life.
- Questions about how the accident took place.
- Questions about the patient's medical condition before the accident.
- Require the patient to take an X-ray examination.
- Questions about the patient's lawsuit.
- Questions about other medical problems the patient may have but are not connected with this lawsuit.

In other words, your patient may be examined but not cross-examined. You may print out this "Bill of Rights" on your clinic letterhead and give it to the patient to take with them when meeting with the insurance company doctor and keep it for their personal reference.

Occasionally a PI lawsuit will go to trial. If you have been treating a patient whose case does go to trial, you may be asked to testify or, more likely, to give a deposition. You may be reimbursed for your time in either case, but the amounts paid will differ. Regardless of whether you have been designated as an expert witness or are giving a deposition as a treating medical provider, you need to know in advance if you will be testifying about some or all of the following issues:

- History and examination of the patient
- Subjective complaints versus the objective findings
- Diagnosis and treatment plan
- Mechanics of the accident and the biomechanical issues
- Whether your treatment was necessary
- Whether your treatment was reasonable
- Opinions made by other doctors
- The possibility of long-term disability
- Prognosis and the cost of future care
- Whether your billing was reasonable and in line with the community

▶ How to dress for a court appearance

Dress and groom yourself in the same professional manner as anyone going to a trial. Anything less than professional attire can give the jury a sense that you and your profession are not credible or reliable. Avoid gaudy jewelry and flashy colors. A business suit, conservative dark shoes, and tie are mandatory for men. Women practitioners should wear a business suit or a conservative dress (not sleeveless, no plunging necklines, no miniskirts), plain stockings (unless you are wearing slacks), and conservative shoes (not sandals). Keep any tatoos covered. Remember, the judge and jury will probably see you only once, and a first impression will be the only impression. Dress appropriately and conduct yourself as a medical professional.

If asked to testify in the court proceedings or in a deposition, below is a list of potential questions:

1. Could you please state your name?
2. What is the address at which you practice acupuncture?
3. You are a doctor of what specialty?

SECTION THREE: GETTING PAID

4. What professional schools have you graduated from?
5. What colleges did you attend prior to your professional acupuncture-Oriental medicine school?
6. When did you first enroll in undergraduate college?
7. What courses did you take at undergraduate schools?
8. How many years were you in attendance at your undergraduate school?
9. What year did you enroll in your specialty college?
10. What year did you graduate?
11. How many years of acupuncture-Oriental medicine college or how many semesters of acupuncture-Oriental medicine college were required to be completed before you graduate?
12. Did you attend acupuncture-Oriental medicine college for three or more years?
13. What degree did you receive upon graduation?
14. Can you tell us, please, some of the courses that you study in a professional acupuncture-Oriental medicine college?
15. Are the books used in acupuncture-Oriental medicine school accepted in other medical or health healing professions?
16. Do acupuncturists have an internship?
17. Are you licensed to practice in this state?
18. What type of license is that?
19. When were you first licensed in this state?
20. Have you been involved in the acupuncture profession as a practicing health care provider since the inception of your license?
21. Are you required to take relicensure classes or do you take postgraduate classes each year?
22. How many cases have you treated involving the spinal column?
23. Approximately how many cervical or neck problems or conditions did you treat in the past year?

24. How many years have you been practicing?
25. During the period of time that you have been in practice from your start until now, approximately how many patients have you treated?
26. What percentage of those patients would you say have cervical or neck injuries?
27. Do you have hospital privileges?
28. So, if you do have a patient that requires surgery, are you able to refer or recommend them for surgery?
29. Have you written or published any articles within the acupuncture-Oriental medicine profession?
30. Has this patient reached the maximum improvement under your care?
31. Have you done all that you can do for this patient?
32. Do you feel that treatment will need to continue or extend beyond this courtroom proceeding?

As a treating medical professional in a PI matter, you may be required to write a *medical-legal report,* especially if there is a court case or insurance mediation. The following is an outline for such a report:

- Written on personal-office letterhead stationary
- For the office of: (name and address of the attorney involved)
- Identifying demographic information:
    Patient's name
    Date of the accident-injury
    Employer
    Insurance company
    Social Security number
- Inside greeting
- History of the accident: how did the accident occur and the mechanics of the injury
- Occupational history, job description: what does the patient do at his or her employment?

- Initial complaints at the scene of the accident
- Presenting complaints: the original subjective complaints, the patient's view of the problem created by the accident
- Past medical history
- Physical examination report
    - Vitals
    - Orthopedic tests
    - Muscle strength
    - Range of motion
    - Palpation findings
    - Acupuncture-Oriental medicine findings/diagnosis
    - X-rays taken, date, views, and report
- Treatment plan administered
- Review of records
    - Emergency room
    - Other doctors
- Diagnosis using ICD-9/10 terminology and criteria as related to Oriental medicine
- Disability—if any
- Lifestyle
- Prognosis, the discussion, summary, and conclusion
- Attachments
    - Accident photographs
    - SOAP notes
    - Police report
    - Laboratory findings and report
    - Hospital report
    - Orthopedic report
    - Psychological report
    - X-ray report
- Closing
- Signature

As you can see, there is, potentially, a great deal involved in caring for PI patients. That being said, if you can create a good relationship with one or more reputable PI attorneys, can find ways to streamline the paperwork involved, and are not uncomfortable with the fact that your reports will be legal documents, you may get many referrals for this type of work.

One word about PI patients—similar to WorkComp patients—you may very well encounter malingerers who choose not to get well no matter what treatment is given. This may be especially true if there is a lawsuit with potentially a great deal of money involved. It can be a sticky business to be involved with such patients. On the bright side, PI patients usually come in for many, many treatments over a reasonably long period of time. And, as acupuncture and Chinese medicine become more and more a part of the medical mainstream, more of us will undoubtedly participate in such patients' cases. Depending upon your situation and personal connections in your town, this type of patient could become one part of your patient mix and should not be denied your care without some investigation.

POINTS TO PONDER FROM CHAPTER 4

- Personal injury (PI) patients have been injured in some type of accident, most commonly auto accidents.

- PI cases require a great deal of paperwork, reporting, and careful chart notes which may become part of a medical-legal record.

- If you consider taking PI cases, do some research about the fault/no fault auto insurance situation in your state. No fault insurance states may be easier to navigate as a PI care provider. Contact your own auto insurance agent and ask questions.

- Know what forms you will need to have on file for PI patients. Most of these will be filled out by the patient, but they need to be completed and in your file.

- If lawyers will be involved in a patient's case, find out the answers to the questions for lawyers listed in this chapter before you decide to treat the patient!

- You may be required to testify in court or be deposed by either the plaintiff or defendant's legal counsel. Find out if you will be paid for your time. If you are asked to appear in court, dress professionally.

- We have included here a list of the things that may be included in required progress reports in PI cases. This list may also be downloaded from the website for you to craft your own reports.

- If you have personal acquaintances who are PI attorneys or can become a part of their referral circle, PI patients often require many treatments and it can be a financially rewarding part of your practice mix.

Working with Workers' Compensation | 5

▶ **Workers' Compensation and your clinic**

Workers' Compensation (Work Comp), also sometimes called Industrial Medicine or Occupational Medicine, is insurance that covers medical services for employees injured on the job. Each state has different laws regulating Work Comp insurance and what types of care must be (or may be) paid for at what rates.

A call to the Department of Insurance for information regarding Workers' Compensation in your state is a good place to begin. The reason to start here is that, in most states, there are one or more private companies that sell Work Comp insurance to businesses of all sizes and these companies are strictly regulated by each state's specific policies and guidelines. If this call does not yield adequate information, follow up by another call to the regulatory body that oversees Industrial Medicine in your state. You can get these phone numbers for every state by visiting the website www.dol.gov/owcp/dfec/regs/compliance/wc.htm or linking to their various websites directly from our website. ● Again, tell the person you speak with that you are new to this game and ask them to help you learn as much as possible, or refer you to appropriate sources of information.

Once you determine that acupuncture services can be covered in your state, ask if they offer seminars to help you learn all the rules for managing Work Comp patients properly. If reimbursement levels are good, it's

> **PRACTITIONER POINTER**
>
> "The most important thing with Workers' Comp patients is that you have to find out all the rules for what and how you can bill in your state, and follow them to the letter."
>
> —Neal Stuart Miller
> Sherman Oaks, CA

SECTION THREE: GETTING PAID

POWER POINT

How to get Workers' Compensation patients

Once you establish that WorkComp in your state will pay for acupuncture treatment and under what circumstances, consider developing a marketing program to meet and work with varying referral sources. There are three general groups of people to network with in this case.

- First, we suggest sending information about why acupuncture is a cost-effective therapy to the Human Resources directors of every company in your area with 25 or more employees. Emphasize the idea that you can save their company money by getting workers back on the job more quickly than other types of medicine. Short treatment duration means their Work Comp insurance goes up less than if the worker needs more treatment.

- Second, this same information needs to be sent to every insurance company that sells Work Comp policies in your state. It is wise to call these companies first and find out who would be the best person in the company to communicate with. If you can find an ally inside one or two companies that carry lots of policies in your state, it will give you someone to call when and if your claims are not reimbursed quickly or to help you know how to navigate the maze the insurance company creates to slow down payments to folks like us.

- Third, if you can find out the names of attorneys who specialize in Workers' Compensation or *employment law*, you should also send them information about your services, since they often have some influence over their clients' choices.

worth the money to go to one of these seminars and really learn the rules and regulations, which can seem Byzantine.

Acupuncture is covered and reimbursed with minimal difficulty in a number of states including Alaska, Florida, New Mexico, Nevada, Arizona, Colorado, California, New York, and others, as long as you follow billing guidelines and you can create reports that support what you are doing *in Western medical terms* (more on what we mean by that in a minute). In most states, acupuncture care is only paid for if there is a referral from a doctor, dentist, or chiropractor. Some states do not require a referral but do require your treatments to be pre-authorized by the insurance company. This may mean filing a report showing medical necessity and will at the very least mean a phone call to the claims adjuster for the company where the patient works. In some states, injured workers may request a specialist of their own choosing after 30 days of being treated by the employers' or insurance companies' specialists. Even after 30 days, however, acupuncturists will still be required to get pre-authorization for their treatments in most cases. Also, most states have a limit to the number of treatments that may be given and a limit that may be given before reports are required. Usually, only certain CPT codes can be billed and these are reimbursed at pre-determined amounts. There will also be requirements for periodic documentation, which you must ascertain from each insurance carrier or the HR department where the patient works.

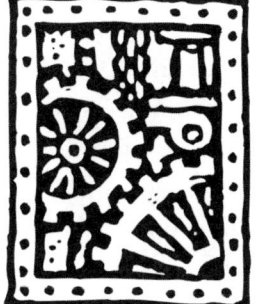

In terms of required documentation, these reports must be written in the same language that orthopedists, chiropractors, and other Western medical providers use. You will not get authorization for six more treatments by saying "the patient feels better" or "the flow of qi and blood is greatly improved." The reports must state specific improvements in function such as "patient's range of motion in shoulder

317

abduction has increased by 30 degrees after two treatments on the following acupoints…" or "after three treatments on the acupoints listed above to increase general stamina, the patient can now work three hours more per day," or "after three treatments to increase blood flow to the lower back on the following acupoints, patient can stand up without leg and back pain for more than four hours."

On your Patient Private or Confidential Information form, there should be a line to fill in when a prospective patient has been injured on the job. When you get a WorkComp case, you need to contact the company that covers the patient, similarly to how you contact any other insurance carrier, and fill out your insurance information form. Even if you already know that they will cover the patient's claim, you still need to find out:

- Do they require pre-authorization for treatment?
- Are there a certain number of treatments that you may do before any authorization is required?
- Are patients allowed to choose their own providers in your state? If not, how can an acupuncturist get chosen for doing treatment? Does the patient require a referral or prescription for acupuncture treatment?
- Is there a limit to the number of treatments allowed?
- What types of reports do they require and how often?
- Do you need to send them an assignment of benefits form in order to get paid?
- Do they have any standard forms they need to send you?
- How long does reimbursement usually take once a claim is filed?
- What is your scope of practice limited to according to the Work Comp system in your state? Do they only allow reimbursement for specific ICD-9/10 and CPT codes? If so, where can you get the list of acceptable codes?
- Do they expect you to use regular CMS forms or do they require some other form for billing?

This is where having a friend or two inside an insurance company can come in very handy. You may be able to get all these questions and more answered if you have already made a friend on the inside of the company you are billing. But we suggest you do as much homework as you can with the Workers' Compensation or Industrial Medicine department in your state. We cannot give you specific answers to the above questions because the answers in each state are different.

If reimbursement levels are low in your state, consider doing somewhat shorter sessions with this type of patient or scheduling more than one patient at a time. If you have more than one treatment room and an assistant, you could treat 2-3 patients per hour and still do a good treatment for each one. Consider scheduling such cases on your quietest day of the week so they don't use the most sought-after times when you want to schedule your higher paying patients. Go back to your figures showing how much your clinic needs to generate per hour to thrive (Section 2, Chapter 3) and see if/how you can make this work. Also, consider that if you do a good job for these patients, others in their company are likely to hear about it. You may get some non-Work Comp patients as referrals and the Work Comp patient may come back to you for a non-work related complaint at a later date. Remember, as we suggest in Section 3, Chapter 2, it is wise to have patients from more than one category of payment, and many practitioners make a very good living caring for people who have been injured on the job.

For far more detail about working successfully with Workers' Comp patients, see *Playing the Game: A Step-by-Step Approach to Accepting Insurance as an Acupuncturist* by Sperber and Hefner-Andersen.

POINTS TO PONDER FROM CHAPTER 5

- Workers' Compensation or Industrial Medicine is the name for insurance that covers people who are injured on the job.

- Many states' policies reimburse for acupuncture. To find out if yours does, go to the website www.dol.gov/owcp/dfec/regs/compliance/wc.htm and call the numbers given.

- Call some insurance carriers that cover Work Comp policies for the industries and large companies in your state. See if you can make a friend or two with claims adjusters inside these companies. Get as much information as you can in advance of taking your first Work Comp case.

- Consider creating a brochure that discusses the benefits of acupuncture for getting people back on the job fast to send to human resources directors at large companies and to adjusters at all the insurance companies that carry policies in your state.

- When you do get a Work Comp case, take a look at our list of questions to ask the insurance company before you take the case.

- If reimbursement levels are low, be creative in how you manage these cases. Can you do shorter treatments, schedule appointments during slower hours, or treat more than one patient at a time in order to accommodate these patients' needs?

- Before you dismiss them, consider other ways that these patients will help you grow your practice if you give them good care.

"Points to Ponder" continues on the next page

- Workers' Compensation patients can be a very nice slice of your income pie and a great source of referrals! But in order to get paid easily for Work Comp, the most important thing is that you find out and then follow all the rules. Consider taking one of the seminars frequently offered by the companies who sell Work Comp insurance.

Selling Products from Your Clinic | 6

Most of the really successful practitioners we know make a significant percentage of their income through product sales. While the most common product lines sold in acupuncture clinics are Chinese herbal medicinals, there are other groups of products that practitioners might consider offering to their patients. We encourage you to consider several possibilities for your clinic depending upon physical space limitations and the kind of products and information that you would like to offer your patients.

Some practitioners do not like the idea of "selling" anything or they feel it is a conflict of interest, like having an MD sell Western pharmaceuticals out of their medical office. To these people we offer the following thoughts.

1. As we discuss in the marketing chapters, think about the fact that, by offering products for people to purchase from you, especially the herbal medicine, you are providing a one-stop shopping opportunity for your patients. This is a convenience to everyone in our busy world. Even if your patient lives across the street from Chinatown in New York City, people may not want to schlep somewhere else to purchase their herbal formulas.

2. In most cities and towns across America, Chinese herbal medicine is not widely available in regular stores or pharmacies, if at all. If you do not provide these products for your patients, they will not be available by other means.

3. You can find herb companies that will take an online order and drop-ship directly to your patient, giving you a share of the profit. In these cases, you will have to place the order and manage the account, but you need not carry inventory. Few reputable herb companies are willing to sell their products

directly to the general public without practitioner oversight due to insurance liability issues and FDA scrutiny. Be aware, however, that there are unscrupulous online sellers who buy and resell herbal products without the permission of the herb company. This is happening more frequently all the time.

4. Studies show that compliance is much better and understanding of how to use products more accurate with patients who receive herbal formulas directly from the practitioner. Thus, patients are likely to get better faster because you were there to educate them about the products you offer.

Also, consider that your pharmacy or other product lines are a profit center that continues to generate income even when you are on vacation or whether you are seeing patients or not. As we say in our live courses, we'd like you to think of your income as a chair with at least three legs, because a chair needs at least that many legs to stand up effectively! Your treatments are, of course, the main leg of the chair. Classes that you teach might be another. Rental of space to other practitioners might be a third, but these two are likely to be relatively small income streams compared to the fees for services that you collect. However, product sales can and should be a steady and profitable source of income, as well as a source of healing for your patients, if managed properly.

▶ Possible product lines to sell

In our chapter on setting up your pharmacy, we suggest that you carry at least one or two good lines of prepared or "patent" medicines as well as either a granule "singles" line or a bulk pharmacy line to create your own formulas. In addition, there are several other types of products that you might consider:

- A vitamin/mineral line if you are allowed to sell these within your scope of practice.

- If you practice either dermatology or acupuncture cosmetology, consider carrying a line of skin care products.

Many people love to use a special product line that was personally recommended for them.

- If you do largely Workers' Comp or PI cases, a line of orthopedic supports and supplies as well as external liniments, patches, and plasters can often be billed to insurance and will sell well in that practice environment.

- In the interest of providing your patients with information about Chinese medicine, it can be effective to sell a small line of books that are easy for patients to read and understand. (See Important Website Tools, Links to Blue Poppy.)

- Aromatherapy products and/or essential oils are a nice adjunct to any practice that treats mostly women. This may include candles, soaps, oils, or creams. Some practitioners do extremely well with products such as these.

- If you participate in any type of multilevel marketing group selling a health-related product, you have a better chance of success given the constant stream of people through your office who will be likely to see your product(s) displayed.

▶ Soft and easy selling strategies

Once you decide what types of products you'd like to sell, how do you go about getting patients to buy them without a great deal of brain damage and without the products sitting around for weeks and months eating up space and cash flow?

While some products are more likely to "sell themselves" than others, it will also depend upon the type of specialty you have and, therefore, the type of patients as well as the physical layout of your space. If you have a nice counter space where people check in and out at your clinic, use this space judiciously to help you sell things. You can find nice plexiglass stand-up frames in varying sizes at office supply stores in which you can put friendly signs about a specific product or group of products that you like. Below is a sample of what we mean by this. If you have a color printer and colored paper, make these signs colorful and attractive. Still, the words can be as simple as, "Ask About Our Aromatherapy Products. They Make Great Gifts," or "Ask Us to Create Your Personalized Essential Oil Formula. Only $6.95 for a one-oz. bottle."

Allergies Got You Down?

Ask Your Practitioner About Our Favorite Herbal Allergy Formulas!

10% Discount During August
(Good for up to four bottles per person)

If you are carrying a good product line, the company may provide you with a sales brochure to give to patients or leave out next to your product display. If not, you might want to create a simple brochure or flyer about your favorite products and their various uses. Keep this simple and conversational. Just make sure it is proofread well and easy to read.

If you want to sell books, you can purchase all types of nice display materials either online or through companies like Siegel Display Company (1-800-626-0322). If you plan to have only one or two books, you can buy small, single bookstands at many office supply stores. A sign next to your book display might say something like, "Easy to Understand Information on Chinese Medicine. Get One for a Friend Today." You can get small stickers that are easy to remove and mark the prices on the front so that people can make a price decision without having to ask anyone, although most books will also have the price on the back cover. We suggest you choose books that are not too large or too complicated. If you are willing to buy in reasonable amounts, say 6-10 copies, many companies will give you a nice discount as long as you have a resale tax ID number (TIN), which you can get from the state government and from the federal government (www.irs-ein-number.com). You will have to have these numbers if you become a corporation or an LLC.

> "Anyone can make soap. It takes a wise person to sell soap."
> —Anon.

If you have a product line that is beautifully packaged or the products themselves are lovely or they smell good, such as candles or soaps, you want to make sure they are out where people can see them without being in a location that makes them tempting to carry away without paying. A small wall display shelf right next to the reception desk can be quite effective in these cases. If you have a line of nice scented candles, you might keep one or more lit in your treatment rooms or in your waiting area. Just be sure not to leave them burning when you leave the office! If you have creams or lotions, an open sample with a sign saying "Try Me" can be all the marketing effort you need to make. Also, be sure to find out from the suppliers you work with whether they have special lines for the holiday season and special display materials or brochures to help you sell the products. Consider changing your product lines or at least the product displays every several months to give things a fresh look.

If you have a great nutraceutical line, you might create a quote such as, "I take such-and-such vitamins and they have doubled my energy level in the last six months. Ask me for more information." Put your name at the bottom and frame the quote to put up in your bathroom.

Last but not least, your various lines of herbal products will sell because you prescribe them for your patients' patterns. If you choose your product lines well, your patients will feel better and be happy to buy them when needed without much convincing. Finally, remember that there are new products coming on the market all the time. Once in a while, we urge you to consider another professional product line than the ones you've been using or the ones you were introduced to in school. You might find better technologies, better crafted medicinals, or something new that works better for you and your patients than what you've tried so far.

▶ What should your markup be?

With the exception of grocery chains and car dealerships, most stores with whom we all do business every day have to mark up their products at least 50% in order to make a profit because of inventory tax, storage and space usage, shipping costs, and because a certain amount of cash flow is always tied up in the product line. Your situation is really no different. You cannot afford to sell products at cost! No retailer can afford to do that. If an 80-100% markup feels like too much, find an amount over 50% that you can live with for most products. A markup lower than 40% will work only if your turnover is really excellent or they are very specialized products and you simply don't feel you can sell them for a higher price. For example, if a product is sold to you for $10 and the shipping per unit is between 50¢ and 75¢, you cannot afford to stock it for more than a few weeks without getting $15.95 or more when you sell it—and $17.95 is better. More than $19.95 is probably unfair to the customer unless you have some very unusual circumstances. Many product lines will give you the suggested retail price. You can, of course, choose to charge either more or less than that depending upon your situation, shipping costs, amount of shelf space, type of market, or other factors.

If you have a real problem with markups or if even having this discussion makes you squirm, I ask you to consider the situation of other retailers from whom you buy. Would you expect them to operate at a loss or in a manner that forces them out of business? Of course you don't. Most of us are more interested in value for our money than we are interested in something being cheap. This is true for the products you sell as well as the services you offer. Price is not the only criteria people have for choosing what to buy. If it were, we'd all be driving around in a Ford Focus or a used Chevy, which is clearly not the case. It does not serve you to price your products or your services too low. It only creates financial stress in your life and a perception of less value to your patients.

Our suggestion is that your markup for herbal products and nutraceuticals should be between 50% and 80%. External herbal products, such as liniments and ointments, usually have a smaller markup . . . say 25-30%. In the world of books, the standard markup for retailers is 20-40%. Be sure to ask publishers how many copies you need to order in order to get a discount of 30-40%. Skin care product lines and aromatherapy products may have different suggested markups. Of course, on any kind of product line you sell, you will be able to get better pricing on larger orders, which will increase your profits. While pricing varies, you need to make sure that you are consistently making some profit on everything that is purchased in your clinic.

In most cases, you need not use a "hard sell" approach, and we don't even suggest that as an appropriate sales method. Good products displayed well will sell without too much effort and can make a real difference in your income as well as the ambience of your clinic. Remember, if you have someone to fill patients' herb orders or deal with other sales, you can be making money on your products even when you are on vacation! If you have a product line that you have done very well with, we hope you'll drop us an email about it so we can share your success story with others.

POINTS TO PONDER FROM CHAPTER 6

- There are many types of products you can sell in your clinic to create another "leg" on your income chair. In addition to herbal medicine, consider skin care products, books, aromatherapy products, and nutraceutical products.

- Some people may consider sales in their clinic to be a conflict of interest, but there are few other options for patients in the world of Chinese medicine than to buy their products from a professional clinic.

- Other advantages are that people prefer one-stop shopping and are always more compliant with products that their practitioner recommends.

- Use small friendly signs and displays to sell products. No hard sell approaches are necessary.

- Make sure you mark up your products enough to make them profitable without gouging. People expect good value but not give-away prices.

- As long as there is someone in your office to fill people's orders for herbs or other products, you can be making money even when you are on vacation.

Buying or Selling an Acupuncture Practice | 7

▶ **Here's what you need to know**

Over the last several years, I [HW] have been asked several times for advice about buying someone else's acupuncture practice. This has become a more common event in the world of acupuncture and deserves an intelligent discussion for those of you who are interested in this option. As with anything in life, it has pros and cons. Here's what you should know no matter whether you are on the buying or selling side of the equation.

First of all, let me say that there are many web resources available on this subject, although all the ones I could find specifically discuss the sale of either a medical (MD) practice or a chiropractic (DC) practice. So the information I am presenting here is as generic as I could make it for acupuncture practices based upon the resources available.

Second, because the information available on this subject is not acupuncture specific, there may be some wiggle room on the numbers I present here, although it's my gut feeling that they transfer pretty well to any medical profession and may be used as a safe rule of thumb for buyers or sellers.

Third, if you have bought or sold a practice, either successfully or unsuccessfully, I'd love to hear from you with your experiences and what you learned from the experience. If we all shared information about business experience with each other, we would all do better as business people. At the end of the day, the more of us who are successful, the better it is for the profession as a whole.

With those things in mind, I have tried to divide the information below into concerns for buyers and considerations or advice for sellers.

▶ Buying a practice

There are many things to consider when purchasing someone's practice. The most important considerations are as follows:

1. What would be the difference in cost between starting and successfully growing your own practice down the block as opposed to buying the practice that is for sale? Be as honest as possible with yourself about start-up and growth costs for a practice.
2. What are you really buying? Are there hard assets such as equipment, furniture, or real estate involved in this transaction? If not, are you buying the accounts receivable or the bank account balances?
3. If there are no cash or hard assets, you are then buying what is called "goodwill." In that case, a medical or chiropractic practice is considered to be worth no more than 30% of the annual gross receipts of the clinic. If there are any hard assets, those are added to the value of the "goodwill."

▶ Practice assessment for a potential buyer

1. Financial records

    There are a few ways to determine or prove the value of gross receipts. Most sources suggest that you require access to two years of tax returns and financial records. If a practitioner selling a clinic cannot provide these records, it is questionable whether they will have kept their patient records in any more organized a fashion! At that point I say, "Buyer beware." If they refuse to give you access to this information, then you certainly don't want to do business with them.

2. **Intangible assets may include:**

    a. The clinic market position (monthly patient visits, positive cash flow, take home pay of the practitioner[s], number of total patient records, income and expense projections, base overhead expenses per month).

    b. Regulatory history (are there any suits or legal problems)

    c. Operational systems in place and quality of patient record keeping

    d. Quality of the facilities and capacity for growth in those facilities

    e. Soundness of the balance sheet and up-to-date financial record keeping

    f. Size and current status of the mailing list

    g. Reputation of the clinic in the community

    h. Staffing situation (will the current staff stick with you)

    i. Visibility of the location

3. **Other considerations you need to research:**

    a. How flexible is the financing and payment structure for this purchase?

    b. How many months is the current practitioner willing to stay in the clinic and work with you? The longer this transition process, the better to introduce you to the client base and the more valuable the practice is to you.

    c. What does an analysis of the local demographics reveal? Is the area gaining or losing population? What is the average age of the population and what was the average age a decade ago? Are there many third party payers serving this community that require you to be paneled in order to serve

PRACTITIONER POINTER

"My advice is don't be afraid to buy a practice. I sold my first practice in 1985 for a very reasonable price. It had supported me well enough, but the new owners expanded it to support two practitioners very quickly. Then they sold it again after a decade or so and now it supports three practitioners. The practice is still there and still growing 20 years later.

For the sale of my second practice, I consulted with a professional business valuation expert to help me come up with a fair price. Again, it is a growing practice with great potential for a good, young, ambitious practitioner.

Remember, if you are buying a practice that has created goodwill, is obviously growing, and the price is fair, it can be so much easier than starting your own from scratch. Get the practitioner to introduce you to as many of the patients as you can and get out into the community and meet people. Tell them you are the person who is taking over so-and-so's practice and you'd love to see them at the clinic. You still have to do your marketing and introduce yourself to the community, but at least you have a potential patient list to start with."

—Don Beans, L.Ac., Ph.D.
Whitefish, MT

the largest segment of the population and what do those panels pay?

d. What does an analysis of the clinical appointment book for the last year reveal? Are there many repeat patients? What is the average number of appointments per patient? What type of hours and workload is the practitioner maintaining and does that work for you?

e. Will the seller send out a letter informing the entire patient list of their upcoming departure and supporting you as their practitioner of choice for referral? Will they pay for that mailing?

f. If you only keep 40-50% of the patients who have come to this clinic, would that be enough to support you while you build the patient base and would the price still be worth it?

g. What is the status of the current lease? Are there opportunities for expansion? Are there any legal or zoning problems with the building that could affect you?

h. What is the seller's definition of an active patient? Is it the same as yours?

i. Who is assuming responsibility for the inactive records and what will it cost you if you must store them?

j. Who owns the clinic name and logo if it is not the person's name? For example, John Smith Acupuncture Clinic is not a name you want to buy as part of the purchase, but you might want to keep the name Whole Woman Health Clinic if it is well established in the community.

If all this seems like too much and you are really serious about wanting to do this purchase, you might consider hiring an independent valuation expert. This is usually a shared expense between buyer and seller whether you end up buying the practice or not.

Finally, buyers, don't ever think that buying a practice absolves you of marketing efforts in the community. Remember that most people who become your patients are buying You. Thus, you will still need to embed yourself in the community in a positive way.

▶ Selling your practice successfully

The first and most important word for sellers is "transparency." If you try to keep secrets from potential buyers or are tempted not to tell the truth about this or that, they will be immediately suspicious and shy away from the purchase pretty fast. If they dig a bit, they will most likely find out what you don't want them to know anyway. So it pays you to be up front about everything, especially anything that is less than the perfect image you wish to project.

That being said, what can you do to help yourself sell the practice smoothly and for the best possible price?

▶ Assess your market position

Before you even think about placing an ad or putting it out in the ethers that you want to sell your practice, you'll be better off if you carefully assess all of the following.

1. How much competition is in the area, and how have you managed that competition successfully?

2. What is your payer mix of cash, fee-for-service insurance, insurance panels, worker's comp, PI, trades, and pro-bono? If you have accounts receivable, what is their average age?

3. Know the local and regional demographic trends (age, income, employment, stability) in advance and make this part of your seller's information package. Cite or footnote your sources with dates.

4. Are there any other practices for sale in your region of the country? If so, can you compare and contrast your practice in a favorable light? If yes, this is a great marketing point.

5. Are there any recent or potential changes in the regulatory climate in your state?

6. Take a close look at your overhead and all expenses and decide if you could be more efficient in your use of resources. Is there anywhere that you could cut costs without losing quality or efficiency? Do you have the best deals on phone service, bank service, draft capture service, laundry service, etc.? If you can do better, you can make your net profit better and your profit/loss statements and balance sheet more attractive.

7. How is cash flow managed in your business? Could you improve internal controls to keep costs even lower, improve the terms on money you owe to vendors, get a better float or a lower interest rate on company credit cards?

8. What are your fixed and variable expenses? Can any of those numbers be improved? If so, do it now.

9. Consider various ways to advertise this sale and write your ad copy carefully. Consider state and national publications, online services, word-of-mouth, your state association meetings and publications, and school newsletters and bulletin boards.

10. Consider carefully your exit strategy. The longer you are willing to stay in the practice and introduce the new practitioner, the more valuable the practice will be and the better the selling price. Also, if you plan to stick around for a while, you can give a potential buyer longer to pay for the practice using their work as part of the pay-off. (They do the work, you get some or most of the income for that work.) Having three years to actually pay off the entire practice price is optimal and may, again, increase the value of your practice. The better the terms and the longer your exit strategy, the more you can charge for the business.

11. When creating a realistic exit strategy, carefully define the patient distribution and work load and how that might/will change over the months of your exiting. Who is responsible for what types and amounts of work by what dates? Be very clear about your final departure date and stick to it.

12. Be clear as to how and how much money needs to change hands and by what specific dates.

13. The more you do to let your patient base know about this transition (letters, postcards, phone calls, open houses, personal introductions), the more valuable the practice is.

14. Give yourself adequate time. If you are planning to retire altogether in, say, five years, start looking for a partner or younger associate now. By bringing someone into your practice, you can avoid selling off your accounts receivable and your equipment for nothing more than their depreciated value.

If this is all too complicated, then you probably are not ready to sell your practice. Even hiring a professional valuator will not exempt you from the work that you must do to assess the value of your practice, because they will require you to provide much of the information listed above.

As I stated at the beginning of this chapter, there are many books and websites that give you information about how medical practices are bought and sold. Whether you are buying or selling, the more you have read on the subject and the more research you have done, the fairer a deal you will be able to create.

POINTS TO PONDER FROM CHAPTER 7

- Buying and selling of practices in our profession is increasing in recent years.

- Buyers need to know that 90% of what they are buying is goodwill and carefully assess the value of that goodwill. In medical practices, goodwill is usually valued at 30% of the last year's gross receipts.

- Before entering into contract negotiations, buyers must carefully assess the following:

  - the clinic market position
  - regulatory history
  - quality of patient record keeping
  - quality of the facilities and capacity for growth
  - soundness of the balance sheet and up-to-date financial record keeping
  - size and current status of the mailing list
  - reputation of the clinic in the community
  - staffing situation, visibility of the location, status of the current lease agreement

- Sellers can sweeten any deal by lengthening their transfer/exit strategy.

- Sellers will gain the trust of potential buyers by total transparency and by having done some serious homework to assess and improve the real value of their clinic prior to putting it on the market.

- Honesty and fair play are the most important qualities to bring to any contract.

SECTION FOUR

Marketing Your Practice

What's in this section:
- First Things First for the New Graduate
- Marketing Inside Out
- Be a Community Team Player
- A Good Mailing List (How to Build One; How to Use One)
- Creating and Using a Presentation Folder
- Writing a Successful Press Release
- Marketing Your Practice on the Internet
- Marketing Odds and Ends

The difficulty of writing about marketing is that you could write an entire book just on marketing, even just on marketing for a private practice in Chinese medicine! Libraries and bookstores have scores of books on marketing, and we encourage you to read one or more from time to time just to keep your head in the marketing mind-set. In "Resources for Going Further" at the end of this section and on the website as well, you will find a list of books that I [HW] especially recommend.

Just to keep things tidy, I have divided this voluminous information into several chapters and done my best not to be redundant. In trying to decide what and how much to include in this section, I've focused on the things that I believe to be the most effective for acupuncturists. These fall loosely into three categories: 1) marketing from within your clinic, 2) marketing outside your clinic, and 3) things that don't really fall into either of those categories. For any excessive cheerleading or mentioning the same idea in a different context more than once, I apologize in advance.

Also, if you have read other chapters of this book, you have probably noticed that marketing is sprinkled throughout it. That is just the nature of marketing. It easily creeps into everything else you do and how you think as a businessperson, as it should. This is another way of saying that marketing is not just a bunch of stuff you do. Marketing is an attitude, a way of thinking about your business to make it as visible as possible and as attractive as possible to the people who might benefit from your services.

Good marketing is not dishonest or slippery. Good marketing does not invite or produce buyer's remorse. Good marketing, fundamentally, is merely having a good thing to say (and the chops to back up your words), saying it well enough for anyone to notice, and saying it often to those who may be interested in listening. Marketing can be as complex as creating a fund-raising event with a cast of thousands or as simple as having a cup of coffee in the same café every morning for six months. So, here we go.

Marketing From Day One: First Things First | 1

What things do you need to consider right away upon graduation with regard to marketing? Hopefully, you have given some thought (and action) to this question well before you receive your diploma. (See Section 1, Chapter 3.) The information below picks up where that chapter leaves off.

▶ Start with a healthy mindset

You have just finished a 3-4 year process to digest a body of clinical knowledge that will allow you to help people be healthier and happier. You deserve to feel good about that accomplishment. Now you need to focus on staying upbeat and positive about sharing your skill and knowledge with whatever community of people you desire to serve. While you cannot usually expect to have a full practice from day one, you can expect success over time, and you can expect people to respond to you and what you are offering in a positive manner. The more you are able to maintain and project this positive attitude, the faster you will find the success you desire. Even on the days when there are few patients or none at all, stay as upbeat as you can. Look at the temporary breaks and slow times in your schedule as opportunities to find more ways to connect with your community, improve the look and feel of your clinic space, write articles or schedule speeches, and take care of yourself. If you start each day asking the universe for what you want and intend to happen and then follow through on your marketing strategy, you will get where you want to go.

As Mark Victor Hansen says in *The One Minute Millionaire,* think, work, and plan "from your dreams, not toward them." That means starting your days visualizing and believing in what you are trying to create. As discussed in the chapter on goal-setting, we further suggest that you write down what you want your practice to look like, what you want your clinic to look, feel, and smell like, draw sketches in your notebook or journal, make a collage, write a poem, or do whatever helps you stay focused on creating what you want in a practice in as much detail as possible. If you can actually keep this discipline of keeping your goals and dreams in your mind, the ways and means of creating it will come if you are paying attention.

▶ Strategic planning

No matter what group of people you plan to serve or whether you will be in a small town or a large city, one of your first tasks as a new graduate is to create a well-organized plan for building your practice or revise the one you (hopefully) created in school or in doing your business plan. This means writing it down and deciding how much work to do on your plan each day and each week. Of course, if it all works really well and your practice grows quickly, your plan must be flexible. You could have a lot worse problems than this! What might this look like? Well, here's what it would look like for me if I were graduating tomorrow.

> "A ship in a safe harbor is safe, but that is not what a ship was built for."
>
> —William Shedd

Start by creating a list of the possible ways you might build your practice. These could include but are not limited to the following:

1. If you already have a location for your practice, call, text, or email everyone you already know who lives or works within a 30-mile radius of your clinic and tell them you are open for business and may you please send them a few business cards to give to friends, family, and coworkers.

2. Send an announcement to the business editors of the local newspapers and let them know you are opening a clinic (or are now working at XYZ clinic that is already in business).

You might also invite those editors as well as the health editors for all local papers in for a free consultation and/or treatment.

3. Walk around the neighborhood of your clinic... four or five blocks in every direction. Who is there and what sorts of businesses are in the neighborhood? How could you serve them? How could you partner with them? Would they let you put your cards up on the employee "break room" bulletin board? Could you do any trades with them for products or services?

4. If you have family in the area, will they take cards and give them out to everyone they know that you don't know? Do they have any influential friends to whom they could introduce you, such as media moguls, hospital administrators, MDs, wealthy socialites, or famous sports figures?

5. If you have any well-known friends such as sports, music, literary, film, or media personalities, organize a grand opening bash with them as the featured speaker or performer, autograph signer, or schmoozer. Send announcements about your party to everyone you can think of. Be as adventurous as you can with this event. The more unusual you can make it in terms of theme, invitation design, food choices, or live entertainment, the more people will come. If you want to create a practice for a certain niche market, make the theme somehow relevant and exciting for those people in particular. Invite the media as well.

6. If you have created a presentation folder, create a list of MDs, DCs, TV and radio personalities, news editors, human resources department heads at local businesses, or anyone else you need to send these to in your area. That part is easy, but here is the hard part: Create a follow-up calling schedule and stick to it. We suggest you get these calls out of the way early in the day so the dread of them does not hang over your

head. When you get the front desk gatekeeper, talk to him/her about who you are and what you do. If he or she sounds at all interested, offer to provide an in-service lunch for their entire office so that you can go and tell them about what you have to offer their patients (or co-workers or employees) and what conditions you can help them to treat more efficiently. (See Chapter 5 of this section about presentation folders below for more on this strategy.)

7. If you are planning to specialize in one area of practice, call every other practitioner in the area and ask them for referrals *for only this type of patient.* You also might consider putting a classified ad in the state newsletter about your specialization. Let these practitioners know that you will refer in turn to other specialties. Offer to trade treatments with them on occasion.

8. If you are planning to specialize in a discipline that you think MDs would find helpful, see if you can find books, brochures, and research (or create your own literature) about your specialty emphasizing how and why your services will help them treat their patients more successfully for less money and time. Send this information to every MD in that field of expertise. Offer to speak to them in person to discuss ways that you can help them treat their patients. Emphasize how you would work with them to benefit *their* patients.

9. Start collecting a mailing/emailing list. This can be used for a wide variety of strategies that we discuss below. A mailing list of interested people is one of your most valuable tools.

10. Join one club, organization, or volunteer group that connects you to the larger community in a meaningful way. This can be anything from coaching girls soccer, Rotary and Kiwanis club, to the planning committee for the local Susan B. Komen 10K fundraising walk. This type of work can be invaluable in the long-term success of your private practice.

OK, there are 10 ideas you could use as is or expand upon and we've yet to even mention the internet. What you have to do is take only a few of these and write them down as an organized plan with a schedule that you can follow through on day by day. At first, this type of work may take up most of your week. As you get patients, it will take up less and less of your week. However, it is our experience that if you create a plan *and follow through on your plan in a systematic manner,* you will build a practice unless you are simply wrong for this work.

Some things will work better than others. Revisions and adaptations to your plan will happen as you go along. You may find that teaching classes at the local community college works better than free talks at the library or that one part of your plan morphs into something completely different. That's great. Be flexible, but be regular and systematic as well. Sometimes this will all be scary and there are always days when everything you try leads down a blind alley. Do your best not to let worry or fear drown you. Remember that failure is always "the path of least persistence" and keep working your plan.

> **"Trust your crazy ideas."**
> —Dan Zodra

I suggest you keep track of your activities other than seeing patients. At the end of each week, make a practice management/practice-building "to do" list for the next week. This helps you avoid chaos, manage stress, and stay on top of your plan. And it feels great to check things off your list throughout the week. See the simple plan on the next page.

This is a pretty sane schedule for the first month out there. Staying organized with ongoing marketing efforts and tracking them each day, this practitioner will have four patients per day next month, and five per day the month after that.

SECTION FOUR: MARKETING YOUR PRACTICE

Week Beginning Monday June 21
To Do List: 1. Write and send letters to all local OB/GYNs 2. Create text for brochure/call designers to create barter 3. Speak to local community college class coordinator, write and send follow-up course description 4. Call herb distributors for new catalogs 5. Create copy for website FAQ 6. Place classified ad for front desk helper/place ad at local acupuncture school 7. Follow-up meeting at All Women's Health Clinic 8. Research case from last Thursday before his next visit
Monday   8AM   Review charts for today's patients
9 AM   Call to follow up with Dr. Jones and Dr. Boswell, offer a lunch meeting; write blog article
10 AM   Patient appointment. Nancy Sinclair (get signed form to her MD requesting records)
11 AM   Patient appt. John Rafferty
1 PM Find research articles to post at website
2 PM   Appointment at All Women's Health Clinic
3 PM Patient appt. Joan Crest; discuss insurance deductible
4 PM   Reminder calls for tomorrow's patients
5 PM   Yoga class at YMCA

▶ **Being remarkable**

In your graduating class and all the ones before you and after you, people mostly took/take the same courses from the same instructors and came/come out with the same skill set. A few

POWER POINT

We have talked to many people about how they got their first patients. While there are variations, of course, most successful practitioners tell a similar story: networking and more networking, which usually started before graduation.

- One new graduate started by treating the guys on her husband's construction crew for various sore body parts at reasonable rates. They came in after work to her small rented clinic space. They told their buddies and wives, and she was off and running.

- Another woman lives in the same city as her family and she had all of them giving out her business cards to friends and coworkers. She had five patients waiting to see her before the paint was dry at her clinic.

- Another new practitioner went to see a local chiropractor and gave him a series of free treatments in exchange for using his clinic on his day off "on a trial basis." The DC is now referring patients to her for care and has put her name on his signage. More important, he is including an announcement of her services in his next newsletter to his 700+ clients. She is expanding to using his clinic on Saturday as well.

- One new graduate has moved back to his hometown of 15,000 folks in upstate New York. Because he knows almost everyone in town, coaches Little League, and has joined the PTO at his children's school, it took him less than a year to have a full practice.

people are "naturals" in both their intelligence and aptitude, but most practitioners have approximately the same skill set and are selling the same thing in the marketplace that you are selling.

> **PRACTITIONER POINTER**
>
> "The marketing never stops. We come back again and again to various ways of getting involved with our community. We are active members of the Historic Olde Town Merchant Association and we participate in all the Olde Town festivals and events. We still do some writing and some talks as well."
>
> —Lisa Lowe and Karen Marks
> Arvada, CO
> www.oldetownacupuncture.com

That being the case, unless you are in a small town or rural area or otherwise the only game in town, you need to come up with other ways to be remarkable. What does that mean?

Remarkable means exactly what it implies: being someone and something worth remarking about... someone that people will tell others about. One place to start is to visit all kinds of professional offices, stores, cafes, museums, restaurants, and retail establishments and take notes. Which ones really light your fire? Why? When you go into a place that really makes you want to spend your money there, try to analyze what is so attractive about that experience. Could you take that idea (the colors, smells, sounds) and "cross-pollinate" it somehow into how people experience your clinic and your services? How can you take the best parts of the limitless possibilities that living in the developed world affords you and make your clinic medically credible and yet so beautiful, interesting, unusual, exciting, soothing, stimulating, singular, or magnetic that everyone who goes there will want to tell all their friends? That's your goal.

There are many possible ways to be remarkable. Could you create the best customer service, the coolest peripheral product options, the best lending library, always-available online research access, the best playroom for kids, the most authentic and beautiful replica of an 18th century Chinese pharmacy, free reflexology for all customers one day per week (choose a day that does not fill up as easily as others), available spa services, walk-in availability, crystal chandeliers, house-calls one day per week, an over-the-counter Chinese herb vending machine (for safe products like Curing Pills®, Cold Quell®, etc.), the most beautiful clinic rooms, an evenings-only practice with a video-game room for the kids, an annual organized fundraiser for the local women's shelter, an ATM machine in your office, low-cost standard Western medical physicals once per month by a young hospital resident, or… ? What would your ideas cost in money, administration, and personal bandwidth? What would be your potential return on investment? Then, try to assess your personal risk tolerance financially, socially, and aesthetically. Once you have done that, pick a marketing "limb" and go out as far on it as your risk tolerance can handle. That's where the fruit is. By this we mean think and dream of the most remarkable, outrageous ideas you can for your clinic. Don't be a clone.

POINTS TO PONDER FROM CHAPTER 1

- A marketing plan is one of the first things to create upon graduation unless you have already created one. It should be flexible and put into effect immediately and carried through day-by-day, every day.
- There are literally as many marketing plans as there are practitioners; consistency and follow-through are what matter most.
- Be flexible with your plan as your patient base grows.
- In a sea of practitioners offering the same services and products, research creative ways to make your clinic remarkable. Assess your risk tolerance, and then go for it.

Marketing Inside Out | 2

At the most generic level, disease causes in Chinese medicine fall into three categories, internal, external, and neither internal nor external. Marketing is similar, *i.e.,* there are things you do inside your clinic, things you do outside your clinic, and then things that don't fall neatly into either category. In this chapter, I [HW] discuss internal marketing—the things you do inside your clinic—to attract and keep new patients.

As stated in other chapters, it is important to keep in mind that you, your clinic, and your services *are* the primary marketing for you, your clinic, and your services. Everything from the cleanliness of the bathrooms, friendliness of the front desk staff, prompt and efficient phone service, and your caring, effective treatments are part of your marketing effort. And those are simply the things that people expect. Beyond that, there are whatever special touches you create as discussed in the previous chapter. Then there needs to be at least a few of the following:

> **Information**

Remember that informed patients usually make better patients and better "sales reps" for your clinic services. When people can understand in simple terminology what you are doing and why, they tend to respond better to treatment and they are more likely to talk to people about what they have learned. So, for the first 3-5 treatments, we suggest that you never send your patient out the door without a book, brochure, research report, flyer, clipping, or some other reading assignment. There are a number of ways to display this information or otherwise let your patients know that they also have online access to information on acupuncture and Oriental/Chinese medicine.

1. **The fun scrapbook**
   Create a scrapbook in your waiting area. Exactly what you think it is, this scrapbook can have all kinds of interesting, fun info and photos in it. Include research or articles from popular or technical media (online or in print), articles you have written, letters from satisfied patients (get permission to share), photos from your recent study trip to China (with captions)—whatever you would like to share with patients. Put each piece in a clear sleeve in the notebook. Make sure it says on the creatively-designed cover that patients may ask for 3-4 (or however many pages you feel you can afford) to be copied for free. Then get a rubber stamp or sticker with your clinic address, phone, email, and website to stamp each page on the top, bottom, or back. That way, when patients ask for copies, your clinic contact info is clearly visible. You never know into whose hands these pieces will fall.

2. **The always-available online database**
   This requires digital cable or wifi in your office and possibly the help of an IT consultant, but is a cool idea given what is available online. Connect this computer to websites with voluminous information about Chinese medicine (like Blue Poppy, Acufinder, or Acupuncture Today). Put a sign next to the computer saying that patients may look up research on their condition at these favorite sites. You may also want to say something like, "Please inquire at the front desk to print out articles." You can charge 5-10¢ per printed page or give the information away. Make sure each page is stamped or stickered as described in #1.

3. **Visible brochure displays**
   There are many types of brochure-holders on the market. These can be attached to the wall or sit on a table or counter. Again, you need to make sure that your card or contact

information is on each brochure. We suggest you either create or purchase at least 4-5 different brochures on various health conditions that you like to treat, as well as more general brochures such as "What Is Acupuncture," "About Chinese Medical Diagnosis," or "How Chinese Herbal Medicine Works." Rotate the rooms these brochures are in for patients to pick up, or take charge of the situation and hand an appropriate brochure to the patient, actively requesting that they read it and write down questions before their next visit.

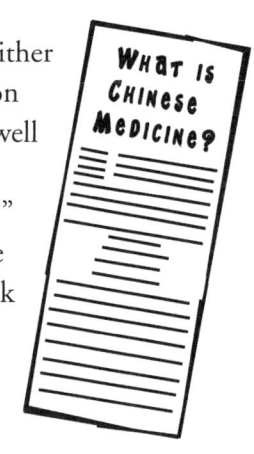

4. **Book-of-the-month displays**

   Educate your patients and create a separate income stream with this idea. A single book holder for a favorite health book on your counter is all you need for this one. Create a sign in a 5x7" plexiglass holder that says this informative book is available for sale and that it will help the patient understand more about our medicine. If you buy several books at a time, you can often get a nice discount from the publisher or distributor and then make the price of the books a dollar-or-two less than standard bookstore retail. Rotate books monthly.

   Another idea is to charge enough on your initial visit to simply give each patient a relevant book and ask them to read it before their second appointment. Patients are impressed with this, you can be sure. Don't mar the books by stamping them, but do put a card in as a bookmark. You don't know where the book or the card may end up.

5. **Monthly or quarterly newsletters**

   This can be a successful way to keep yourself in your patients' minds. It does not have to be long. Indeed, people don't want it to be long. One or two pages are enough. You can offer a free healthy recipe for the season, an article about in-the-news healthcare issues, an interesting bit of research on acupuncture, articles about Oriental medical politics in your state (if the issue will affect your patients' lives), special upcoming classes or events you are offering, seasonal preventive health tips, or information about specific herbs or formulas. These should be very short articles, by the way. Bullet-pointed articles usually get read... things such as, "Five Tips for Preventing Seasonal Allergies." Put a newsletter sign-up form in with other new-patient forms that people fill out when starting care. Many will want the information as long as you agree not to rent or sell your mailing list. Also take newsletter sign-up forms when you do public lectures or classes. Finally, be sure to mention how to sign up for your newsletter with your author info at the end of any articles or blogs you publish.

The cheapest, easiest way to do a newsletter is by email. There are lots of software options and online services for creating a nice email newsletter. You can also use very simple text-formatting with live links that go back to pages on your website. If you do a print version and send by U.S. mail, it costs quite a bit more money and brain damage, but, if your list is not large this may be no problem, it looks classy, and can also be used as a handout at live events.

Remember, in every newsletter, to tell readers how much you appreciate their referrals; it is the best way for them to thank you for your services. It is okay to actually ask them for this assistance. If you do an email newsletter, you can put this message into a small "box" in a different color than the rest of the text. If you are doing this on paper, make your request stand out with bold or italic text in a different color.

6. **Clipping/research files**

   Put up a small sign in your waiting area stating that you have a research archive and patients may ask to see the list of articles currently available. You could also simply post the list of articles and state that people may request copies at a few cents per page. Again, make sure your stamp is on at least one page of each article that goes out the door. This does require you to keep adding to your research articles on a regular basis so that information remains fresh. One clinic I know combines this idea with the scrapbook idea and has over 100 articles in clear sleeves in a notebook with a notice on the front saying that patients may buy copies at 25¢ per article.

7. **Framed clippings on specific diseases**
   This is especially good if you only want to treat a certain range or type of conditions. Take short articles about Chinese medicine or acupuncture and specific conditions and frame them as information "art" in your treatment rooms, bathroom, and next to your front desk. Keep 2-3 extra copies in a file if anyone requests one for a friend.

8. **Signage throughout your clinic**
   Especially important and so easy to do, I've put this last on the list because I want you to remember it! Signs can be about all sorts of things. You could start with simple "did you know" signs; something like "Did you know that insomnia is the most common condition suffered by Americans? Research shows that acupuncture and Chinese herbal medicine can help people with this often difficult condition. Ask me about treatments for insomnia for yourself, friends, or family." Consider a small poster of the WHO list of what conditions acupuncture can treat. (Yes, it's out of date and incomplete, but it's all new information to your patients.) How about regular flyers for classes and lectures you are doing, special product or service offers, or community volunteering and fundraising events in which you are participating? And, last but not least, a sign telling people that you appreciate their referrals right next to your card holder is always a good idea.

> "If you give people what they want, you will get what you want."
>
> —Zig Ziglar

▶ Artistic touches

- Think about the image you want to project in your clinic: medical efficiency, warm and homey, ancient esoteric China, sleek Euro-chic, or...? Every piece of furniture, the art on the walls, the picture frame style, the wall colors, even your biz card colors, can project the same image throughout.

- Add artistic pieces selectively. Spare is usually better than cluttered. You want people to notice a few beautiful things rather than be overwhelmed by visual excess. Also, if you have important signage around your office, clutter may keep people from noticing what you have to say. (Unless, of course, you go for a cluttered, 19th century antique Chinese pharmacy look with lots of fun esoteric visual stimulation. There is always a reason to break almost any rule.)

- Whatever look you choose for your clinic, make sure it communicates a healing message. You want your clinic to be a haven, a place that, by its very nature, supplements and nourishes yin, warms but calms yang, and rectifies stagnant qi.

- One way to connect with the community and use an element of artistic surprise in your clinic is to offer a local artist(s) a place to exhibit their work. Displays can change quarterly or semiannually. While there is a hassle factor with this idea, you get some potentially nice art in your clinic while becoming known as a team player in your community. Consider working with a group of local artists to organize a fundraising art-show event for a local non-profit. Everybody gets some free publicity, there are many people to help publicize the event, and lots of new folks visit your clinic!

▶ One-stop shopping

Some practitioners say that they don't want to have the hassle of selling things in their clinic or managing inventory. They may believe it is a conflict of interest to prescribe and then sell herbal medicinals in their clinic. While I applaud good ethics, the truth is that until Chinese herbal medicine is available by prescription in drugstores across North America, your patients have nowhere to go to acquire Chinese medicine other than your office. You are providing a service and helping your patients sort from among dozens of products at the health food store that may or may not be right for their pattern(s) of disharmony. See Section 3, Chapter 6 for considerable detail on this subject.

▶ An effective phone system

In the same way that an acupuncture channel connects outside stimuli to the inside of the body, your phone is one of your company's lifelines from the outside world to your checkbook, the "spleen-stomach" of your practice. The presence or absence of prompt, effective phone access can make or break your clinic. It does not matter how well you do the rest of your marketing or how good a clinician you are if no one can reach you by phone promptly or if the phone part of patient management is handled poorly. While I freely admit that the lack of availability and effective phone communications within our practitioner community is a pet peeve of mine, it is, truly, a vital element in your success or lack of it!

There are several elements to an effective phone system.

- **Availability**
  If you are not available by phone easily and reliably, you will lose business to those who are. Period. If you believe that you cannot afford office help for answering phones, confirming appointments, marketing assistance, and product ordering, get an answering service, a call-forwarding service that vibrates the cell phone which never leaves your body, or some other method of being able to get back in touch with callers within 10-15 minutes at the longest. That being said, we have heard the same story from practitioners ad infinitum

> **POWER POINT**
>
> **What can a skilled phone-answerer-office-manager do for your clinic?**
>
> We cannot stress enough what we hear from practitioners who have hired a staff person to help them manage their business. You are trained to treat patients and the power of your treatments is based on being able to focus. This is also where you can make the best income. Think about how much better work you could do if there were someone to answer your phone, manage product inventory, keep the office clean, help with outbound patient contact, help with insurance forms and other business correspondence, proofread anything you write before it goes out the door, greet your patients, handle patient payments, and make copies of charts, articles, and promotional materials. A really good office assistant can do all these things, allowing you to practice the skills you worked so hard to learn. Most seasoned practitioners tell us that they pay their office help as much as they possibly can because that help is so valuable. The $25-$40K this person costs you per year could earn you twice that much. Really. If you don't have any office help, make a short-term goal of hiring someone to help you as soon as possible. You won't be sorry.

that, "After I hired someone to manage my office and answer the phone, my practice doubled in a month." Think about it.

- **Courtesy**
  If you have never studied acting, sales, or patient management specifically, we suggest you consider taping yourself or your office staff and listening to how you sound or even taking some online courses in medical patient management.

Learning how to script your calls with potential new patients, angry patients, persistent telemarketers, and missed appointments, all while remaining absolutely courteous on your busiest days, is an acquired skill. Letting each caller know that you care about their needs and issues without being a pushover to everyone who calls requesting that you come in early, stay late, give a discount, buy their product, or otherwise make a special case for them is not something most of us are trained to do. However, we can tell you from personal experience that courtesy to every person who calls, every time, and effective patient management on the phone will go a long way toward helping you build your business. Just think about the last time you ordered a product from a catalog and the person on the other end of the line was tired, short, or monotone-voiced. Then think of a time when you spoke to someone on the phone who was helpful, knowledgeable, and you felt like they were in the room with you. Which company are you more likely to order from again?

- **Adequate numbers of lines**
  Online all the time? Go wifi and get fax software so that your computer becomes a fax. If a high-speed modem is your only option, those are usually separate from your phone line, but you still need two lines. That way, if you are on the phone with one patient, have an incoming fax or email, and another patient calling in all at the same time, the second phone line will at least ring. The important thing is that patients have as easy a time as possible getting in touch with you.

- **Using your phone to market directly**
  If you have a hold function on your phone, it is great to record a hold message to be played while someone is waiting. In many businesses this is merely music, but you could also tell patients about an upcoming class or event, a new herbal product you are selling that will help allergy or cold sufferers, or why they should schedule a treatment at the spring and

> **POWER POINT**
>
> When you or anyone on your office staff answers the phone, it's nice to say something like, "Thank you for calling White Crane Clinic. This is Sarah. How may I help you?" Or "Good afternoon. White Crane Clinic. Sarah speaking." Also, speak clearly and not too rapidly so people can understand what you said the first time. When your phone answerer (you or a staff person) speaks too fast, without good enunciation, or with a strong foreign accent, people may think they have reached a wrong number and hang up!

fall equinox. This same information could also be part of your after-hours answer recording as well as a link on your website home page.

- **Calling (or texting) your patients**
  Outbound calls (and texts) are an effective way to keep you and your services in your patients' minds. There are several legitimate reasons why you might call them, and most will appreciate the attention as it is not something they are used to from health professionals.
  - Courtesy calls (also called "bonding" calls) within 24 hours after a first treatment just to see how they responded to the treatment and if they have any questions.
  - A call after they have been using herbs for 3-5 days to see how they are doing or if they are responding as you feel they should (you may also ask them to call in for the same reason). This call also allows you to make dosage adjustments or schedule a short follow-up appointment.
  - A call after someone has not been in for six or more months to tell them about a new procedure you think could help their condition, just to check in and say hello, or tell them about a lecture you will be giving or a class you are going to teach that they might find interesting.

On the companion website you will find the names of several companies that offer business telephone-marketing tips, classes, and related services. One of the best is www.teldoc.com.

▶ Other internal marketing tips

- This one we got from an award-winning realtor. Whenever she sends out anything to a client, she closes the envelope with a colorful small sticker that says, "I always appreciate your referrals." Notice this is active, not passive voice, *i.e.*, it is personal from her to her client, visible but not aggressive. Or, you could make stickers that say something like, "Cold season is here! Ask about my favorite cold remedy." These little messages help keep you in your patient's mind in a pleasant way.

- Books and toys for children can make a mother's visit easier. Many of us have had the experience of the young child who wants to be on Mommy's lap and is inconsolable that she is on a table with pins sticking out of her. A good toy corner can be very helpful in such cases.

- Good signage is really important for people to find your clinic easily. It is always unfortunate when someone is twice as stressed as normal when they arrive five minutes late for their

---

POWER POINT

Make sure your patients know that you want and need their referrals and that referrals are as important as the checks they write! You can put up a sign in your waiting area or give out cards to satisfied patients and ask them to refer their friends and colleagues. Then find a way to reward your best referrers. (Yoga class coupons, movie certificates, free herbs or a free foot massage with their next appointment, a free book on Chinese medicine... Be creative.)

first appointment because there were no signs outside, in the lobby, on the door, or anywhere that helped them find you easily. We've all been through this type of annoying experience. Make sure this does not happen to your patients. Good signage prevents liver qi!

- If you use a cell phone to keep in contact with patients, keep it on silent vibrate and keep in on your body. That way you can leave the treatment room at the first convenient moment without disturbing your current patient's experience. Get a landline as soon as you can.

- A spotless, shiny bathroom is not optional. Give it a quick once-over every day and a serious cleaning at least once a week.

- Keep your reception area as tidy, artistic, and uncluttered as possible. That way people are more likely to experience your clinic as a calming and healing haven from start to finish.

- Remember that the way a patient is spoken to on the phone, as they enter, if they have to wait, and, most importantly, when they are paying and leaving is most effective if at least somewhat "scripted." This topic is discussed in more detail in the patient management chapter (Section 2, Chapter 13).

- Make sure the last thing each patient hears when departing from your clinic is, "Thank you for coming in." Remember that they don't have to be your patient. People like to know their business is appreciated.

- Ask each patient to sign a Release of Records form to get their records from other care givers. Some won't want to do it, but those who agree to do it have given you a good excuse to contact their doctor(s), which is a marketing opportunity. See the Power Point on page 420 for more detail on this subject.

HOW TO DO A FREE, 15-MINUTE CONSULTATION

A short, free consultation can serve a number of good purposes and can be a powerful marketing tool.

- Start with a link on your website saying "click here to ask about a free consultation to see if acupuncture may help you." You can also put this statement on your business card or offer these to attendees at lectures you give.
- If possible, schedule consultations during clinic hours when at least one patient will be coming or going.
- Use a standard form with very little on it: name, phone, and email address, major complaint, duration of complaint, what other therapies they have sought for the complaint.
- Keep "diagnostics" short. Perhaps take the pulse or just look at the tongue to confirm/deny your hypothesis based on person's age, sex, body type, and complexion.
- Ask if they have questions they'd like to ask. Keep your answers short and simple. Don't let yourself or your visitor ramble.
- If this is a patient you feel comfortable with and think you can help, make a simple statement like, *"I have treated people with your condition successfully in the past. (or) Your condition is definitely treatable by acupuncture. We start with a thorough diagnosis and a course of 6-8 sessions over a month. I can give you a brochure/some research to take home about what OM says about your condition and information about our clinic. Would you like me to see how soon we can get you an appointment?"*
- If the person's energy feels strange to you, you can tell them you don't think you can help them!

Then show them around the office (if there is anything else to show), give them appropriate educational literature, and send them on their way or introduce them to the front desk person to make an appointment. If they don't schedule on the spot, send them an occasional email with a link to some research, your e-newsletter, or an invitation to your next free lecture.

▶ You are your marketing

As we are fond of saying, "Every minute is a marketing minute." This is especially true when you are working in your clinic. Your services, your skill, your demeanor, and the way your clinic feels, smells, looks, and acts are the most important part of any marketing effort you can create. You cannot afford to be lazy with regard to any of these points. Take classes and continue to improve your skills. Make sure people feel that coming to your office is like entering a safe and healing space. If your clinic is humane, yet run as an efficient, clean, well-oiled machine with just a touch of magic, you are ahead of the game as a marketer. That is why I always tell graduating students that running a private practice requires the passion of a Romeo, the patience of a Saint Francis, and the intellectual curiosity of a Socrates.

POINTS TO PONDER FROM CHAPTER 2

- You and your clinic itself are the most important aspects of your marketing. Don't skimp on how your clinic feels, looks, or operates.

- There are lots of other ways to market from inside your clinic: lots of available educational information for your patients, excellent and prompt telephone customer service, engaging artistry and aesthetics in your clinic, one-stop shopping convenience, good signage, spotless bathrooms, and toys for kids.

- Your telephone is your lifeline. Make sure you are easily available, your phone patient management skills are honed, you have adequate incoming lines, and your hold message or after-hours recording includes simple marketing messages.

- A successful clinic is both humane and run like a well-oiled machine, but with just a touch of magic.

Community Team Builders and Marketing 3

This chapter is about "outside" marketing, which means everything from pounding the pavement in your neighborhood handing out cards, volunteering for community projects, using the same service people and companies in your town over and over and getting to know them well, to writing articles for the local media or giving free speeches to every possible organization that will let you in the door. While we truly believe that inside marketing (Chapter 2 in this section) is fundamentally the most important in your overall marketing efforts, few new practitioners can grow a full practice without ever doing any outside marketing. No matter how great your clinic or your skills, you have to do some things to let people know about you in the initial few years of your professional life.

> **PRACTITIONER POINTER**
>
> "My experience has shown me that networking is very important. I tend to be shy, but I've forced myself to be as social as possible, and every event I attend helps my practice to grow. I took an acupuncturist out to dinner when I first arrived here, which was a big investment for me at the time. That relationship has grown since and now her office regularly refers patients to me. And she provides moral support and encouragement!"
>
> —Elizabeth Liddell
> Philadelphia, PA

Below we have included all the ideas we can think of or have heard about that can be effective for practitioners of Chinese medicine and acupuncture. Not every idea will work for everyone, but there are some very effective marketing ideas here. Unless you are really not meant for this work, some of these ideas will appeal to you and bring patients in your door.

▶ Effective pavement-pounding methods

Above we said that one good strategy is to walk concentric circles around your clinic in a five block radius and see what is there. Take a notebook and pen with you. There are all types of marketing possibilities here. You could:

- At every business location find out if you can post a flyer on the staff break room bulletin board.

- Is there a service or product from a business down the street that you can help promote? See if you can create a you-scratch-my-back-I'll scratch-yours relationship, where you can sell their products in your clinic or give out their cards and vice versa.

- At every company that has more than 25 employees there is likely to be a human resources (HR) person who is in charge of medical insurance, Workers' Comp referrals, payroll cafeteria plans, and other personnel services. It's a great idea to meet these people, offer them a free treatment, provide them with educational materials and brochures, or bring them a complete presentation folder about your clinic services.

- If you are specializing in any specific niche market, note every business that has any relationship to your specialty. For example, if you do acu-facelifts or dermatology, you want to make sure that any and all day spas, beauty salons, or beauty supply retail outlets have your cards and brochures. Perhaps you could do a trade with the owner… treatments in trade for putting your cards out next to their cash register? Perhaps you could do a free in-service lecture for their entire staff on how your services complement theirs?

- Introduce yourself to the wait staff at every restaurant and coffee shop that you can. Give them cards and tell them you'd love their referrals. Then pick one or two that you frequent as often as you can. Get to know everyone there on a first name basis. Go whenever it is the least busy and start conversations with them. That is to say, become their friend. One practitioner we know gets over 50 referrals per year from one coffee shop near his clinic.

- If you are in a large office building, make sure every receptionist at every office in the building has your card and that you take the time to learn about all his or her aches and pains and anything else he or she is willing to share. If there are MDs or DCs in your building, are there ways that you could enhance their services to patients without being a threat? Find out if the office staff would be interested in a lunchtime in-service about acupuncture. Provide sandwiches, drinks, (maybe some *ju hua* tea?) and let the staff convince the MDs in their clinic to let you educate them about your services.

- If you are in a residential neighborhood, write a short letter of introduction about your clinic and leave it in every screen door. Offer them a "good neighbor" discount on their first treatment or a free consultation. Put a smiling photo of yourself on this letter or brochure. Or, even better for more courageous souls, knock on every door, introduce yourself and offer them a brochure and a free consultation at the new clinic in the neighborhood.

▶ Corporate marketing strategies

If you are in an area with a few large companies (100+ employees), it is really useful to find ways to connect with them. Again, the HR department is a good place to start.

- Find out the name of the head of the HR department and send or bring in a presentation folder to them. Try to get an appointment to find out what ways you might serve the company's employees. Find out what insurance company they use and whether their policy reimburses for acupuncture. What Worker's Comp insurance carrier do they use? Will they share their insurance rep's name with you?

- Do they have a company newsletter and would they like some free, short articles on relevant topics?

- Do they have any in-service lectures on health for their employees? Could you give one of these on stress management, repetitive strain injuries, managing low back pain, graceful aging, preventing the common cold and flu, etc.?

POWER POINT

Tips for writing for corporate newsletters
- Keep your article to a half-page unless the editor asks for something longer.
- Use bullet points for things like, "Five Tips for a Healthy Holiday Season."
- Don't use jargon, Chinese words, or difficult-to-read words and sentences.
- Don't write in long sentences with lots of commas, clauses, phrases, etc.
- Keep articles friendly and think about the "what's in it for the reader" message.
- All you want in return is your name and contact info at the bottom of the article.
- If they don't ask you for a follow-up article for next quarter, take the initiative and call the editor to see if there has been any feedback and if they want another article. Better yet, bring them three or four short articles all at one time.
- Find out what digital formats they prefer and send them both a digital file and a hard copy for proofing.

▶ Community participation

Almost every city and town in the U.S. has a myriad of opportunities for community involvement. You can get yourself on all sorts of committees for fundraising, riverfront cleanup, hospital auxiliary, homeless shelter, school music program, AIDS relief, battered women, humane society... the list goes on and on. The more you can participate in the community, the better known your name will become. People instinctively like to buy products and services from people they know and trust. While you also must create trust by running a really great clinic with effective services humanely and efficiently delivered, in your early years of practice you will also need to find ways to weave yourself firmly into the warp and weft of your chosen community. And who knows, you may make some wonderful friends while you are building your practice. Here are just a few ideas.

Health fairs or community fairs

These are tricky, but they can be effective if you really work them and don't just stand around behind your table under your pop-up tent, smiling. If you live in a small town or city, these are probably more effective than in a large city. Here are a couple of ideas that have appeal.

One woman gets her patients to come and be treated for free. She actually sets up appointments for them as if it were a regular day, each one 45 minutes apart. She gives simple pro-forma treatments, nothing complicated and she does not do an interview with them, just a treatment. But there's lots of rubbernecking as people stop to talk to her and to her patients while they are on the table with needles sticking out. She then gets the benefit of on-the-spot referrals from her patients telling passersby how great she is as well as the fascination-with-needles curiosity factor working in her favor. She has people to talk with all day, gives out lots of cards and brochures, and definitely gets patients from these events.

Consider bringing a fishbowl and put a sign on it saying "put in your business card for a prize drawing." You should give away something really good, not just a free treatment. A great piece of Chinese artwork that you brought back from China could be attractive, a package of wonderful general health-promoting herbs that you normally sell in your clinic, or a set of Chinese medical self-care products. Your prize should be worth at least $100. Also have some second or third place prizes that you display on the table, such as an interesting book on Chinese medicine for the general reader or two bottles of AllerEase® for hay fever sufferers if it happens to be either spring or fall. This is all to create traffic at your booth and build your mailing list. What you will find is that if you have 2-3 people hanging out at your booth, more folks are likely to stop to see what the other people stopped for. After you pick your prize-winners at the end of the weekend, you use the rest of the business cards as contact information for later. After the fair, send a postcard to each person who stopped by your booth and left a card or signed up for the newsletter. Thank them for stopping and let them know that they did not win the prize but that, if they have any more questions about Chinese medicine or acupuncture, you'd be most happy to hear from them on the phone during regular business hours. If you want to be really aggressive, you can tell them that the card is good for their first bottle of herbs free when they come in for an initial examination and treatment.

These events are easier (and cheaper for the booth rental!) if you share the booth with three or four other practitioners working in two-by-two shifts of a few hours each. Here are some more ideas for creating traffic and conversation.

- Stand in front of your booth, not behind it. Wear an easy-to-read name-tag and a shirt with you clinic name monogrammed on it. Keep your cards or a basket of giveaway goodies (pens, herb samples, magnets, etc.) handy. Smile and start as many conversations as you can.

- Bring an acupuncture doll and different sizes of needles in a case or laminated onto something. A display of various bulk Chinese herbs can be a visual attraction.

- If you have a newsletter, make sure to have a sign-up sheet on your table for anyone interested. Put up an easy-to-read little plexiglass sign that says, "Sign Up Here for a Free Health Tips Newsletter."

- Give out gingersnaps and licorice ropes, explaining that they have Chinese herbs in them or have a large dish of Chinese "trail mix" with lycium berries, black date pieces, and walnuts.

- Invest in some brochures on different conditions that you treat well. Don't just leave them on the table but actively hand them to people. (Make sure your contact info is on each one!)

- If your fair is near Thanksgiving or Christmas, you might give away little tubes of Curing Pills and put up a sign explaining how to use them after consuming a large meal to avoid indigestion.

- If there are several practitioners sharing a booth, you can do pro-forma treatments on each other because people like to see the needles. They will inevitably ask, "Doesn't it hurt?" to the person on the table.

- Consider giving free pulse diagnosis sessions for 10 minutes each, explaining just one simple thing to each person about their health.

- If you put up a large sign above the booth, don't make the sign say "Ace Acupuncture Clinic." The sign should have a what's-in-it-for-me-the-passerby message like "Acupuncture Works! Any Questions?" or simply "Improve Your Health Today!"

- Make sure all your current patients and friends know that you are doing the fair. Ask them to stop by with their friends and family.

CHAPTER 3 | Community Team Builders and Marketing

POWER POINT

Script for a health fair

"Hello, I'm Honora. I'm an licensed acupuncturist here in Boulder. I see you're looking at the low back pain brochure. (Hand them the brochure if they did not already pick it up.) Do you have back pain?"

Then you let the person talk for as long as they need to and don't interrupt. When they have finished, ask several questions:

1. How long have you had this?
2. How frequently do you get the pain (or other symptoms)?
3. When did the problem start?
4. On a scale of 1-10, what is the intensity of your pain?
5. What do you think is causing this problem?
6. What other doctors have you seen about this condition?
7. Did their treatment help you?
8. What else have you tried?
9. What will you do if this gets worse?
10. Is it bad enough that you want to solve the problem if you could?

Then, if it is a condition that you feel capable of or have experience treating, tell them that you think you may be able to give them some relief. Give them your card and a brochure and take their name and phone or email in order to follow up if they are not willing or able to schedule an appointment right then and there.

The key here, no matter how you set up your booth or how you staff it, is that you have to really "work" the event. If you do this right, you will be tired after a few hours, but you will get lots of people stopping by, signing up for your mailing list, asking questions, taking cards, and, hopefully, becoming your patients. One final word, don't do this type of event if you are shy.

Volunteering our way to success

Are you a great organizer? If so, consider organizing an event (walk-a-thon, food drive, acupuncture fundraisers at your clinic) for your favorite charity. Involve other local acupuncturists or even your state association. This is a great way to get media coverage and, as a group, promote our profession! If you cannot find the juice to create an event yourself, participate in as many such events as you have time for. All the people you work with, march with, run or walk with, call on the phone, and raise money from are prospective patients. People want to do business with others who are active in promoting good things in their community. So get out there and get some other acupuncturists to join in with you! This is how we all succeed together!

After any committee or event that you work on, follow up on those connections. After you've worked on the breast cancer walk-a-thon committee (or whatever), send follow-up notes to everyone you worked with that say something like:

Dear Sally,

Just a note to tell you how much I enjoyed working with you in the last month on the walk-a-thon. I feel great about what we were able to accomplish together. If I can ever be of service to you or your family when it comes to your health, or if you ever have questions about my acupuncture services, please don't hesitate to call. I'd be happy to speak with you. Thanks again for your great energy working on the walk-a-thon committee.

Yours sincerely,
Honora Wolfe

Remember to include your business card.

> **POWER POINT**
>
> Be paranoid in reverse. Assume that people are plotting to make you happy and help you to fulfill your dreams. What you believe matters!

Playing the media card

There are lots of ways to interact effectively with the media. Get the names of every health editor, feature editor, city editor, or Sunday magazine editor at every newspaper in your area you can find. Send them a presentation folder with a cover letter or an email with a link to your blog or website offering your services as an authority on TCM and acupuncture. Tell them you are always happy to hear from them or write an article or column for their section of the paper. If you have had any articles published elsewhere (like those corporate newsletters we mentioned above), send them copies. Offer to have them come to your clinic for a tour or a treatment.

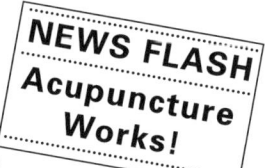

Always had a fantasy about your own TV or radio show? It is not so very hard to get on cable TV or public radio. With a short, effective audio-video demo (YouTube?), you could have a talk show on the radio about health-related issues. If someone in your town already has such a show, you can at least get booked in as an expert once or twice a year. The same is true of cable TV. Call the local public TV stations and talk to the manager about what the possibilities are and what hoops you'd need to jump through to do this. Even if you get taped for a show that airs at 2 AM, you could do "Health Tips for Insomniacs" as your theme! If you want to get on a local or even a nationally syndicated talk show as a guest, do some digging on the internet and send out information to every producer you can find. Of course it helps if you are a published author or have some special expertise about a relevant in-the-news topic, but it could be worth it to fish in this pond. Somebody has to be the expert the next time Oprah wants to talk about Chinese medicine, so why not you?

If you want to contact media folks by phone, use odd times of the day. These people often work weird schedules, but the gatekeepers who work for them work regular 9-5 schedules. Thus, if you call at 7:30 AM or PM, who knows who will answer and what access you may have? If using email, keep messages short and to the point. This may be a good time for snail mail, by the way, which might get noticed since it is less and less commonly used.

If you have something really exciting to share and the chops to do it well, you can contact every syndicated columnist in the U.S. (almost). *Editor and Publisher* magazine has a list they sell very inexpensively (949-660-6150). Just make sure whatever you send them is professionally done. You can also go to www.radio-locator.com for a list of radio stations and then contact producers with your great idea.

If you want to be an expert on a specific subject (improved sports performance, preventing anorexia, treating PTSD or brain injuries, whatever is currently the hot health topic), go to your local/regional paper and TV station websites and find the names of relevant editors (health, special features, modern living, etc.) and send them a short, powerful email message. Keep it to three paragraphs max and use powerful words and sentences to get across your message. If possible, it's even better to reference or tie to a previous story that this journalist has written or covered. So do some homework first... and never use attachments. Give them the guts of what you have to say in a sound bite. Deliver it in a way that makes their job easier and, who knows, you might become their main contact for alternative health for years to come.

What skills could you teach?
Can you teach t'ai chi, yoga, qi gong, cooking, calligraphy, or anything related to health or Chinese medicine? If so, find a way to teach it in your community. This could be through the local community college, YMCA, the city recreation department, a lifelong learning clearinghouse, or a local related business. If you are good and you do this regularly, at least some if not most of your students will become patients at some point. Remember,

everybody will be somebody's patient someday. Why shouldn't they be yours?

> **POINTS TO PONDER FROM CHAPTER 3**
>
> - At least when you are starting out, you will need to do some proactive outside marketing. This may include events, committees, health fairs, volunteering, writing articles, teaching classes, becoming a media darling, giving lectures, and following up on those contacts.
>
> - Search out and make contact with the human resources departments of all companies with more than 100 employees. Can you write for their newsletter, give free classes or talks to their employees, post your business cards on the break room bulletin board? Find out what type of insurance they have and if it reimburses for acupuncture. How can you get regular Worker's Comp referrals from these companies?
>
> - People like to do business with people they know and like. (Repeat this phrase to yourself regularly!)
>
> - Media folks are always looking for a new story and a new angle. If you find ways to help them write the story or gain access to something of interest, you will get in the news and could become a regular 'source' for articles on complementary and alternative medicine.
>
> - Do you like to write, teach, organize events, or give public lectures? Consider your talents carefully and how you can give your best back to your community. That's how new patients will find you.
>
> - Never go anywhere without your business cards, don't be shy, and remember that everyone is someone's patient someday.

Building & Using a Mailing List | 4

Whether you are a tiny one-person show or a large, multi-practice clinic, a good mailing list is an important asset to your business. This, of course, means both an email and regular mailing list. You can and should start on this very early ... even while you are still in school. Your goal should be a minimum of 200 names for a postal mailing list and as many names as you can get your hands on if you use an email list. In either case, more is always better.

➤ Where to start

There are several ways you can collect mailing list names and contact information.

- Ask your friends or family in the area where you are going to practice for likely referrals. Ask your patients for referrals of friends who would be happy to receive information about your newsletter, classes, lectures, etc.

- When you give a free lecture, do a health fair, or attend any other public event where it is possible, put out a mailing list sign-up sheet. Be sure to put on the top of the sheet what kinds of things you will be sending. Also put a statement saying that you never rent or sell your mailing list to other companies or organizations.

- When you teach a class for a community college, pass around the same type of sign-up sheet as described above.

- Your intake forms packet should include one giving you permission to send cards, emails, or other general information from your clinic (HIPAA requires this now anyway). Explain on the form the kinds of things you will be sending and that you don't sell or rent your list to any other company or organization. If a patient signs this form, you have been given permission to include them on your list.

- Are there local businesses that serve the same niche of people that you serve? If so, include these businesses on your mailing list. The same is true of local MDs or other health providers. While you might not send them every single card, blog, or newsletter that you publish, there will be occasions when you want to include them in a mailing/emailing.

- Look for the names of local/regional newspaper editors, TV and radio producers, or other media folks who should be on your list. Keeping in regular touch with these types of people can lead to all sorts of unforeseen marketing opportunities.

- Mailing lists grow faster than you might think. Keep a hard copy file for cards and sign-up sheets, but put them in a digital file as soon as you can and always keep a backup!

- If you write articles for a local paper, parenting newsletter, corporate newsletter, chronic fatigue support group website, or wherever, your contact information and the fact that you publish a newsletter, recipe-of-the-month, health tips articles, etc. should be at the end of every article. Say something like, "Honora Wolfe is a licensed acupuncturist in Boulder, CO. You can sign up for her free Health-Tip-of-the-Month newsletter by sending your contact info to honora@bluepoppy.com or calling 303-447-8372."

The point I'm making here is that there are lots of ways to build a mailing list. Now let's discuss what to do with those names and addresses.

➤ Using your mailing list

This makes me think of the statement, "Vote early and often." The greatest mailing list in the world won't do you any good if you don't use it. On the other hand, you need to consider

> **POWER POINT**
>
> Even when people sign up for something, they may change their mind or not even remember that they signed up. If it feels like spam or they decide they are not interested, you are required by web etiquette to give them a way to opt out. When you do email newsletters, always include a "Click Here if you wish to unsubscribe from this newsletter" link at the bottom of your letter, article, or announcement. Make sure you or your staff takes care of any opt out requests promptly… the same for your postal mailing list.

timing your mailings for budgetary reasons, as well as in relationship to what is happening in your community.

- Divide your list into categories. You may do a mailing to MDs or DCs that does not go to patients. You may want to do a media-only mailing of a press release or offer yourself for interviews on a timely, in-the-news subject. Try a corporate mailing offering free lectures for their brown-bag lunch series. You may want to divide your list based on whether people are or are not already patients. This is true whether the list is for postal mailings or email blasts.

- Speaking of dividing your mailing list into specific groups, if you use Microsoft Access or Excel or another major database or mailing list program, there are many ways to subdivide or segment any list. You can create various categories when you set up your digital file. Then, when you want to print labels or envelopes or merge a letter, you can choose from those specific categories whom to include in the mailing.

- Of course emailings are cheaper by far than postal mailings even if you use an email service. Make sure all your sign-up sheets and forms have a line for email addresses. Most online interface software such as Firefox, Explorer, Outlook, Safari, etc., provide a way to create large email groups. However, remember that online privacy is a huge issue for everyone. Whatever software you use has to be able to send to each person as if they were the only one, while all the other people in the group are receiving "blind" copies. There are lots of companies that will manage your email list and send mass emailings for you, on a schedule or one-time only. (Check out MailChimp, ConstantContact, iContact to start.)

- Start using your mailing list right away. One of the most important principles of marketing is to have a good message, say it well, and say it *often*. Not all the plums on any tree ripen at the same rate. But shame on you if you are not there when each one does ripen. The only way to "be there" is to stay in touch regularly with anyone and everyone who has given you permission to do so or who is a public entity and does not have to give you permission. Ideally, that means you send out a postcard, email, e-newsletter, course announcement, or other missive every 8-12 weeks to some segment of your mailing list.

- Keep these cards, emails, press releases, and newsletter articles short and sweet, at least most of the time. People don't have time to read a lot. And, very important, always try to craft a headline that explains what's in it for them if they do read the whole thing. Headlines should be as funny, compelling, dynamic, poignant, or outrageous as possible. Then you can explain (quickly and to the point) the message you really want to get across.

- Here's a fun email newsletter idea for good cooks or nutrition aficionados (we mentioned this idea in Chapter 2 of this section). Create a Recipe-of-the-Season newsletter or a Nutrition News newsletter. The entire newsletter is simply a recipe with an introduction on why you like this recipe, its nutritional or Chinese medicinal qualities, etc. Or you can write about a specific herb or formula (in easy-to-understand layman's terms) and why you like it for the current season. This type of message allows you to send out something fun and useful while simply staying in the patient's (or potential patient's) mind... no advertising at all here. As we said before, everybody becomes someone's patient someday.

- Mail out an autumn email about preventing the common cold and winter flu. Something like, "Why Does Everyone Need Three Bottles of XYZ Chinese Cold Remedy?" or "What Chinese Medicine Makes a Great Stocking Stuffer?" This is followed by something like, "You can stop a cold or flu before it starts if you have one bottle at work, one in the medicine chest, and one in your car's glove box. Buy three bottles and get 10% off. This offer is good through 12/15/XX." This could also be a reminder to come in for an autumn constitutional strengthening/flu prevention treatment or treatment series.

- You can do the same thing for spring or fall allergies, post-Halloween sugar blues, or post-holiday digestive tune-ups. Or you can tie your reminder to Breast Cancer Prevention Month or Diabetes Month. The possibilities are endless.

As you can see, the point here is to find reasons to stay in touch with your patients, your possible future patients, people with businesses related to the niche market you want to serve (bicycle clubs, women's groups, skin care spas, etc.), the media, possible referrers such as MDs, DCs, DOs, PTs, CMTs, and RNs, and make your messages something they will be happy to receive because of useful content, humor, or because they already love you. A mailing list is a very powerful and important part of your marketing toolkit!

CHAPTER 4 | Building & Using a Mailing List

POINTS TO PONDER FROM CHAPTER 4

- A good mailing list is one of your best communication tools to potential patients or referrers.

- There are lots of ways to build up a mailing list. We've listed eight possibilities.

- A mailing list does you no good unless you use it often. We list lots of ideas and you could easily come up with a dozen more.

- The chapter is only five pages long; we suggest you read the whole thing.

Creating Your Presentation Folder | 5

A presentation folder (PF) is a public relations tool with many uses. It describes, formally, beautifully, and in organized detail, everything you want any specific group or person to know about you and your clinic services. There are several things that should always be included in a PF and many optional pieces. A PF can be formal and slick, like a corporate media kit, or done more simply on your office computer and inkjet printer. Either way, we encourage you to create one and update it regularly as your professional situation changes. You will find many uses for this tool.

➤ What goes in a presentation folder?

Your folder should include at least the following pieces:
- A cover letter explaining why you are sending them this information and how you hope they will respond to it.
- A curriculum vitae (CV)
- Information flyer or brochure about your clinic and the services available, hours of operation, and prices
- Your business card
- A map with directions to your facility
- Letters of reference from a patient or another practitioner (MD, DC, PT, DO, JD, other professional)

Optional pieces for your presentation folder:
- A short, nontechnical book on Oriental medicine
- Prescription pad
- Articles from magazines or newspapers about acupuncture or Oriental medicine
- Articles or research papers you have written on any subject related to Oriental or alternative medicine
- Your clinic mission statement

- Articles or brochures about specific conditions (*e.g.,* sports medicine if you are sending the PF to an orthopedist)
- Printed research supporting the ability of acupuncture and/or Oriental medicine to treat a specific condition effectively
- Any other relevant or interesting information about you, published articles about your clinic from the newspaper
- Copies of any letter received from a satisfied patient regarding how much your services helped their condition
- A small notepad with your name and phone number
- A magnet with your clinic name and phone number or a business card magnet
- Evidence of malpractice insurance for your practice

Remember, most of these pieces can also be used for a website!

Okay, let's go back and talk about each of these elements separately.

> **Writing an effective cover letter**

A cover letter should be short and to the point. A good cover letter can mean the difference between someone actually reading through your PF or not bothering to look further. Below is a sample cover letter. This same letter and others specific to different audiences are on this book's website and can be downloaded and tinkered with to your heart's content.

What you will notice about this and other letters on the website is that these are one page, to the point, specific, and friendly. They tell the reader exactly how you hope they will respond, *i.e.,* they give the reader a next step to take that is low risk: look through the PF and call for more information. Other options in this type of letter are to offer a free luncheon in-service, times that you are available by phone, or references upon request. Proofread! Consider creating different cover letters for different uses. Letters to the media, other acupuncturists, or corporate HR managers would, of course, be completely different in content.

VITAL HEALTH ACUPUNCTURE CLINIC
SARAH SMITH, L.AC.
1234 FOREST STREET
DES MOINES, IA 60000
515-123-4567

August 14, 20XX

Des Moines Health & Orthopedics
Attention Dr. John Doe
4444 Main St.
Des Moines, IA, 60000

Dear Dr. Doe,

My name is Sarah Smith and I am a Licensed Acupuncturist in the state of Iowa, certified by the Iowa Board of Medical Examiners.

I have recently relocated my clinic to the above address and would be happy to accept referrals from your office for patients whose conditions may not be responding well to traditional healthcare options. I offer safe, competent, and effective care with acupuncture, Chinese herbal medicine, and nutritional counseling to help people with problems in the following areas:
- pre- and post-surgical care
- pain management
- migraines and chronic headaches
- chronic insomnia
- environmental sensitivities and food allergies
- fibromyalgia and chronic fatigue immune deficiency syndrome

Enclosed is a packet of information about the benefits of acupuncture and Chinese medicine. I would love to offer my services to your patients and to work with you to improve their chances at full recovery from the conditions listed above. My clinic is also able to provide documented research on a variety of other healthcare concerns and proof of malpractice insurance upon request.

I believe that the integration of our two medicines is the future of modern health care and I look forward to being of service to you and your patients. Please feel free to contact me at any time with questions or requests for further information.

Yours sincerely,

Sarah Smith, L.Ac.

▶ The curriculum vitae or CV

A curriculum vitae means, basically, the "curriculum" of your life or what you have done with it. It is short, preferably one page long, and mentions only the most important aspects of your professional history. There is a sample CV in the Marketing Examples on the website that you can download and imitate. There are also websites and books that can help you do a really good CV. Basically, you need to include the following:

1. Your name and contact information at the top.

2. Educational history. This includes your BA or BS undergraduate degree, any advanced degrees, your acupuncture school certification, and other professional training certifications that are relevant. Do not put dates, but do put them in chronological order.

3. Licenses and credentials. Here you will list your NCCAOM certification, your state license, Red Cross first aid training, certification in Clean Needle Technique, and any other licenses (nursing, massage, midwifery, psychotherapy) that you have.

4. Professional experience. If you are a brand new graduate, you may use the college clinic as one listing. Again, put no dates. If you have other professional experience in another field put that down. If you are young and were waiting tables or tending bar, we suggest putting down something like, "Consultant to the Food Industry." If you were cleaning hotel rooms, put "Consultant to the Hotel Industry." You may need to be a little creative if you don't have a lot of professional experience at anything.

5. Societies and memberships. Are you a member of Rotary, Kiwanis, Big Brother, or the Chamber of Commerce in your town? If so, by all means include that information here. Have you joined your state professional association or a national professional association such as AAAOM? It looks very good

to be a member of a few associations, so consider joining. Many associations get discounts from various professional product suppliers, which could easily pay for the membership each year.

6. Publications. At least list a couple of papers you wrote in school. If you have written for your state professional association newsletter, a corporate newsletter, a local newspaper, regular blogs, or any other publication, list it here.

That's it. Be concise, spell out acronyms such as NCCAOM because no one outside the profession knows what they mean, and leave out dates. Proofread everything to make sure spelling is correct. If you are a lousy speller, get someone(s) else to proof it for you. Actually that advice goes for every piece you create for your PF!

▶ What is the definition of a good business card?

I get asked to critique a lot of practitioners' business cards, and have created a list of what's helpful and what's not from a marketing point of view. There is still lots of room for interpretation here, but these are the basics.

1. Your business card is your calling card and should be easy to read. Don't make people work to find the information they want. That means using an easy-to-read typeface. We suggest that you stay away from *Flowery*, **Chinesey**, or 𝔥𝔦𝔤𝔥𝔩𝔶 𝔰𝔱𝔶𝔩𝔦𝔷𝔢𝔡 typefaces. Pick fonts that allow people to find and read the information immediately. Don't use more than two different typefaces on one card.

2. Your name is the most important piece of information.

3. Your phone number is the second most important piece of information. Don't make it smaller than 11 point type and make its placement on the card prominent enough to find in an instant.

4. Email address, regular address, and website address if you have one, are the next most important pieces of information on your card. If you have a fax number, include it as well.

5. If you have a logo, a color scheme, or a USP (see Section 2, Chapter 1) for your clinic, these help identify your clinic, especially if they are repeated on your signage, brochures, or other written promotional pieces.

6. On the back of the card, you might include a map to your clinic, hours of operation, or a "Your Next Appointment Is" section.

7. If you don't have a logo, it's really nice to do a photo of yourself on your card. When people meet you at a public fundraising event or health fair and find your card two months later, your photo helps them remember the conversation they had with you.

8. In terms of papers, use a nice textured card stock or high gloss stock for your card. If you put your photo on the card, always use high gloss stock.

9. We don't suggest plastic cards. They're cute but people cannot write on them.

▶ Creating a prescription pad

Most of us have had the experience of being in a doctor's office and the doctor wanting to refer us to a specialist. Behind their appointment counter, the office staff person checking you out looked through a pile of prescription pads and tore off one saying, "Here is the name of the specialist Dr. Smith wants you to see." They may even have made the appointment for you right while you were there.

In the world of medicine, practitioners refer patients to each other all the time. It is simply standard operating procedure. If a

SECTION FOUR: MARKETING YOUR PRACTICE

referring office has a prescription pad from your office, you are more likely to be able to participate in this network.

What should be on a prescription pad?
These are pretty simple. We have included one sample below and a couple other samples on the website. Basically you want "Acupuncture Prescription" at the top, your name and contact information next, then the patient's name, date of the referral, diagnosis, space for any specific requests from the referring practitioner, and the name and contact phone for the referring practitioner. It should not be larger than one-half page, but one-quarter page is also fine. If you don't want to list all the modalities and procedures, just leave an empty space for the physician to write something like "evaluate and treat."

Once you have a digital file for a prescription pad, take or email the file to your chosen printer and have them print 100 pads, 20-25 sheets to a pad. Like your business cards, give these out liberally to any other practitioner who will refer to you, even if you have not sent them or don't need to send them a PF.

Your name and address here
Acupuncture Prescription

Patient Name: _____ Phone: ( ) _____ Date: ___/___/___

Primary Diagnosis: _____

Secondary Diagnosis: _____

Instructions/Precautions: _____

Frequency of Treatment: _____ /wk   Duration of Treatment:: _____ wks   Re-check with Doctor: _____ wks

Treatment Plan   Evaluate and Treat as Necessary ☐

Modalities ☐	Procedures ☐	Exercises ☐	Functional Rehab Prog ☐
☐ Heat	☐ Myofascial Release	☐ Flexibility	☐ Knee
☐ Ice	☐ Massage	☐ Strength	☐ Cervical
☐ Electrical Stimulation	☐ Traction (Mechan/Manual)	☐ Endurance/Cardio	☐ Shoulder
	☐ Cerv ☐ Lumb ☐ Spinal	☐ Trunk Stabilization	☐ Lumbar
☐ TENS Trial	☐ Acupuncture	☐ Posture/Body Mech	☐ Hand
☐ Interferential Trial	☐ Pilates	☐ Home Program	☐ Other:
		☐ Gait Training	
		☐ Therapeutic Exercise	Evaluations ☐

Referring Physician: _____

➤ **Clinic brochures. The byword is keep it simple!**
Your clinic brochure needs to grab the reader's attention within a two-second perusal. That really is all the time you have. Following a few simple rules will make it more likely that anyone will actually read what you spent so much time to write.

1. Your headline must be a what's-in-it-for-me statement that grabs attention because it responds to a need or problem. That means don't put the name of your clinic or a picture of your clinic on the front. Or, if you must put your name on the front, put it at the bottom of the front panel. A headline like, "Post-op Patients Return to Normal in 50% Less Time with Regular Acupuncture," "Chinese Medicine Treats Insomnia with No Side Effects," or, "Modern Research Shows Relief for Menopausal Women with Chinese Medicine," is likely to get the MDs or HR folks you are trying to reach to actually read the rest of your words. Of course you will need to quote some research to support your statements, but such research is available on a wide variety of subjects.

2. On your general clinic brochure, put a photo of you treating someone on the inside or the back. If you don't have enough text for a three panel fold brochure, a two panel fold can be just as effective.

3. Use a serifed typeface for the body copy of your brochure (such as Times Roman, Century Schoolbook, Garamond, or Goudy) and a sans serifed typeface for the headlines (**Futura,** Arial, **Univers**). Serifed faces are easier to read for lengthy body copy, sans serifed faces pop out if used sparingly for headlines and subheadlines.

4. It is usually easier to read text lines that are at least three inches across and not more than four inches across and at least 11 points tall. Also, the longer the line, the larger the typesize and the more space between lines (called leading)

you will need. It is also easier to read text that is flush left or right, not justified on both sides (see below).

Notice that the headline below is bold, large, and sans-serifed. The body text in the first paragraph below is flush left, ragged right, and 11 points tall. It is easy on the eye.

What Is Chinese Medicine & How Does It Work?

Chinese medicine is the oldest, professional, continually practiced, literate medicine in the world. This medical system's written literature stretches back almost 2,500 years. And currently 1/4 of the world's population makes use of it. One can say that modern Western and traditional Chinese medicines are the two dominant medical systems in the world today.

Notice that the paragraph below is justified on both sides, causing "rivers" of uneven white spacing between the words, as often seen in the newspaper. It is harder to read than the paragraph above.

Isn't Chinese Medicine Just a System of Folk Healing?

No. This system has been created by some of the best educated and brightest scholars in Chinese history. These scholars have recorded their theories and clinical experiences from generation to generation in literally thousands of books...

The message here is, as much as you can, design your brochure to make it easy to read.

5. Bullet points get read first. Short paragraphs are more likely to get read than long ones.

6. Don't use too much Chinese medical jargon. On the other hand, don't write as though you were speaking to a first-grader.

7. Proofread by reading forward for context errors, then backward for spelling errors, because the eye tends to see the spelling of words the way the mind thinks they should be.

8. It is useful to have one brochure about your clinic and others about specific subjects or disease conditions.

9. If you cannot do your own clinic brochure, see if you can trade for treatments with a graphic designer, copywriter, and proofreader. For brochures on specific diseases or other topics, Blue Poppy and Acupuncture Media Works as well as other companies have many from which you may choose for use in presentation folders and at public events.

Letters of reference from patients

If you don't get any of these spontaneously, ask your best patients if they would be willing to write one for you to use in your presentation folder. Tell them exactly to whom the folders will be sent. Many, if not most, will be happy to do so if they have seen good results from coming to you. Tell them you are trying to get more referrals from MDs, DCs, or whatever and would they mind you using their letter of referral to send to their family doctor (or specialist, etc.) as well? They might or they might not want you to do this, but you won't know if you don't ask. If you ask three or four patients these questions, you are likely to get one letter by the next week. If you ask a second time to the patients who initially said yes but then forgot to bring in or send a letter, you are likely to get at least one more, and that's all you need. You should try to get one or two new letters each year, minimum.

▶ Articles and research

There are many sources for articles on Chinese medicine, alternative medicine, and acupuncture specifically. Web-based sources are almost endless. If you have to use paper only sources, then clip the article (if it is not from a magazine or newspaper owned by the library!) and make neat, clearly visible copies that are not crooked, smudged, or difficult to read and that you can scan to fit on normal-sized pieces of paper. If you print out articles from the internet, put your clinic stamp or sticker on them so it's clear where they came from if separated from your PF.

Other things that we have listed for inclusion in your PF do not really require any explanation. So, let's discuss how to put this all together and what to do with it when completed.

▶ Putting your presentation folder together

If you go to any good paper supply store, you will find a wide variety of papers and presentation folders. Choose a tasteful color combination and buy some matching large envelopes. Start with purchasing only 10-15 of these.

If possible, design your pieces so that they are easy to see in the folder. Perhaps some can be taller and others shorter so that they are staggered in height, the taller ones behind the shorter ones. If you do this, cut them carefully or get that done at a professional copy shop so they are not crooked across the bottom. We have seen some very classy looking folders that used some variation of this technique. Use the same paper and choose consistent colors and typefaces throughout as much as possible. Obviously some pieces will not "match" and that is OK as long as many (at least all the ones that you create yourself) of them do. If you have a color printer, be a little conservative on your use of colors unless you are marketing yourself as wild and outrageous on purpose, or if your specialty is pediatrics.

Once you are sure that there are no spelling errors, print out one set of all your pieces and put it together. Get some feedback from a friend before you make all the remaining copies. Then organize your cover letters depending upon where you are sending them. Obviously, a media person cover letter would emphasize your knowledge about a hot topic they have recently covered or that is being covered a lot in the news. A letter to an assisted reproductive technologies clinic would be different from a letter to an orthopedist. A letter to an HR department would emphasize fast and effective remediation of injuries.

Final steps

You can handwrite your envelope labels but consider using labels that can go through your inkjet or laser printer. Get relatively large-sized labels. MS Word has label specs for almost all sizes of labels. Type in the addresses for where you want to send these or pull them from your mailing list (see Chapter 4 in this section).

Take one completed presentation folder to the post office, get it weighed for postage, and buy some beautiful stamps, the largest sized ones that work. Don't have your folders metered! People love beautiful stamps and are more likely to take notice of your folder. If you are hand-delivering any of these (and that is quite okay), dress your best for this sojourn. When you are well dressed, you look and feel more confident. When you feel more confident, others notice it and respond accordingly.

Who gets your presentation folders?

If you are on a budget, choose carefully to whom you will send these. They will have cost you a lot of time and a couple of bucks (at least) apiece. However, one good medical referral relationship, one supportive HR director, one interested hospital director, or one great media contact can make a $250-$300 expenditure completely worth your while. And, once sent out, you never know under whose eyes your folder will pass. Send them to:

- Local MDs and DCs in your community who, according to your research are likely to be friendly to alternative medicine or who have been referred to you by family or patients. How about your own family practitioner?

- All of the media people discussed in Community Marketing, Chapter 3 of this section.

- Call the local hospital(s) in-service or community coordinator and see if there is an opportunity to connect. If there is an interest or you can actually talk to someone who has an open mind, send that person a folder, or deliver it in person.

- If you are interested in working in a very specific medical niche, definitely send folders to all the medical practitioners who specialize in that niche. Remember, in this case, give them evidence of malpractice insurance.

- If you happen to live in a town with one or more large corporations or unions, find out the names of the medical insurance provider PPO or HMO, Workers' Comp insurance provider, or human resources directors and send a folder. Do your homework first. Call and see if you can get a specific decision maker's name. Make your cover letter specific to the kinds of injuries or health complaints you believe to be most common in their world.

- During political campaigns to expand your scope of practice, you may want to send your PF to some governmental body or to specific politicians.

- Remember, again, that much of the content of this piece can also become content on your website.

Also, keep a digital backup of all these files and a few extra hard copies in reserve for spur-of-the-moment public relations opportunities. Add to or change items in your folder as your professional situation evolves. Presentation folders are a great way to help grow the use of acupuncture and Asian medicine in the U.S. by educating the people who are most likely to either influence or control where people go for medical care.

> **POINTS TO PONDER FROM CHAPTER 5**
>
> - Presentation folders (PF) are a useful component in your outside marketing toolbox. They have many components, some optional, some mandatory.
>
> - When designing a PF, use consistent design elements such as papers, fonts, colors, and logo as much as you can.
>
> - Write several different cover letters for different audiences—the media, specific healthcare professionals, hospital directors, corporate human resource directors, Workers' Comp administrators, or politicians. Keep your cover letter to one page with a specific request for a follow-up step.
>
> - Make sure you have at least 5-6 different pieces in your PF.
>
> - Plan to spend a minimum of $2 and a maximum of $10 per unit on a good PF.

Using Press Releases | 6

Press releases are how the media get a lot of their news. Either the media run the release with their own editing or follow up on the release to develop their own story. Press releases are a way of garnering free advertising and are typically the first step in getting your name in the paper or a piece done about you on radio or TV. Press releases are easy to write and send and should be a regular part of your overall marketing plan. Below are some keys to writing a good press release—one that will get read and translate into free media coverage for your clinic.

1. **Use an active headline to grab the reporter's attention.**
   Your headline should be short, active, and descriptive. For instance, instead of "Honora Wolfe Receives Award," use "Honora Wolfe Named Boulder's Best Acupuncturist."

2. **Put the most important information at the beginning.**
   The reporter needs to know who, what, when, where, why, and/or how in the first two paragraphs. In a busy newsroom, that's often all that gets read.

3. **Avoid hype and unsubstantiated claims.**
   If you make a claim, be sure you have evidence to back it up. It is illegal for a licensed health professional to promise a cure. Whatever you say, be sure it's true.

4. **Be active and to the point.**
   Try not to use passive voice. Get to the point quickly. Don't meander. All you really need to do is answer the questions: Who, What, Where, When, Why, and How.

5. **Keep your release to maximum two pages. One is better.**
   Reporters tend to be busy people. They're not going to hunt through a poorly written, meandering four page release. The

only file such an unfocused, poorly written release is going to go in is the circular kind.

6. **Include a contact.**
   If your release strikes an interest, the reporter will want to know how to get more information. Every release should have the name, email, phone, and fax numbers of a contact person (usually you) on the bottom. This is another reason for good phone service at your clinic.

7. **Keep jargon to a minimum.**
   Technical Chinese medical terms are a no-no here. You know what qi, yin, and yang are, but the general public does not. Also try to use more simple Anglo-Saxon words and fewer words that come from Latin. Remember, journalists write for the average 8th-grade reader. So keep it simple. Communication is more important than showing off your education.

8. **Stress benefits (WIIFM).**
   Everyone wants to know what's in it for me. Don't say that Chinese medicine is 2,000 years old, wonderful, or the best. People want to know what benefits they are likely to experience. A better approach is to tell them about freedom from side effects, low cost, proven healing effects, or anything that expresses a benefit to the prospective patient. Maybe it's something as prosaic as convenient parking and weekend office hours. Telling them how good Chinese medicine is or how good you are is not a direct benefit to the reader.

9. **Proofread.**
   Be absolutely sure you *and someone else* proofread your press release before sending it off. Proofread your release for spelling and also for grammar. Then proof it again to check to see if you've followed the previous nine pieces of advice. Nothing can sink a press release faster than a sloppy, unprofessional presentation. As a corollary of this, don't use

fancy typefaces, emoticons (smiley faces) or cutesy graphic symbols. They're hard to read and look amateurish.

10. **Who should you send it to?**

This is a bit more of a discussion and the answer depends upon who you want to see and respond to the information. That said, you can start with daily newspapers in your community. Contact the city editor or the editor in charge of the section that relates to your content. If there are weekly newspapers in your area, send to the editor or managing editor. The same is true for magazines, whether local or national. For radio stations, send to the news director or public service director (*e.g.*, if you are doing some event or activity that relates to a non-profit in your community). For TV stations, send to the news director.

Generally, your contacts will prefer to receive news releases by email unless they say otherwise on their website. Send your release the way that the publication wants it sent. When using email, don't send an attachment (other than links to photos or videos); copy the release directly into the email. Attachments won't get opened.

Send your press release to one publication at a time or blind copy (BCC) the recipients to make the news release submission more personal.

Some outlets may prefer that you upload the press release directly to their website over a secure submission platform.

Don't worry too much about finding out which exact individual you should send your release to if you don't have a lot of time. Whomever you send it to, get the person's title right, and that should be sufficient. If your release is interesting, it is likely to get into the right hands.

On the following page is a sample press release.

Stillwater Health Clinic
3001 Baseline Ave.
Boulder, CO 80301
303-447-8367

Press Release

For immediate release.

Honora Wolfe Named Boulder's Best Acupuncturist

July 19, Boulder, CO: Local acupuncturist, Honora Lee Wolfe, received the Best of Boulder Award as acupuncturist of the year for 2014. This award was given by the Daily Camera Newspaper yesterday at a ceremony held at the Broker Inn. Each year, the Daily Camera holds a contest for determining the Best of Boulder in 35 different categories. Ms. Wolfe, who is also a Fellow of the National Academy of Acupuncture and Oriental Medicine, has won this award two times before, in 2002 and in 1995. Ms. Wolfe has practiced acupuncture and Chinese medicine in Boulder since 1988. She attended trainings at the Shanghai College of Chinese Medicine in the People's Republic of China in 1984, 85, and 87. Besides having the support of her many satisfied patients, Ms. Wolfe has taught at the Southwest Acupuncture College in Gunbarrel and is the author or translator of several books on Chinese medicine, including Better Breast Health Naturally with Chinese Medicine and Managing Menopause Naturally with Chinese Medicine. Ms. Wolfe currently conducts a private practice at Stillwater Health which is a multipractitioner alternative healthcare clinic located at Baseline and 30th in Boulder. For the last several years, Ms. Wolfe has specialized in the treatment of chronic pain and sports injuries.

END-END-END-END

For further information, Ms. Wolfe can be contacted at: 303-447-8367 or by email at: honora@stillwater.com.

SECTION FOUR: MARKETING YOUR PRACTICE

➤ **Formatting**

Standard format for a press release done on paper is double-spaced on one side only of white 8 1/2 x 11" paper. Put your name and address on the top of the page. On-paper releases are fine unless they prefer email or have a submission form on their website. If only sending to one publication, tell them it's "first run" in addition to "for immediate release." If it's going to be on paper, use a computer to compose the release. No handwriting!

In terms of topics for press releases, there is no end to the things you can announce. If you go to a seminar, tell people what you learned and how it could potentially help them. If you go to a convention or symposium, tell them about the new techniques, information, or instruments you've brought back. If you and a group of local acupuncturists are volunteering to clean up a local derelict field, are raising money together for a local non-profit by

---

P O W E R   P O I N T

Resources for writing press releases:

1. *Six Steps to Free Publicity* by Marcia Yudkin, Plume, 2008. As the title describes, this book provides practical advice for a small business' publicity campaign.

2. *The Associated Press Stylebook and Libel Manual,* Addison-Wesley, 2011. A guide for spelling and punctuation, as well as information on avoiding libel and respecting copyright.

3. *The Elements of Style, 4th Edition* by William Strunk & E.B. White, Macmillan, Revised 1999. This little book is the time-honored guide to clear writing.

4. Public Relations Society of America, 33 Maiden Lane, 11th Fl., New York, NY 10038; 212-460-1400, www.prsa.org. National organization for PR professionals sponsors educational seminars.

running an evening donation-only clinic, or are doing the Ride-the-Rockies bicycle fundraiser as a team, that's news. If you receive an award or certificate for anything, for sure tell people about that. Let's say you were recently elected as secretary of your state acupuncture association. You and I know that's mostly a lot of work and an honor of dubious distinction, but it sounds good to those who don't know any better. You might think these things are no big deal, and they aren't if that's the way you couch them. But put another spin on them and they're news with benefits for you to market. Instead of telling people that you address and lick the stamps of your state association's newsletter, tell them you've been elected to the Board of Directors. Now you're one of the head honchos of acupuncture in your state.

POINTS TO PONDER FROM CHAPTER 6

- You can help out the local media, become a local expert, get free publicity, and build your business, using press releases.
- Create a good media mailing list.
- Whenever you do anything that is interesting, remarkable, even a seminar with an interesting topic, write a press release and send it to all the local media.
- Follow the rules: one page, double-spaced, or emailed using the submission form on their website, with Who, What, When, Where, Why, and How statements.
- Is it Breast Cancer Awareness Month or National Diabetes Week, or The Great American Smoke Out? Find a timely hook, create a marketing activity in your community, and let the media know you are a mover and shaker in your town.

Marketing Your Practice on the Internet | 7

Here are some revealing statistics about computer and internet usage. More than 80% of US households were connected to the internet by the end of 2012. At the time of this writing, over 85% of U.S. businesses are connected, there are over 2.4 billion internet users worldwide, Facebook is the 2nd largest "country" in the world, and over 355 million computers were sold worldwide in 2012. Sales of products and services on the internet were up by 3.7% in 2012 (and are expected to reach $327 billion by 2016). Perhaps more important, *over 62% of all off-line purchases are influenced by online research.* Throughout 2014, there will be over 1 billion Google searches per day and that number is likely to increase each year. This chapter is an attempt to give you the basics of what you need to know (at this swiftly-changing moment in time) to maintain some type of internet presence, create a simple website, and/or do basic internet marketing.

➤ A website is no longer optional

No matter how you get it done or how sophisticated you need it to be, most of us need to have a website, at least a basic one, for any type of business we wish to operate. There are three basic ways to get a website built. 1) Use online web creation tools that walk you through the process. (See Web Resources listed below for leads.) 2) Take a community college class in Dreamweaver or html code writing. 3) For the technologically faint of heart, I suggest you hire a good web designer and create a long-term relationship with them. Tech-nerds need acupuncture, too, so at least a partial trade may be possible! Lets look at the pros(+) and cons(-) of these in a little more depth.

Online website creation tools:
- +Mostly free
- -Require a learning curve for most of us
- -May lack flexibility of design
- +Often come with cheap site-hosting
- -There is often little or no tech support
- +Great if you are computer savvy. VistaPrint, Weebly, Yahoo, and Wordpress are some of these. Find tons more with a websearch or look at software review sites such as http://www.top10bestwebsitebuilders.com/.

Learn sophisticated website-creation software:
- +If learning something like Dreamweaver® turns you on, you can pretty much create anything you want.
- -Time, money, and a steeper learning curve required
- +You can keep your site updated on your own and don't have to wait until your webmaster can fit you in to their queue

Hire a web designer:
- ++With a good webmaster, you can get exactly what you want as well as good search engine optimization (SEO)
- + A good contract should have good tech support
- - Costs $$ (but less than you might think). I [HW] suggest you try www.Elance.com and ask for bids from the freelance web designers. You can also look at their work and read references about them at this service.

Check references and look at the company or person's work!! You should be able to get a simple 5-page site for $500-$1,000. You can also get a simple, low-cost website with hosting at Acufinder.com, AcupunctureClinicWebsite.com, TCMDirectory.com, and ChineseMedicineTools.com, but these may or may not meet all your criteria. More of these pop up all the time, so search and compare prices, services, tech support, and long-term contracts.

SECTION FOUR: MARKETING YOUR PRACTICE

▶ What about my domain name?

- A domain name is not expensive. You should be able to get a good domain for $10-$15 per year. You may already have done this after reading Section 1, Chapter 3 in any case!
- Pay a visit to fatcow.com, godaddy.com, or justhost.com and see if the domain name you want is available.
- Try to choose a domain name that includes key words, *e.g.*, www.DallasAthleticAcupuncture.com says exactly what you do and where you are.
- Names like www.crazyhorseclinic.com are fun but will not help your search engine rankings.
- .com and .net are better than other designations; .org is only for non-profits; .edu is only for schools
- It's cheaper and easier to buy a multi-year contract if you are fairly sure you will be keeping your domain name for a while.

▶ What about hosting?

Online website creation software like Weebly or Wordpress and domain sellers like GoDaddy offer hosting and marketing packages along with other services, but, perhaps, little or no customer service. Prices start as low as $6-$10 per month for minimal services (static pages + an email account) and go up from there. Get more of what you need for $25-$30 per month, *i.e.*, a decent bulk email feature to send newsletters and capture names. Again, sites like justhost.com or fatcow.com have decent packages.

There are lots of smaller local and regional companies that do hosting. Start with price shopping, but mostly ask about their tech support, which is a good reason to stay local. You can always visit with the people in person and keep your money and networking in your city or town.

The main features you need are to be able to capture visitor information, especially email addresses, and to send bulk emails.

You may also want to sell a few products online (there is more about that later in this chapter). Also ask about marketing support costs, such as key words on the homepage, metatags, and search engine optimization and submission.

▶ What should my site include?

A good website is meaningful, unique, succinct, and laced with key words and calls-to-action for visitors. If you are not a good writer, hire a copywriter to help you create the content and proofreading services to minimize typos. Remember that "content is king" is practically a mantra for web gurus. Your web designers will be easy to work with if you can create the content you have agreed upon and that they require for building your site, and on the schedule to which you both agree. I suggest checking out a few practitioners' websites and see what they have included. If you have an outline, some files written (already proofread, of course!), photos taken, color scheme ideas, etc., completed before you start, it will help you save money when you visit a designer or even if you build a site yourself.

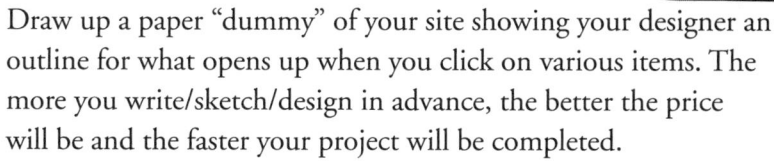

Draw up a paper "dummy" of your site showing your designer an outline for what opens up when you click on various items. The more you write/sketch/design in advance, the better the price will be and the faster your project will be completed.

Calls-to-action are there to tell your visitors how to interact with your site. "Click here to read about what acupuncture can treat" or "Click here to see a video of exercises to enhance digestive health" or "Click here to send me a question about your health" are all good types of calls to action. Use as many as you can.

The first sentence or two at the top of your home page should have all the **key words** that you think people would use to find your site. For example, "Back to Life Acupuncture Clinic in

Boulder, CO, specializes in treating people with all types of back pain." This has the words "acupuncture," "Boulder," and "back pain" that will help search engines and, thus, your prospective customers find you easily. Write a list of key words you want on your home page and as many other pages on your site as possible. Use them in your text as much as you naturally can. A photo or two of you working, or of the inside and outside of your clinic, or of your pharmacy, are good additions and give visitors a sense of who you are and what your practice feels like.

Your site should look/read like your biz card, company brochure, letterhead, etc. In other words, it should have an integrated look and feel in terms of colors, fonts, photos, and design elements. This goes for everything that you produce to promote your practice.

If you really cannot afford to have a website, maybe you can sell ad space to related, local businesses to help pay for your site. For example, if you sell facial care or herbal products, ask the manufacturer of those products to place an ongoing ad at your site to pay for the hosting fees. If that sounds unlikely, at least consider doing trades with other related local businesses, putting their logo and link on your site if they do the same for your site.

▶ Building link popularity

Speaking of links, one of the best ways to get higher search engine rankings is for your site name to show up on lots of other people's sites. One way to do that is to provide content for other people's sites in exchange for a mention of your URL (web address) at the end of each piece. If you like to write, offer your content for free to as many other websites as possible. For example:

- *Boulder Parents Magazine* has a website. Most magazines do. Offer to write a health-wellness piece for their website every

POWER POINT

Examples of good site content

People want and expect some value-added content. For example, on my Back to Life Clinic website, I want a short article (I really mean short) such as the following:
"Research on Back Pain and Chinese Medicine"
- 3-5 bullet points on things to do at home and what to avoid.
- Maybe some photos or a link to a YouTube video of you demonstrating a couple of exercises.
- At the end of the article describe how acupuncture has proven in research to help many types of back pain.
- At the very end is your phone number, email address, and an "Ask the Acupuncturist" form for questions or to book an appointment.

I might also include the following:
- Several articles on different, related subjects, especially conditions you prefer to treat.
- A "Links" page allows you to request to trade links with other people's sites (as many as possible). Link trading is a good way to increase "link popularity," which helps you get higher in search engine lists. More on that below.
- An "opt-in" email sign-up form that gets them something free (a quarterly video newsletter on health, discount coupons for classes you teach, specials on seasonal herbal products, a free consultation). Opt-in means they choose to sign up or not. This is vital because it gives you an inexpensive way to stay in touch with potential patients! By the way, each communication you send out must have instructions at the bottom on how to unsubscribe if they so choose.
- Information on any products you are selling on your site.

- other month in exchange for mentioning your name and URL address on their website (and perhaps in their print magazine as well?).
- Do the same thing with as many other publications and websites as you have time to contact. If you really want to use the web as your main marketing medium, this is how you do it without spending lots of cash.
- Get your name/URL on as many listing services as possible. See below for details.
- Offer to trade links with other practitioners' websites in other cities. The more of these links you can create, the better your "organic" search engine placement (good search engine placement that you have not paid for) will be.
- If you can create short articles or videos about acupuncture, Chinese medicine, alternative health, the benefits of exercise, etc., all day long, offer these articles to other people for their websites in trade for your URL link appearing with the article.
- Search for health blogs where you are allowed to leave a comment. There are thousands of these out there. Every time you leave a comment, put your URL and maybe a link to your own blog, at the end.

▶ What are listing services?

There are lots and lots of these out there! Your website can be listed at your state association website, the AAAOM website, AcuFinder.com, AcupunctureToday.com, www.gancao.net, www.byregion.net, http://alternative-doctor.com/links, www.citysearch.com, and www.Chinesemedicinetimes.com. Look for local, regional, and national places to list your website. Some are free and some not. It's worth it to spend some cash here if you are serious about web marketing, but do a Google search for "Alternative Health Listing Services" and only pay for ones that come up on the first page of your search or you are wasting your money.

CHAPTER 7 | Marketing Your Practice on the Internet

➤ Search-based web ads

The best of this type of advertising is probably small ads through Google Business and Yelp (check out this site if you have not already done so). The way this works is that when someone searches for acupuncture in your city, your little ad appears along the side of the page and your little "bubble" appears when the local map pops open. You choose the keywords that relate to your ad and the amount you are willing to pay for each appearance or if someone clicks your ad. This is not cheap, but if used over time, it can be very effective. This type of ad can be done on Facebook and other social networking sites as well, with costs per click-through.

➤ Google Places

One absolutely vital place for you to be listed on the internet, irrespective of having a website, is claiming your business on Google Places. To see what that is, go to Google and do a search for acupuncturists in your town. See the map that comes up with the little bubbles for various clinic locations? You need to be there, too. This is easy and need not cost you money, although you can enhance placement of your listing through the use of AdWords on Google if you want more exposure.

Google gives you all sorts of straightforward tutorials for creating and enhancing your listings and advertisements. Just do what they say, create the listing as per their instructions and then search on Google by using the key words you'd expect potential patients to use. Remember that over 60% of non-internet purchases are made after people did internet research! In other words, they may call you to get information or make an appointment, but the research that made the decision about who and where to call was done online! So check this out and do it as soon as you have a physical address, a decent website, and are ready to spend a bit of cash on advertising!

SECTION FOUR: MARKETING YOUR PRACTICE

▶ Using bulk email blasts

You could purchase opt-in email lists of people interested in alternative health. However, as mentioned in the chapter on mailing lists, it is more effective to collect email addresses from your patients, anyone who attends a class or lecture, and from business cards that you collect here and there; these addresses go in your web database. The two most important website hosting features totally worth paying for are visitor data collection and group emailing for you to easily and accurately keep track of and stay in touch with interested visitors. As stated above, all outbound communication from you must have an opt-out statement of what people do if they are no longer interested.

Even if you have no website but do have an email "address book," you can hire an online bulk-email-sending company to send e-communications for you. These are easy to find online (MailChimp, ConstantContact, iContact), or your email service

---

Resources for going further with your website marketing

Books to help you with web-based marketing
The Zen of Social Media Marketing: An Easier Way to Build Credibility, Generate Buzz, and Increase Revenue by Shama Kabani and Chris Brogan
Successful Website Marketing by Peggy Ridgway
Self-Promotion Online by Ilise Benun
Internet Marketing for Less than $500 a Year by Marcia Yudkin
Get Clients Now: A 28 Day Marketing Program for Professionals by C.J. Hayden

Online promotion services
While you can find hundreds of these by doing an online search, I would start with local companies. That way you can interview both the owners and get local referrals to see how they have measured up to expectations and how well they fulfill their contracts.

CHAPTER 7 | Marketing Your Practice on the Inernet

provider (Safari, Firefox, Thunderbird) may already include this service. Be sure to include one or two reasons for people to get back in touch with you, your contact info, and unsubscribe info every time you send anything.

Keep email communications short. People don't scroll down very far unless they are *really* interested in something. A basic formula is a good intro headline to capture interest, then some bullet points, and then a call to action (call you, attend a class, watch your new video, attend a webinar, etc.) No more than one or two of these emails per month or people will start to tune you out or unsubscribe altogether.

➤ **Blogging and vlogging**

A blog or vlog and a social network profile at places such as Facebook are your virtual representatives. These are where people can maintain anonymity yet make that first contact in a potential relationship with you. It's important to remember that, especially for many non-Asians, coming the first time for acupuncture for Chinese medicine requires a great deal of trust. Few people will come to you without some belief that they can trust you. A blog is a great way to help you establish credibility and enough trust for people to make that first call or send you that first email. The best news is that there are ways to create an internet presence in the blogosphere for free (at the time of this writing), notably at Wordpress or Blogger, which are easy enough to use that some people adapt them as a basic "website" as well. I suggest you poke around and check out various blogs at both sites for samples of how to use this software to the best advantage. Another good thing about both these sites is that they allow you the

POWER POINT

For more help with blogging and how to do it really well, you might check out articles to get you started at sites like Thoughts.com, Blogspot.com, and ProBlogger.com. There's a ton of help out there for almost any online activity such as blogging.

411

opportunity to use the margin of the screen as a "brochure" about you and your services. This includes your contact information, what services you offer, general information about acupuncture and Chinese medicine, etc.

Besides creating a Blogger or Wordpress brochure, you should actually post blogs there! On other people's blogs (as mentioned on page 408), you can post guest entries or comments. There are tons of health-related blogs out there. For example, if you do a search for "hay fever blogs," "fibromyalgia blogs," "infertility blogs," or "GI disease blogs" (you get the idea) you will come up with pages of blog sites where your knowledge would be appreciated and well received. But don't just make your comments "ads" about yourself. With your (hopefully regular) posts on yours and others' blogs, potential clients get a chance to "meet you" and know a great deal about your personality as well as your skills, history, and knowledge. Your posts can establish you as an expert (or not) and create a virtual person for people to relate to directly. If people feel like they know you through your posts, you'll greatly increase your success in attracting clients. You might say to me, "People from anywhere on the planet could read my blog. How do I know if any of them will become my patient?" True. Still, I would respond that the world is getting smaller every day and you never know where the next patient or referral will come from. Also, if you put your web address in every blog post and comment on others' posts, you are improving the natural positioning of your website without paying anyone to do search engine optimization for you.

Another positive thing to remember is that blog posts do not have to be long or scholarly. They can be short, personal, simple informational tidbits or even questions, about which people are encouraged to comment and dialog with you. Do try to spell correctly and use complete sentences, however, since your purpose is to sound both personable *and* intelligent!

Sites like Blogger, Blogspot, CafeMoms, Wordpress, Squidoo, and other large blog centers are also great because search engines love blogs. Having a blog that you post at regularly helps your rankings in the search results when someone searches online for what you do or what you blog about. So, if you want to create a web presence in less than an hour and for no cost, try Blogger, Wordpress, or Squidoo. And remember, if you already have a website, a blog increases your opportunities for communication with potential clients, gives them a way to get to know you, and increases site traffic in the search engines.

Squidoo is another free and easy website-alternative or internet-promotion tool, created by the marketing genius Seth Godin. Because of Mr. Godin's insight and communication skill, Squidoo includes almost everything you need to get started marketing yourself on the internet, website or not. On Squidoo you build what is called a "lens" on any subject, as broad or narrow a subject as you want, and including as much or as little as you want. For example, there could be a lens on "My Acupuncture Practice in Miami," or one on "Everything You Wanted to Know About Acupuncture," or whatever subject you think might interest the clients you want to attract. The lens is actually a collection of absolutely anything digital that you want to share on this subject. In addition to blog or vlog posts about you and your practice, you can link to any web-based resource that seems useful, informative, fun, or relevant. This should include YouTube videos (yours and others), books reviews, blog posts by you and others, photos, and your and others' websites. Your Squidoo lens can even serve as a website alternative until you decide to create one of those as well.

The marketing value of Squidoo is that search engines love it the way they love blogs. From a potential client's perspective, your presence here can establish you as an expert and someone they may want on their healthcare team. For example, if you are a tai chi teacher, you would insert links to your favorite tai chi books, your personal tai chi teachers, tai chi videos on YouTube, other tai chi websites or blogs, articles about tai chi you find in the online press, and anything you yourself write about tai chi. While this may seem like potentially giving business away, usually the contrary is true. For example, videos absolutely don't compare to working with an actual tai chi teacher and most people visiting your Squidoo lens are likely to be seeking something beyond video instruction. By referring to related, useful resources beyond yourself, you make it clear that you know the industry and that your motivation is client-centered and all about providing great content to people whether they buy from you or not. That makes you the open-hearted and generous sort of person people want to study with. Squidoo is also free, user-friendly, and fast.

> **POWER POINT**
>
> To see a comprehensive list of social networking opportunities, check out "social networking sites" at Wikipedia.com. There are literally hundreds of them, many quite subculture-specific. An interest in treating children or families, for example, might lead you to join networks such as CafeMoms.com. Check this out for sure! 200,000 moms talking to each other about everything; join the conversation!

▸ **Social network (SN) marketing**

I thought about making this topic into its own chapter, but decided not to. While it may be true that all the patients you could ever need are friends, colleagues, and acquaintances of all the people that you already know, after years of working with several SN sites, I remain unconvinced that, other than YouTube, they will help you grow your business to any great extent. If you believe otherwise, here are some ideas. Sites like YouTube, Facebook, Twitter, LinkedIn, Pinterest and others give you potential access to several degrees of separation through all your friends and acquaintances. On Facebook you can do things as simple as write Chinese-medicine-specific messages or quotes on your newsfeed and those of your friends, let all your networked friends know about upcoming classes, speeches, volunteering, events, special offers you are giving, or review great books on CM that you read recently. Start a fan-club for yourself; ask your Facebook friends for referrals; create Facebook events. You can, for a small amount of money that you control, also avail yourself of Facebook advertising opportunities, although you must follow their rules quite specifically or your ads will not be placed. Similar possibilties exist at LinkedIn, Twitter, and others. To use YouTube effectively, create a channel and record lots of short videos (2-5 minutes) on relevant subjects like a qi gong exercise for each season, how to make an herbal decoction at home, how to use a hot herbal compress, cooking or self-massage demos, or a tour of your clinic. Post a new video each week and link it to your home page, your blog, your Facebook page, your Twitter feed, and to comments you post on other people's blogs. Video is over 60% of internet use, so don't ignore video if you seek online marketing success.

This discussion could be endless. If you have a real interest in it or if you already have a healthy social network presence on the web, I suggest you read lots of articles on SN marketing at sites such as www.ehow.com, www.geeknews-central.com, www.hubspot.com, and similar websites. Type in something like "grow your business using Facebook." There are tons of articles, ebooks, classes, and blogs on these subjects, so poke around, read stuff, and decide how to connect. One thing I suggest is to keep your personal SN presence separate from your business presence, *i.e.*, have two Facebook or Twitter pages.

▶ Other online opportunities

People love to talk about things and services they like. Online this has been "formalized" through websites such as Yelp and Angie's List. You can ask your best patients to "yelp" about you, but do not be tempted to fake another name and do it yourself.

You'll get "busted" for this by Yelp in a heartbeat. Go to Yelp, type in "acupuncturist" for any city and see who your competition is. *Yelp is also a better place to buy ads than Facebook.*

If you want to know what the press and online world is saying about acupuncture, Chinese medicine, your clinic name, your name, or any other subject, go to Google Alerts and sign up be alerted by email any time these subjects appear in the news. This is an excellent way to collect articles for your waiting room scrapbook and see what new research is being reported in our industry. You'll be surprised how often we are in the news!

Got photos of your trip to China to study medicine or video of you teaching qi gong or working in your clinic? Share them at Flickr, Instagram, Pinterest, or YouTube and link them to your website, Facebook page, Twitter feed, and blog. State that these are open source (*i.e.*, anybody can use your photos as long as you are given attribution using your YouTube or website address). More people visit YouTube than most of the other sites put together in the whole online universe. Pinterest could also be useful if you create a product line that is highly photogenic.

▶ Prefer live contact?

Prefer face-to-face marketing opportunities? I sure do and believe it to be way more effective than dinking around all day on Facebook! Go to Meetup.com and see what's happening in your area in the coming days (or hours!) that you might attend for fun or volunteering and networking. Or, create an event yourself and post it there. This can be really easy… something like "Interested in the Politics of Food (or March Madness, or whatever subject you like)? Meet me at the XYZ Bar (or offer your clinic space as a Meetup location!) at 5 PM for a rousing conversation."

▶ The wonderful world of e-commerce

If you want to sell anything on your site, the easiest way to do it is to create a "merchant account" at PayPal. That way, people can pay you either with credit cards or their PayPal account. All the tools you need in order to add the PayPal information and capability to your site are available at PayPal. They have both online and telephone help (unlike Facebook, Google, or YouTube!) if you get stuck. You can sell books, herbal products, facial or personal care products, aromatherapy candles, soap, CDs or DVDs, or offer sign-up for live or online classes.

If, by any chance, you are a shy person, selling yourself on the internet may be a great place to start. While you still must try to find some comfort level with people when they call, write, or come in to see you, there is a huge potential audience out there on the web, just waiting to find out about you and your services, without the requirement of standing up in front of groups and giving lectures.

▶ Conclusion

This chapter could go on for many, many more pages. It may also be the case that, within a year (or even a few days!) of the publication of this book, something in this chapter will no longer be accurate or there will be new services that we should have discussed. The main thing to know is that the internet is a huge and constantly growing resource for almost all types of businesses. Don't be overwhelmed and don't hang out online all day(!!!); pick a couple of these suggestions to start and add on as something seems relevant. Schedule time to work on this type of marketing the same as you would for anything else, do the work, and close your browser. Being lost in cyberspace all day won't get you patients. In my opinion, the internet is no easier as a marketing tool than any other type of marketing. Still, if you are comfortable with it, this is one tool that many practitioners are using successfully to get new patients. You can, too.

POINTS TO PONDER FROM CHAPTER 7

- Since the use of the internet is growing exponentially, there are many opportunities to market your services.

- There are many ways to get a website built. The easiest is to hire someone to do it for you ($500-$1500 for the least expensive and simplest sites). You can do all or part of it yourself with software such as Dreamweaver or free online resources for the more techno-savvy.

- Domain names (your URL) need not cost more than $10-$15 per year.

- Hosting services can cost as little as $10 per month, but make sure you have three things:
  1. Opt-in information gathering ability
  2. Group email blasting ability
  3. Ability to add PayPal® or other e-commerce options

- Blogging is an effective way to market yourself online for free. Get started at Blogger or Wordpress and "disease-specific" blogs. Use Squidoo to create digital credibility.

- YouTube videos can be easy to create, give you visibility and credibility, and link to every other place on the internet you are using for marketing.

- Social network sites can also be a source of patients through your friends and your friends' friends, but choose carefully how you spend your time here. It can be a huge time-sinkhole for little return.

- Consider ads on Google Places and Yelp as your first choices if you spend money on internet marketing.

Marketing Odds and Ends | 8

As I said at the beginning of this section, it is more difficult to decide what to exclude than what to include when talking about marketing. Marketing is, from one point of view, the sum total of everything you do. As Seth Godin, one of my favorite marketing gurus, says, it can be the way you answer the phone, launch a new service, paint your rooms, or organize your schedule that will make the positive difference. Getting in the habit of excellence and of exploring the limitless possibilities for a great clinic should be a daily goal. Being the most expensive instead of the least, the fastest or the slowest, the hottest, the easiest, the most efficient, the oldest or the newest, or just the most, you should test the limits of what works to grow your practice every chance you get. If you can think of a way to overwhelm those you serve with your remarkability, you're there.

Meanwhile, here are a few more tips.

- Silent auctions are an opportunity to use your services to market your services and support your community at the same time. Donate a series of treatments. Think how many people will walk by the bidding tables deciding what to bid on.

- When you do a speaking engagement, after the lecture, follow up with a thank you card to the person who was in charge. Let them know they can contact you any time for lectures on other related subjects.

- Donate the proceeds of one treatment per month to a specific local cause. Send a press release to the local media announcing that you are doing this and what the cause of the month is.

- Never go anywhere without a stack of business cards in your pocket. Take every opportunity to talk to anyone who will listen about what you do.

SECTION FOUR: MARKETING YOUR PRACTICE

POWER POINT

A path to getting more MD/DC/DO/ND referrals!

Ask each new patient to sign a Release of Records form for any practitioner they've seen for their current complaint. Send the form with a nice cover letter stating that you are treating Mary Jones with acupuncture for her condition, will be seeing her for X weeks of treatment, and will be asking Mary to return to his/her office for occasional reassessment. State that you are happy to speak with him/her at any time or may be in contact to discuss the case. Include a couple of your cards and perhaps a brochure about your clinic services.

Repeat this process as Mary's condition improves. Use appropriate medical language ("Mary's range of motion for left shoulder adduction has increased from 30° to 70°.") Repeat again when Mary is released from your care. Include another business card each time your send something.

This strategy is one way to begin building rapport with medical professionals in your area. The next time this practitioner is asked, "What do you think, doc, should I try acupuncture?" your name is the one they may remember.

- Develop an "elevator speech," 2-3 sentences about what you do so that, in line at the grocery store, you've got something compelling and interesting to say to anyone who asks, "What do you do for a living?" Practice until you have it memorized.

- During "The Great American Smoke Out," give free treatments to people trying to quit. Send a letter to social services offices in the city health department as well as doctors in town citing the success of acupuncture for dealing with addictive behaviors and offer to help their patients quit. Remember to include a few business cards.

- If you are giving a lecture somewhere that you've never been before, go and check out the room in advance. You'll be more comfortable when you arrive for the talk and do a better job.

- Start and maintain a support group of businesspeople and related professionals. Meet once per month for an early breakfast. At each meeting, two people get to discuss an issue or problem they have and ask for everyone's opinion. This is very powerful and can energize your business in ways you can't imagine. Napoleon Hill calls this your "mastermind" group.

- When there are no patients, don't just sit and read clinical books. Go out and meet others in your building or on your block. Introduce yourself and pass out your cards. If you practice in a high-rise office building, does every receptionist in that building know you on a first name basis?

- Speaking of high-rise offices, what about the building janitor and the guy who runs the coffee shop in the lobby? These people talk to a large percentage of the people who work in your building. They both should have some of your cards in their pocket or by the cash register!

Finally, as much as you can for as long as you can, keep your intellectual curiosity alive. This will help you stay interested in and passionate about what you are doing professionally. Go to seminars, read books, research what is out there. Really learn and understand this medicine to the limit of your ability. Don't be lazy. This type of passion and true skill are magnetic and seductive. The universe supports it and will support you because of it. At the end of the day or the end of a career or the end of a life, you have only yourself and your own integrity to answer to. If you truly love and understand this medicine and you can communicate that love to your patients through everything that you and your clinic embody, you will be successful. That, exactly that, is the essence of good marketing.

Growing Your Life... Avoiding Burnout | 9

OK, let's say you have your practice off the ground enough to pay yourself, the rent, heat, insurance, and phone bill. Most of your practice days are pretty busy and referrals are good. Now you have to decide how large and busy a practice you want to create. The point of a private practice is to help your patients and support yourself financially and emotionally, not to create practitioner burnout. If this is you or if it will be you in another several months, your situation is pretty good and you should feel proud of yourself. You are in the minority in our profession, though we hope this book will help more practitioners be effective and successful businesspeople. With that in mind, we feel it is important to talk about handling a large, busy, and successful practice so that the growth is managed in a way that supports you and doesn't make you crazy.

So how do you keep a balance and how do you keep growing without making yourself sick? Here are several ideas to consider:

➤ Raise your prices

This is one way to make sure that the patients who are coming to see you really want to be getting their therapy from you. Send out a notice to all your active patients or put a flyer in their herb prescription bags announcing that, on the first of the following month, your prices will go up $5-$10 per treatment, exam, and/or intake, or that you will charge $25 for a 15 minute phone consultation. State gently that, if these prices are too high for anyone, you are happy to refer them to one of a number of other practitioners in the area. You may lose a few people, but probably not many. At least this may slow your growth for a while.

▶ Hire an assistant

In the chapter about getting a job (see Section 1, Chapter 8), we discussed all the reasons it might be great to hire a new graduate to work with you. Another reason is that you may be able to have one or more assistant practitioners to whom you refer specific types of ailments without your clinic losing any income. This help may be supervised or not, but, even if and when it is unsupervised, as the boss you can set very clear guidelines about patient care in your clinic. That way, if you are charging $65 for your treatments and $55 for your assistant's treatments but paying the assistant $40, you are still making money. You will, of course, have to figure out what other costs may be incurred by having an assistant to make certain that there is profit for you in the deal. Such an arrangement may also require that you have some type of corporate structure because fee-splitting is illegal in many states. Still, if you are growing at this rate, it is probably time to consider incorporation or an LLC if you have not already done so. That means your helper(s) have to be employees unless they are merely renting space from you on a per hour basis, which is a completely different sort of arrangement.

POWER POINT

Tips for hiring an associate (sample contract at website)

- Make sure you hire someone who is as like-minded as possible when it comes to patient care and general habits.

- Pay them enough that they will want to stay with you for at least one year. Two years is better.

- Run the numbers carefully to make sure that you are making some money from the assistant's work. One key to capitalism is hiring other people's labor to make you money. Giving jobs to people is also a wonderful thing to be able to do.

▶ Hire a professional associate

Another way to hire help and lighten your load is to find a specialist who offers services completely different from your own. If you wish to move your personal practice largely in the direction of gynecology, for example, and have fewer other types of patients, you might hire a new practitioner who does not wish to specialize in anything specific but, instead, wishes to get a wide range of experience for a while. If you pay them a fair wage and provide a pleasant working environment, this can be a good solution for limiting the growth of your own practice while providing more services to patients. Such an arrangement also gives you someone to cover patients when you want to take time off or need to go out of town. You may need a lawyer-written contract that discusses the minimal length of time the practitioner must work for you, how the relationship will be severed, or how a future partnership may be created, what benefits in addition to salary you will pay, and who gets the profits from herb and product sales.

In this case, you would contact your existing clientele to announce that you will only be taking gynecology cases in the future and that you are proud and happy to have so-and-so as the new practitioner joining your practice to take care of all other types of complaints, also describing what if any new skills or services you will now be able to offer at your clinic. They need to feel assured that they will still be well taken care of and that you will be there to consult with the new practitioner about their personal history and specific needs. While you may lose a few patients through this type of transition, you will keep most of them if you market it well. You could also manage this slowly, only channeling new patients to the new practitioner while keeping your current patients and allowing natural attrition to take care of slowing the growth of your practice.

Another possibility is to hire a young MD who is still a resident and looking for a moonlighting job. This may cost less than you think and will add prestige to your clinic and allow you to offer some basic medical screening services that could be very valuable to your patients. See Section 1, Chapter 9, page 81 for more information about a practitioner who has had success with this option.

We also realize that such a plan may require a larger space and more treatment rooms, but, if your practice is growing, you may consider moving into a larger clinic space in any case.

▸ Interns or treatment aides

Another possibility is to hire a new graduate or even someone who has not yet graduated from school to assist you directly in treating your patients. This intern's jobs may include doing moxa, tuina, removing cups, taking out needles, cleaning up the treatment rooms after each patient, checking on patients while you are off doing an intake on the next patient, taking blood pressures or doing other basic intake and exam procedures, pulling out files, making follow-up phone calls, or whatever else you feel you can legally delegate. This person is not the same as your receptionist or front desk staff. They help you directly in the treatment room, streamlining each patient's therapy and, thereby, allowing you to see more patients without losing quality of care. At the same time, this new practitioner is receiving excellent on-the-job training. Pay scale can be $14-$18 per hour for such work.

> **PRACTITIONER POINTER**
>
> "Follow through with what you say you will do. Arrive on time. Look people in the eye. Make it easy for people to come to see you. Don't forget to get treatments and take herbs yourself. You can be much more effective in marketing Chinese medicine when you are doing the things you'd like your patients to do."
>
> —Elizabeth Liddell
> Philadelphia, PA

SECTION FOUR: MARKETING YOUR PRACTICE

▶ **Close your practice for a specific period of time**

This is an extreme measure, but we have heard of it. Alternatively, you may have your front desk tell people that you are not taking new patients until such-and-such a date and then create a call-back system for anyone who wants to be put on a waiting list.

Want to sell your practice? Get a free quote and selling ideas from Professional Practice Specialists, Inc., www.practicesales.com, 800-645-7590. See Section 3, Chapter 7 for more on this topic.

▶ **Conclusion**

Of course it is our hope that all practitioners will become so successful that they need to consider options for limiting or channeling the growth of their practice or hiring a younger practitioner to work for them in order to maintain their personal health while still growing their income. We hope that any practitioner out there who has managed this phase of their professional life in some creative way that we have not discussed here will get in touch with us. I [HW] might post your story on my blog and include it in the next edition of this book. It is our personal goal that thousands more acupuncturists become financially and personally successful beyond their wildest dreams.

> **PRACTITIONER POINTER**
>
> "I am so grateful to be an acupuncturist! I want to develop a therapeutic relationship for life with each patient, so I try to bring my A-game to my work every day. When each patient leaves my office, I hope I gave them as much as they gave me!"
>
> —Lori Gritz
> San Diego, CA

CHAPTER 9 | Growing Your Life... Avoiding Burnout

POWER POINT

Want more ideas? Cruise over to my blog at http://successfulacupuncurepractice.blogspot.com/. Mostly I write about practice management and success issues and there is an archive of my blogs as well. Maybe I can give you a bit of inspiration from time to time! I wish you a successful and happy professional life. Think more, do good work, and stay in touch!

POINTS TO PONDER FROM CHAPTER 9

- Once you are running a full, successful practice, you need to think about how to keep your patients happy and your income growing without leading to personal burnout, which does neither you nor your patients any good.

- You can raise your fees significantly and see who drops out of your practice. This will only work for a short while if you are good, so do this first.

- You can hire an associate, a specialist, or an MD to serve some of your patient overload.

- You can hire a treatment assistant to take out needles, do tuina, cupping, and/or moxibustion.

- You can limit your hours and take a waiting list for new patients.

- You can close your practice altogether for a month or two, taking no new patients until you feel there is space in your schedule.

- Take care of your health while you are taking care of others.

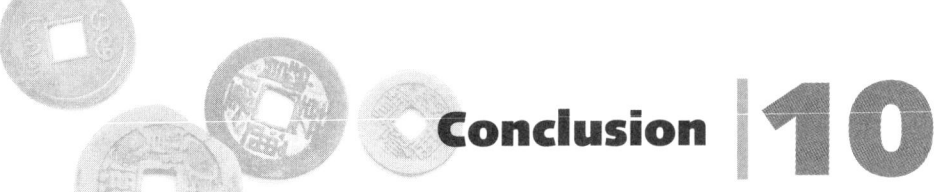

Conclusion | 10

At the beginning of this book we suggested that you try to think and work "from your dreams," visualizing the life, working environment, and income that you desire with as much clarity and intensity as you can. Everything included in this book is created to help you do just that. If you are clever, hardworking, and persistent enough to become wealthy (and we really hope you are), we'd like to suggest that you also take some time to consider how you will use that resource.

We believe that being a wealthy person carries with it great responsibility. There are only so many ways to spend money on yourself, and, ultimately, that is not what makes for a truly successful and happy life. So, what would you do with your money, time, or both if all your own needs and wants were met? How would you go about leaving the world a better place than you found it? What we are suggesting is to also formulate some meta-goals for after you have become materially comfortable and secure—in other words, reasons for becoming wealthy beyond simply materialism.

We leave you with those thoughts and we thank you for purchasing and, hopefully, reading and using this product to help you fulfill your goals and dreams. Best wishes to you for great and happy success. Live long and prosper.

Honora Lee Wolfe
Marilyn Allen

Resources for Going Further (books, classes, websites)

• Also go to http://pointsforprofit.bluepoppy.com •

▶ Resources for entrepreneurship
Websites
http://www.youngentrepreneur.com/forum Young Entrepreneurs Organization has a really good business plan template

http://www.weainc.webs.com/ Women Entrepreneurs of America has a blog, local chapters for business, referral, and moral support

www.entrepreneurship.org articles, resources, hot links, bookstore, glossary, media resource center

www.tannedfeet.com resources, legal forms, marketing, PR, human resources, humor

www.entrepreneurs.com resources, articles, web guide, marketing services

www.startupjournal.com Wall Street Journal Center for Entrepreneurs, business plan tools, trademark search, bookstore, articles, how-to, financing, running a business

Books
Steps to Small Business Start-up by Linda Pinson & Jerry Jinnett

The Entrepreneur's Guide to Finance & Business: Wealth Creation Techniques for Growing a Business by Steve Rogers et al.

Entrepreneurs: Talent, Temperament, Technique by John Thompson & Bill Bolton

What No One Ever Tells You About Starting Your Own Business by Jan Norman

Start Your Own Business: The Only Start-up Book You'll Ever Need by the staff at *Entrepreneur Media*

Thinking Like an Entrepreneur by Peter I. Hupalo

Working for Yourself: Law and Taxes for Independent Contractors, Freelancers and Consultants by Stephen Fishman

How to Start and Run Your Own Corporation by Peter I. Hupalo

The Young Entrepreneur's Guide to Starting and Running a Business by Steve Mariotti et al.

Defying the Odds by Marcia Israel-Curley

Free Money and Help for Women Entrepreneurs by Matthew Lesko et al.

Entrepreneur's Ultimate Start-up Directory by James Stephenson

Think & Grow Rich by Napoleon Hill

▶ Resources for writing a business plan
Web resources
www.bplans.com sample plans, software, legal advice, market research, "ask the experts," web directory

www.sba.gov/ business plan basics and tons of other stuff besides!

www.businessplans.org software, resources, consulting, examples, tools
www.planigent.com customizable, downloadable, do-it-yourself plans
www.morebusiness.com/templates_worksheets/bplans/ templates, tools, books
www.planware.org software to try and buy, white papers to read, things to do
These sites come and go, but you can find dozens of sites and blogs on this subject. Some online sleuthing will help you get exactly the help you are looking for.

Books
Anatomy of a Business Plan by Linda Pinson
Successful Business Planning in 30 Days by Peter J. Patsula
Business Plan Kit for Dummies (with CD-Rom)
   by Steven J. Peterson & Peter E. Jaret
The Ernst & Young Business Plan Guide by Ernst & Young LLP
***The One Page Business Plan* by Peter J. Patsula, highly recommended!
The Successful Business Plan: Secrets & Strategies by Rhonda Adams
Business Plans for Dummies by Paul Tiffany & Steven J. Peterson
How to Write a Business Plan by Mike McKeever
The Complete Book of Business Plans by Joseph A. Covello
The McGraw-Hill Guide to Writing a High-impact Business Plan
   by James B. Arkebauer
Writing Business Plans that Get Results by Michael O'Donnell

▶ Resources for lowering taxes & legitimate business deductions
Websites
www.Kiplinger.com
http://taxes.about.com/od/taxplanning/Lower_Your_Taxes.htm
http://www.wikihow.com/Save-Money-on-Taxes
www.articlesbase.com/business-articles/

Books
422 Tax Deductions for Businesses and Self-employed Individuals
   by Bernard Kamoroff
The Complete Idiot's Guide to Tax Breaks & Deductions by Lita Epstein
Lower Your Taxes—Big Time! by Sanford C. Botkin
Your Federal Income Tax (Publication 17), *Tax Guide for Small Business*
   (Publication 334), and *Guide to Free Tax Services* (Publication 910) are all free from your local IRS office online or at 800-829-1040
The Confident Indie: A Simple Guide to Deductions, Income and Taxes for The Creatively Self-employed by June Walker

RESOURCES FOR GOING FURTHER (BOOKS, CLASSES, WEBSITES)

▶ Resources for finding a job
Job search websites
www.acupuncturetoday.com
www.alternativehealthjobs.com
www.monster.com
www.postdocjobs.com
www.tcmstudent.com
www.pocacoop.com
www.careerbuilder.com
www.job.com
www.overseasjobs.com
http://www.indeed.com/
www.nationjob.com
www.jobsonline.com

Books
Push: 50 Secrets on How to Land a Job by Creating Social Media Buzz by Nelson Wang
Get a Life, Not a Job: Do What You Love and Let Your Talents Work for You by Paula Caligiuri PhD

▶ Resources about "buzz," word-of-mouth marketing
Websites
www.womma.org/ WOMMA (Word of Mouth Marketing Association)

Books
The Anatomy of Buzz by Emmanuel Rosen
What Clients Love: A Field Guide to Growing Your Business by Harry Beckwith
Tribe by Seth Godin
The Tipping Point: How Little Things Can Make a Big Difference by Malcolm Gladwell
How Customers Think by Gerald Zaltman
Why We Buy: The Science of Shopping by Paco Underhill
Creating Customer Evangelists by Ben McConnell & Jackie Huba
Love Is the Killer App: How to Win Business and Influence Friends by Tim Sanders
The Secret of Word-of-Mouth Marketing by George Silverman

▶ Resources for learning the art of negotiation
Websites
At any given time, there are many blogs and online articles to give you inspiration for negotiating anything: a job offer, a lease deal, a buy/sell agreement, a partnership.

Books
Getting to Yes: Negotiating Agreement Without Giving In by Roger Fiske *et al.*
The Only Negotiating Guide You'll Ever Need: 101 Ways to Win Every Time in Any Situation by Peter B. Stark & Jane S. Flaherty

431

Getting Past No: Negotiating Your Way from Confrontation to Cooperation by William Ury
Secrets of Power Negotiating by Roger Dawson
A Woman's Guide to Successful Negotiating by Lee E. Miller & Jessica Miller

Resources to improve and inspire your marketing
Websites
www.marketingtips.com
www.successmagazine.com
www.marketingsurvivalkit.com
www.clickz.com
http://www.insights-for-acupuncturists.com/lisa-hanfileti.html
www.acupunctureclinicmarketing.com/
www.acupuncturemarketing360.com/Free

Books
How to Give a Damn Good Speech by Philip R. Theibert
Chase's Calendar of Events published by McGraw-Hill
Purple Cow: Transform Your Business by Being Remarkable by Seth Godin
The Icarus Deception: How High Will You Fly? by Seth Godin
The Art of Possibility: Transforming Professional and Personal Life by Rosamund Stone Zander & Benjamin Zander
Raving Fans: A Revolutionary Approach to Customer Service by Kenneth Blanchard and Sheldon Bowles, *et al.*
Marketing Outrageously by Jon Spoelstra
Don't Worry, Make Money: Spiritual and Practical Ways to Create Abundance in Your Life by Richard Carlson

Resources for hiring and managing employees
Websites
www.entrepreneur.com
www.assessmentspecialists.com
www.businesstown.com/hiring
http://www.irs.gov/Businesses/Small-Businesses-&-Self-Employed/Hiring-Employees
www.entrepreneur.com/humanresources/index.html

Books
Finding & Keeping Great Employees by Jim Harris and Joan Brannick
Perfect Phrases for Performance Reviews by Douglas Max and Robert Bacal
1501 Ways to Reward Employees by Bob Nelson and Kenneth Blanchard
Why Employees Don't Do What They're Supposed to and What to Do About It by F. F. Fournies

RESOURCES FOR GOING FURTHER (BOOKS, CLASSES, WEBSITES)

First, Break All the Rules! What the World's Greatest Managers Do Differently by Marcus Buckingham & Curt Coffman

Resources for working with your money neuroses
Websites
http://www.successwithmoney.com/debt/debtfreemind.php
www.flyingsolo.com.au/
www.growingwealthy.com
www.artofabundance.com

Books
The Millionaire Course: A Visionary Plan for Creating the Life of Your Dreams by Marc Allen
The StartUp Garden: How Growing a Business Grows You by Jim Collins & Tom Ehrenfeld
Making Peace with Money by Jerrold Mundis
Peak Vitality: Raising the Threshold of Abundance in Our Material, Spiritual and Emotional Lives by Jeanne House
Money and the Meaning of Life by Jacob Needleman
Your Money or Your Life by Joe Dominguez, **highly recommended

Resources for billing insurance
Books
Playing the Game: A Step-by-Step Guide to Billing Insurance as an Acupuncturist by Dr. Greg Sperber and Tiffany Andersen-Hefner
The Acupuncture Code Book by H.J. Ross & Co.

For lots more resources and links, go to:
http://pointsforprofit.bluepoppy.com

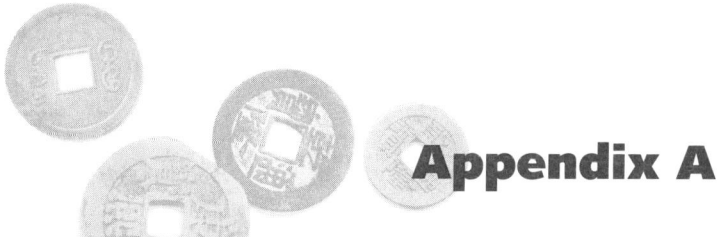

Appendix A

Getting a National Provider Identifier (NPI) Number

All healthcare providers, whether an individual or a group practice, that provide medical or other health services or supplies, must now be assigned an NPI 10 position numeric identifier. This NPI is a unique identification number that will be used by all health plans. It will be required on all CMS-1500 forms, on superbills, and may be required on some HIPAA-related forms as well.

There are three ways to apply for an NPI:
- Online at https://nppes.cms.hhs.gov
- Mail to request an application from NPPES, PO Box 6059 Fargo, ND 58108-6059
- Phone NPPES to request that an application be sent to you at 800-465-3203 or 800-692-2326

Healthcare providers must notify NPPES within 30 days of an office relocation. Since your NPI will be used for billing purposes and other transactions, it should be kept private and secure.

Appendix B

10 Things to Consider When Creating a Work Agreement with a Hospital

These questions need to be at least discussed, and better yet written in your contract or work agreement with any hospital or other public health facility.

1. How much should you charge? If you had no overhead at all, how much would you need to make per patient or per hour to be comfortable? That's where you might start. If most of your patients will be billing insurance, discuss how much you will be reimbursed for various codes.
2. Who will order supplies and who will pay for them? How will needles and other biohazard materials be handled? If you are required to pay for these items, could you be reimbursed?
3. How many treatment spaces do you want or need to work efficiently? If you need more than one treatment space at a time to be efficient or make an adequate living, will that always be available?
4. Be collegial and neither arrogant nor intimidated. If you value what you do and start from a position of building a positive relationship with the other practitioners and administrators on the hospital team, trust is likely to be easier to build. Also remember that, to get along most effectively, you need to dress in professional medical style and speak medical-speak comfortably.
5. How will your services be marketed and who will be responsible for that marketing? Will you have access

Appendix B continues on the next page

to other departments to put out brochures, put up signage, give in-service lectures, attend meetings, and meet others who are potential referral sources? Will you be allowed to use the hospital name on your card to help you market outside the hospital?

6. How long will you work there before your contract is up for renewal? Under what conditions can you terminate the contract legally? Is it transferrable to another practitioner?
7. Are there any other duties for which you will be responsible in addition to doing acupuncture? Do any of these require training?
8. Will you be permitted to prescribe herbal medicine in appropriate situations? If so, how will it be paid for?
9. Will you be salaried, an independent contractor, paid by the hour or by the patient? Will you have any benefits such as health insurance or paid vacation? If not right away, when might such benefits begin and how do you apply for them?
10. If most or all patients are billing insurance for your services as well as other services in the hospital, how will that billing be handled and how does it relate to what you are paid?

A simple online search for hospital jobs for acupuncturists will get you pages of results from all over the U.S. If this is a goal of yours, check out these leads now. For more in-depth information on working in hospitals and negotiating with hospitals, search the archive of issues at *AcupunctureToday.com*.

Index

A
aborm.org, 22
accident report, 306
accountants, 54, 56, 147
accounts receivable, 61, 331, 335, 337
active listener, 230
acu-facelifts, 365
acupuncture care, 19, 84, 97, 105, 109, 133, 184, 263, 303, 317
acupuncture cosmetology, 323
aesthetics, 363
Affordable Care Act, 48, 262, 275, 281
Allen, Marilyn, 1
alternative care coverage, 262
alumni newsletter, 71, 79
American Acupuncture Council, 40, 42
Americans with Disabilities Act (ADA), 148-149, 178
annual gross receipts, 331
anorexia, 374
answering services, 28, 241
Appointy, 26
arbitration, 67, 228
arbitration agreement, 228
aromatherapy, 167, 324, 328-329, 417
articles of incorporation, 239-240
artistic touches, 355
assignment of benefits contract, 279-280
Associated Press Stylebook and Libel Manual, 400
attitudes about money, 251-252, 254
auto accident information form, 305-306

B
barter, 240, 270
barter arrangement, 240
billing services, 111, 243
Blogger, Blogspot 411-413, 416, 418
blogging, 410-411, 413, 418
bonding call, 231, 234, 237
bookkeepers, 238-239
Brand, Eric, 221
brand identity, 19
brochures for your clinic, 389
brochure displays, 351
bulk herb preparation services, 245
bullet points, 367, 391, 407, 410
bulletin boards, 72, 336
business associate agreements, 195
business bank, 246
business cards, 19, 21, 25, 57, 105, 107, 109, 117, 244, 342, 347, 369, 374-375, 386, 410, 419, 421
business phone hours, 225
business plan, 2, 87, 92, 144-146, 155-161, 342, 429-430
business structure, 49, 140
buying an acupuncture practice, 330-331
by-laws, 64, 66, 239

C
CafeMoms, 413
call forwarding services, 28
cash flow, 14, 131, 160, 324, 327, 332, 336
C-corporation, 53
certification, 37-38, 40, 285, 385
Chambers of Commerce, 16
Chinese pharmacy, 349
choose advisors, 28
Clean Needle Technique, 40, 385
clearinghouse, 375
clinic brochures, 389
clinic market position, 332, 338
clinic mission statement, 385
clinic partners, 81, 200
clinic software, 179, 184, 190, 194
Cliniko, 26
CMS, 116, 197, 206, 294, 296-297, 300, 318, 435
cold sufferers, 361
community acupuncture, 1-2, 7, 14, 22, 70, 93-94, 96-97, 125-126, 132-134, 166, 204, 257, 271, 274
community college, 29, 345-346, 374, 376, 402
community participation, 368
compliance manual, 194-196, 198
comprehensive patient examination, 288
computer geek, 238, 243
concentration ratio, 234
confidence and communication, 237
confidential information form, 185, 296, 304
conflict resolution procedure, 63
continuing education, 11, 97, 137
co-pay, 264, 270, 276, 278, 281-282
corporate HR managers, 383
corporate marketing strategies, 366
corporations, 52-53, 56, 58, 146, 394
course of therapy, 232
court appearance, 309
covered entity, 193

439

CPT codes, 197-198, 264, 269, 287, 290, 298, 301, 317-318
Craigslist, 72-73, 105, 112, 210, 307
credentialed panel, 278
credit card machines, 259-260, 274
credit report, 214
current procedural terminology, 197, 282, 287
curriculum vitae, 74, 382, 385
customer service, 127, 199, 209, 260, 281, 282, 348, 363, 404, 432

D
day-to-day operating tasks, 116, 141, 156
death or incapacity, 67
deferment, 33
demographics, 16, 31, 332
dermatology, 77, 100, 221, 323, 365
Direct loans, 34, 36
disclosure form, mandatory, 185
diversified cash base, 258
documentation, required, 317
domain name, 404
don't be lazy, 421
Dreamweaver, 402-403, 418
dropped patient, 236

E
E&M codes, 287-289, 298
e-commerce, 417-418
electronic medical records (EMR), 1, 2, 47-48, 111, 184, 189-190
elevator speech, 420
email blasts, 378, 410
employee maintenance, 209
employee manual, 205, 207-208, 210
employees, 30, 128, 141, 176, 192, 199-200, 205, 209, 216-217, 240, 262-263, 268, 279, 281, 315-316, 344, 365-367, 375, 423, 432
endangered species, 252
energy exchange, 253
equipment for your practice, 31
exit strategy, 151-152, 336, 338
expenses, log of 131
experienced retirees, 134

F
Facebook, 30, 72, 74, 91, 152, 174, 273, 307, 402, 409, 411, 414-417
fax log, 24, 116
featured speaker, 343
federal audits, 52, 56
Federal Perkins loan, 33, 36
fee for services, 262
fee-splitting, 423
FFEL, 33
fibromyalgia, 294, 384, 412

financial policy form, 186
financial success, 254
first right of refusal, 66
Flaws, Bob, 43, 219
follow-up phone calls, 72, 425
forebearance, 33
forms, designing your own, 23
Free Health Tips, 370
front desk gatekeeper, 344
Frostad, John, 261

G
Genbook, 26
general clinic brochure, 389
general partnership, 52, 55
get out of town, 99
goals, setting, 4-6, 9-11, 13, 157
Godin, Seth, 413, 419, 431, 432
going rates for similar services, 134
golden rule of medical charting, 46
goodwill, 49, 331, 333, 338
goals, setting, 10, 12-13
Google Alerts, 416
Google Places, 409
Grad PLUS loans, 32-33
graphic designer, 238, 244, 391
greed, 252
gynecology, 77, 84, 100, 221, 424

H
Hansen, Mark Victor, 8, 341
hard assets, 331
hardship waiver forms, 24, 271
healthcare operations form, 187
Healthcare Providers Service Organization, 42
health editor, 373
health fairs, 368, 375
herbal dispensary, 30, 111, 218, 222
herbal inventory, 112
herbal practitioner, 233
Hill, Napoleon, 421, 429
HIPAA compliance forms, 184-189, 192-198
HIPAA regulations, 116, 192-198
hiring and firing procedures, 63
HMO, 30-31, 123, 394
hospital administrators, 343
hourly income requirements, 156
hourly wage, 200
human resources (HR), 30, 205, 263, 281, 316-317, 320, 343, 365-366, 375, 393-394, 429
HVAC, 238

I
IBR, 33-35
ICD-9/10 codes, 293, 295, 301

INDEX

improvements in function, 317
independent contractor, 89-90, 437
individual patient identifiable health information, 197
industrial medicine, 315, 319-320
information scrapbook, 351, 354
informed consent form, 185
initial phone conversation, 237, 304
Instagram, 416
insurance benefits, 276, 280, 305
insurance claim form, 297
insurance patients, 111, 113, 186, 193, 257, 262, 275, 284, 292, 301, 305
insurance tracer letter, 284, 300
intake form, 184
intangible assets, 332
intellectual curiosity, 421
interact effectively with the media, 373
internal marketing, 164, 350, 360
International Classification of Disease, 293
internet marketing, 2, 14, 402, 411
inventory management, 63, 118
IRS rules, 211-212

J

janitorial services, 28, 195
job description, 201, 208, 223, 310
job qualifications, 201
joint venture limited partnership, 55-56

K

key words, 404-406, 409
Kiyosaki, Robert, 50

L

laissez-faire, 39
laundry service, 238, 242, 335
lawsuits, 40-41, 46, 53, 66, 210
lazy, don't be, 421
lease agreement, 242, 338
lectures, giving, 375, 417
legal protection, 53, 58, 210
legal representation, 306
legalzoom.com, 38, 63
lending library, 165, 349
letter of denial, 267-268
letters of reference, 382, 391
liability waiver, 24, 114
lifetime goals, 10
limited liability company (LLC), 55, 140
limited partnership, 55
liniments, 167, 324, 328
LinkedIn, 72, 91, 112, 307, 414-415
link popularity, 406-407
listing services, 408
loan forgiveness, 32, 36
logo, 25, 31, 107-109, 117, 122, 334, 387, 395, 406

M

mailing list, 266, 332, 338, 344, 353, 369, 371, 376-381, 393, 401
maintaining an herbal pharmacy, 119
malpractice insurance, 22, 28, 37, 40-42, 45, 48, 50-52, 56-57, 83, 85, 87, 129, 137-138, 179, 181, 228, 246-247, 285-286, 383-384
managed care network, 257, 264, 270, 276, 278, 281-282
managed-care organizations, 278
managerial experience, 70, 74
mandatory disclosure form, 24
marketing, good, 165, 420
marketing plan, 156, 349, 396
marketing, the essence of good, 420
markup, 63, 327
mastermind group, 421
media coverage, 372, 396
media moguls, 343
Medicaid, 265-266, 278, 296, 298, 301
medical history form, 184
medical-legal report, 311
medical lien, 306
medical malpractice insurance, 245-247
medical transcription, 238, 242
Medicare, 49, 54, 56-57, 211-213, 217, 267, 278-279, 296
Meetup.com, 416
mentoring opportunities, 70
merchant services providers, 261
metatags, 405
methods of payment, 257, 259, 262, 264, 266, 268, 270, 272
MIEC Group, 42
mission statement for you clinic, 385
money neuroses, 251, 433
money, the love of, 252, 254
movie certificates, 363
multi-discipline treatment facilities, 21

N

name availability, 20, 106
National Diabetes Week, 401
NCCAOM, 17, 37-40, 72, 137, 385-386
negotiating a lease, 141, 148-149
negotiation, 74, 431
networking, 15, 80, 83, 92, 347, 364, 404, 409, 414, 416
new patient FAQ, 24
newsletters, 44, 79, 336, 352, 367, 373, 378, 404
niche market, 30-31, 146, 165, 343, 365, 380
no fault insurance, 314
no fault or tort liability, 302
nonprofit corporation, 56
Norcal Mutual Insurance Group, 42

441

National Provider Indentier (NPI) number, 298, 300, 435

O
Office Ally, 111, 119, 190, 206, 243, 300
office manager, 241
off-peak-hours, 75
Old Testament, 254
One Minute Millionaire, The, 8, 341
online promotion, 411
operating agreements, 62
operational procedure guidelines, 63
Oriental medical jargon, 391
orthopedic surgeons, 80
OUM Healthcare Professionals Program, 42
overhead expenses, 332

P
paralegal, 238, 240, 306
paranoid in reverse, 375
PARQ form, 186
partnership, 9, 50, 52, 55, 58, 60, 64-65, 69, 212, 239, 424, 432
partnership return of income, 52
partnerships, 52, 57, 78
part-time position, 73
patient abandonment, 245
patient charting requirements, 46
patient health history, 24, 114
patient management, 24, 63, 74, 112, 224-225, 227, 229, 231, 233-235, 237, 294, 356-358, 361, 363
patient management software, 294
patient medical records, 45
patient, the disappearing, 234
paying taxes, 45, 49, 55
Paypal, 417, 418
payroll company, 205, 214, 216, 217
personal budget, 129
personal injury patients, 195, 270, 303, 306, 308, 310, 312
personal injury questionnaire, 306
phone questions people ask, 237
phone system, effective, 356
phone verification for acupuncture, 305
phone verification of insurance coverage, 282
physical examination, 289, 312
pills, powders, tinctures, 234
Pinterest, 414, 416
plastic cards, 387
POCAcoop.com, 29, 93, 94, 96, 431
postcards, 44, 73-74, 260, 336
post-op patients, 389
potential patients, 19, 25, 28, 59, 86, 105, 124-125, 243, 381, 407, 409
poverty, 132, 252, 271

power of attorney, 284, 305
practice management, 1, 3, 14, 17, 257, 345, 427
pre-authorization for treatments, 317-318
preferred provider organization, 264, 435
prescription pad, 382, 387, 388
presentation folder, 74, 92, 107, 343, 365-366, 373, 382, 384, 386, 388, 390-394
privacy officer, 194
privacy practices notice, 44
prize-winners, 369
pro bono, 335
professional corporation (PC), 58
professional disclosure form, 185
professional medical care providers, 42, 435
Professional Practice Specialists Inc., 426
progress reports, 303, 314
prospective patient interactions, 106-107, 132, 163, 191, 225-226, 283, 318, 372, 397
Protected Health Information (PHI), 43-44, 196
provider services department, 283, 292
public lectures, 353, 375
Public Relations Society of America, 400
publicity, free, 355, 400-401
pulse diagnosis sessions, free, 370

R
radio personalities, 343
raise your prices, 422
range of motion, 304, 312, 316, 420
realistic budget, 134
reduced pricing, 232
reflexology, 349
regulations regarding acupuncture, 16
regulatory climate, 16, 335
release of patient information form, 186
religious affiliations, 17
renewal requirements, 21, 38
rent-free clinic, 75
requirements for documentation, 21, 28, 38, 40, 193, 196, 211-212, 226, 317
rescission of attorney assignment of benefits, 305
research, printed, 383
return on investment, 349

S
Sandler, David, 7
satisfied patients, 60, 351, 360, 399
Schedule C, 51
Schedule K-1, 52
Schedule SE, 51, 55, 213
Schedulicity, 26
school diploma, 48
scope of practice, 50, 187, 281, 318, 323, 394

SCORE, 106, 134, 240
S corporation, 53-54
Scott Danahy Naylon Co., 43
scribble or erase, don't, 47
script for a health fair, 371
search engine, 14, 403-408, 412
secrets of negotiation, 74, 338, 431
self-care products, 369
self-employment taxes, 51, 212-213
selling an acupuncture practice, 331, 335-337, 426
setting goals, 4-6, 9-11, 13, 157
sliding scales, 271
Smoke Out, The Great American, 401, 420
SOAP notes, 185, 312
social network marketing, 418
software for your clinic, 179, 184, 190, 194
software programmer, 110
sole proprietorship, 50-53, 55, 136
specialization, 19, 100-101, 344
Squidoo, 413-414, 418
Stafford loans, 33, 36
standard decocted formula, 234
start-up capital, 37
state acupuncture board, 16-18
state sales tax, 16, 38, 56, 211, 215-217
statute of limitations, 45-46, 48
Strand, Eric, 1, 221
student loan debt, 32-36
subrogation, 151, 303
suggested retail price, 328
surviving partner, 67

T
tax preparation, 239
teaching classes, 1, 345, 375
The Elements of Style, 400
The Great American Smoke Out, 401, 420
third-party payers, 41, 47
three-month trial period, 76
tourists, 273
treatment aides, 425
treatments, free, 144, 266, 267, 272, 273, 347, 420
trust your crazy dreams, 12
Twitter, 32, 414-416

typefaces, 386, 392, 398
typical business plan, 158
TV shows, 343, 373-374, 377, 396, 398

U
unemployment compensation, 207, 210
unique selling proposition, 109
urinalysis, 229

V
vacation, 59, 63, 69, 77, 90, 129, 173, 175, 177, 204, 245, 323, 328, 329, 437
valuation expert, 333, 334
visual symbol, 25, 109
voluntary simplicity, 256

W
web ads, 409
web designer, 238, 243, 402-403
web marketing, 405, 408
website content, 224
website creation tools, 403
Western diagnostic intakes, 81
Western medical providers, 229, 317
Western medical system, 2, 38, 41-42, 80, 84, 91, 179
what can you call yourself, 39
Wood Insurance Group, 43
word-of-mouth, 14, 336, 431
Wordpress, 411-413
Workers' Compensation, 28, 46, 49, 100, 195, 315-321
  in California, 291
writing articles, 364, 375
writing press releases, 400
written promotional pieces, 387

Y
Yahoo, 403
Yelp, 105, 152, 240, 260, 307, 409, 414, 416

Z
Zazzle.com, 108

Honora Lee Wolfe

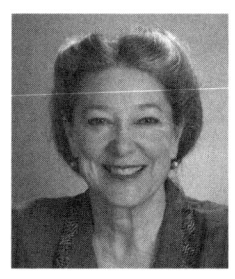

Honora Lee Wolfe has been involved in professional health care education since 1976. Director at the Boulder College of Massage Therapy for five years, Ms. Wolfe went on to study tuina massage at the Shanghai College of TCM and completed her acupuncture training in 1988. She teaches regularly at national and regional acupuncture colleges and conferences in North America and Europe and is the author or co-author of several books, including *Prince Wen Hui's Cook: Chinese Dietary Therapy*, *How to Have a Healthy Pregnancy Healthy Birth with Chinese Medicine*, *Managing Menopause Naturally with Chinese Medicine*, *Better Breast Health Naturally with Chinese Medicine*, *Points for Profit: The Essential Guide to Practice Success for Acupuncturists*, *The Successful Chinese Herbalist: How to Prescribe Correctly, Gain Patient Comliance, and Operate a Profitable Dispensary*, and most recently *Western Physical Exam Skills for Asian Medicine Practitioners*.

Marilyn Allen

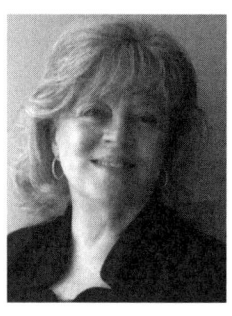

Marilyn Allen is a practice management consultant for the acupuncture profession, with expertise in practice building, office management, marketing, and professional ethics and jurisprudence.

With a M.S. in Management and Administration from Pepperdine University, she has honed her skills in several large complementary medicine clinics. Marilyn serves as the Public Relations and Marketing Director for the American Acupuncture Council. She has been appointed to the Acupuncture Advisory Committee for the Little Hoover Commission in the State of California. She has recently represented the American Association of Acupuncture and Oriental Medicine at the Meeting of the World Health Organization for the standardization of patterns and syndromes. Marilyn also serves on the Chairman's Advisory Group, and is a member of, the US Delegation for the International Standards Organization, to standardize herbs and medical devices used in Acupuncture offices.

Marilyn has been a contributor to three different Oriental Medicine journals and in 1999 was named as the Editor of Acupuncture Today.

OTHER BOOKS ON CHINESE MEDICINE AVAILABLE FROM:
BLUE POPPY PRESS
1990 North 57th Court, Unit A, Boulder, CO 80301
For ordering 1-800-487-9296 PH. 303\447-8372 FAX 303\245-8362
Email: info@bluepoppy.com Website: www.bluepoppy.com

ACUPOINT POCKET REFERENCE
by Bob Flaws
ISBN 0-936185-93-7
ISBN 978-0-936185-93-4

ACUPUNCTURE, CHINESE MEDICINE &
HEALTHY WEIGHT LOSS   Revised Edition
by Juliette Aiyana, L. Ac.
ISBN 1-891845-61-6
ISBN 978-1-891845-61-1

ACUPUNCTURE & IVF
by Lifang Liang
ISBN 0-891845-24-1
ISBN 978-0-891845-24-6

ACUPUNCTURE FOR STROKE REHABILITATION
Three Decades of Information from China
by Hoy Ping Yee Chan, et al.
ISBN 1-891845-35-7
ISBN 978-1-891845-35-2

ACUPUNCTURE PHYSICAL MEDICINE:
An Acupuncture Touchpoint Approach to the
Treatment of Chronic Pain, Fatigue, and Stress
Disorders
by Mark Seem
ISBN 1-891845-13-6
ISBN 978-1-891845-13-0

AGING & BLOOD STASIS:
A New Approach to TCM Geriatrics
by Yan De-xin
ISBN 0-936185-63-6
ISBN 978-0-936185-63-7

AN ACUPUNCTURISTS GUIDE TO MEDICAL RED
FLAGS & REFERRALS
by Dr. David Anzaldua, MD
ISBN 1-891845-54-3
ISBN 978-1-891845-54-3

BETTER BREAST HEALTH NATURALLY
with CHINESE MEDICINE
by Honora Lee Wolfe & Bob Flaws
ISBN 0-936185-90-2
ISBN 978-0-936185-90-3

BIOMEDICINE: A TEXTBOOK FOR PRACTITIONERS
OF ACUPUNCTURE AND ORIENTAL MEDICINE
by Bruce H. Robinson, MD   Second Edition
ISBN 1-891845-62-4
ISBN 978-1-891845-62-8

THE BOOK OF JOOK: Chinese Medicinal Porridges
by Bob Flaws
ISBN 0-936185-60-6
ISBN 978-0-936185-60-0

CHANNEL DIVERGENCES Deeper Pathways of the
Web
by Miki Shima and Charles Chase
ISBN 1-891845-15-2
ISBN 978-1-891845-15-4

CHINESE MEDICAL OBSTETRICS
by Bob Flaws
ISBN 1-891845-30-6
ISBN 978-1-891845-30-7

CHINESE MEDICAL PALMISTRY:
Your Health in Your Hand
by Zong Xiao-fan & Gary Liscum
ISBN 0-936185-64-3
ISBN 978-0-936185-64-4

CHINESE MEDICAL PSYCHIATRY
A Textbook and Clinical Manual
by Bob Flaws and James Lake, MD
ISBN 1-845891-17-9
ISBN 978-1-845891-17-8

CHINESE MEDICINAL TEAS: Simple, Proven, Folk
Formulas for Common Diseases & Promoting Health
by Zong Xiao-fan & Gary Liscum
ISBN 0-936185-76-7
ISBN 978-0-936185-76-7

CHINESE MEDICINAL WINES & ELIXIRS
by Bob Flaws   Revised Edition
ISBN 0-936185-58-9
ISBN 978-0-936185-58-3

CHINESE PEDIATRIC MASSAGE THERAPY: A
Parent's & Practitioner's Guide to the Prevention &
Treatment of Childhood Illness
by Fan Ya-li
ISBN 0-936185-54-6
ISBN 978-0-936185-54-5

CHINESE SCALP ACUPUNCTURE
by Jason Jishun Hao & Linda Lingzhi Hao
ISBN 1-891845-60-8
ISBN 978-1-891845-60-4

CHINESE SELF-MASSAGE THERAPY:
The Easy Way to Health
by Fan Ya-li
ISBN 0-936185-74-0
ISBN 978-0-936185-74-3

THE CLASSIC OF DIFFICULTIES:
A Translation of the *Nan Jing*
translation by Bob Flaws
ISBN 1-891845-07-1
ISBN 978-1-891845-07-9

A CLINICIAN'S GUIDE TO USING GRANULE
EXTRACTS
by Eric Brand
ISBN 1-891845-51-9
ISBN 978-1-891845-51-2

A COMPENDIUM OF CHINESE MEDICAL
MENSTRUAL DISEASES
by Bob Flaws
ISBN 1-891845-31-4
ISBN 978-1-891845-31-4

CONCISE CHINESE MATERIA MEDICA
by Eric Brand and Nigel Wiseman
ISBN 0-912111-82-8
ISBN 978-0-912111-82-7

CONTEMPORARY GYNECOLOGY: An Integrated
Chinese-Western Approach
by Lifang Liang
ISBN 1-891845-50-0
ISBN 978-1-891845-50-5

CONTROLLING DIABETES NATURALLY WITH
CHINESE MEDICINE
by Lynn Kuchinski
ISBN 0-936185-06-3
ISBN 978-0-936185-06-2

CURING ARTHRITIS NATURALLY WITH
CHINESE MEDICINE
by Douglas Frank & Bob Flaws
ISBN 0-936185-87-2
ISBN 978-0-936185-87-3

CURING DEPRESSION NATURALLY WITH
CHINESE MEDICINE
by Rosa Schnyer & Bob Flaws
ISBN 0-936185-94-5
ISBN 978-0-936185-94-1

CURING FIBROMYALGIA NATURALLY WITH
CHINESE MEDICINE
by Bob Flaws
ISBN 1-891845-09-8
ISBN 978-1-891845-09-3

CURING HAY FEVER NATURALLY WITH
CHINESE MEDICINE
by Bob Flaws
ISBN 0-936185-91-0
ISBN 978-0-936185-91-0

CURING HEADACHES NATURALLY WITH
CHINESE MEDICINE
by Bob Flaws
ISBN 0-936185-95-3
ISBN 978-0-936185-95-8

CURING IBS NATURALLY WITH CHINESE
MEDICINE
by Jane Bean Oberski
ISBN 1-891845-11-X
ISBN 978-1-891845-11-6

CURING INSOMNIA NATURALLY WITH
CHINESE MEDICINE
by Bob Flaws
ISBN 0-936185-86-4
ISBN 978-0-936185-86-6

CURING PMS NATURALLY WITH CHINESE
MEDICINE
by Bob Flaws
ISBN 0-936185-85-6
ISBN 978-0-936185-85-9

DISEASES OF THE KIDNEY & BLADDER
by Hoy Ping Yee Chan, et al.
ISBN 1-891845-37-3
ISBN 978-1-891845-35-6

THE DIVINE FARMER'S MATERIA MEDICA
A Translation of the Shen Nong Ben Cao
translation by Yang Shouz-zhong
ISBN 0-936185-96-1
ISBN 978-0-936185-96-5

DUI YAO: THE ART OF COMBINING
CHINESE HERBAL MEDICINALS
by Philippe Sionneau
ISBN 0-936185-81-3
ISBN 978-0-936185-81-1

ENDOMETRIOSIS, INFERTILITY AND
TRADITIONAL CHINESE MEDICINE:
A Layperson's Guide
by Bob Flaws
ISBN 0-936185-14-7
ISBN 978-0-936185-14-9

THE ESSENCE OF LIU FENG-WU'S GYNECOLOGY
by Liu Feng-wu, translated by Yang Shou-zhong
ISBN 0-936185-88-0
ISBN 978-0-936185-88-0

EXTRA TREATISES BASED ON INVESTIGATION &
INQUIRY: A Translation of Zhu Dan-xi's Ge Zhi Yu
Lun
translation by Yang Shou-zhong
ISBN 0-936185-53-8
ISBN 978-0-936185-53-8

FIRE IN THE VALLEY: TCM Diagnosis & Treatment of
Vaginal Diseases
by Bob Flaws
ISBN 0-936185-25-2
ISBN 978-0-936185-25-5

FULFILLING THE ESSENCE:
A Handbook of Traditional & Contemporary
Treatments for Female Infertility
by Bob Flaws
ISBN 0-936185-48-1
ISBN 978-0-936185-48-4

FU QING-ZHU'S GYNECOLOGY
trans. by Yang Shou-zhong and Liu Da-wei
ISBN 0-936185-35-X
ISBN 978-0-936185-35-4

GOLDEN NEEDLE WANG LE-TING: A 20th Century
Master's Approach to Acupuncture
by Yu Hui-chan and Han Fu-ru, trans. by Shuai Xue-zhong
ISBN 0-936185-78-3
ISBN 978-0-936185-78-1

A HANDBOOK OF CHINESE HEMATOLOGY
by Simon Becker
ISBN 1-891845-16-0
ISBN 978-1-891845-16-1

A HANDBOOK OF TCM PATTERNS
& THEIR TREATMENTS   Second Edition
by Bob Flaws & Daniel Finney
ISBN 0-936185-70-8
ISBN 978-0-936185-70-5

A HANDBOOK OF TRADITIONAL
CHINESE DERMATOLOGY
by Liang Jian-hui, trans. by Zhang Ting-liang
& Bob Flaws
ISBN 0-936185-46-5
ISBN 978-0-936185-46-0

A HANDBOOK OF TRADITIONAL
CHINESE GYNECOLOGY
by Zhejiang College of TCM, trans. by Zhang Ting-liang
& Bob Flaws
ISBN 0-936185-06-6 (4th edit.)
ISBN 978-0-936185-06-4

A HANDBOOK of TCM PEDIATRICS
by Bob Flaws
ISBN 0-936185-72-4
ISBN 978-0-936185-72-9

THE HEART & ESSENCE OF DAN-XI'S
METHODS OF TREATMENT
by Xu Dan-xi, trans. by Yang Shou-zhong
ISBN 0-926185-50-3
ISBN 978-0-936185-50-7

HERB TOXICITIES & DRUG INTERACTIONS:
A Formula Approach
by Fred Jennes with Bob Flaws
ISBN 1-891845-26-8
ISBN 978-1-891845-26-0

IMPERIAL SECRETS OF HEALTH & LONGEVITY
by Bob Flaws
ISBN 0-936185-51-1
ISBN 978-0-936185-51-4

INSIGHTS OF A SENIOR ACUPUNCTURIST
by Miriam Lee
ISBN 0-936185-33-3
ISBN 978-0-936185-33-0

INTEGRATED PHARMACOLOGY: Combining Modern Pharmacology with Chinese Medicine
by Dr. Greg Sperber with Bob Flaws
ISBN 1-891845-41-1
ISBN 978-0-936185-41-3

INTRODUCTION TO THE USE OF PROCESSED CHINESE MEDICINALS
by Philippe Sionneau
ISBN 0-936185-62-7
ISBN 978-0-936185-62-0

KEEPING YOUR CHILD HEALTHY WITH CHINESE MEDICINE
by Bob Flaws
ISBN 0-936185-71-6
ISBN 978-0-936185-71-2

THE LAKESIDE MASTER'S STUDY OF THE PULSE
by Li Shi-zhen, trans. by Bob Flaws
ISBN 1-891845-01-2
ISBN 978-1-891845-01-7

MANAGING MENOPAUSE NATURALLY WITH CHINESE MEDICINE
by Honora Lee Wolfe
ISBN 0-936185-98-8
ISBN 978-0-936185-98-9

MASTER HUA'S CLASSIC OF THE CENTRAL VISCERA
by Hua Tuo, trans. by Yang Shou-zhong
ISBN 0-936185-43-0
ISBN 978-0-936185-43-9

THE MEDICAL I CHING: Oracle of the Healer Within
by Miki Shima
ISBN 0-936185-38-4
ISBN 978-0-936185-38-5

MENOPAIUSE & CHINESE MEDICINE
by Bob Flaws
ISBN 1-891845-40-3
ISBN 978-1-891845-40-6

MOXIBUSTION: A MODERN CLINICAL HANDBOOK
by Lorraine Wilcox
ISBN 1-891845-49-7
ISBN 978-1-891845-49-9

MOXIBUSTION: THE POWER OF MUGWORT FIRE
by Lorraine Wilcox
ISBN 1-891845-46-2
ISBN 978-1-891845-46-8

A NEW AMERICAN ACUPUNTURE By Mark Seem
SBN 0-936185-44-9
SBN 978-0-936185-44-6

PLAYING THE GAME: A Step-by-Step Approach to Accepting Insurance as an Acupuncturist
by Greg Sperber & Tiffany Anderson-Hefner
SBN 3-131416-11-7
SBN 978-3-131416-11-7

POCKET ATLAS OF CHINESE MEDICINE
edited by Marne and Kevin Ergil
SBN 1-891-845-59-4
SBN 978-1-891845-59-8

POINTS FOR PROFIT: The Essential Guide to Practice Success for Acupuncturists 5th Fully Edited Edition
by Honora Wolfe with Marilyn Allen
ISBN 1-891845-25-X
ISBN 978-1-891845-25-3

PRINCIPLES OF CHINESE MEDICAL ANDROLOGY: An Integrated Approach to Male Reproductive and Urological Health by Bob Damone
ISBN 1-891845-45-4
ISBN 978-1-891845-45-1

PRINCE WEN HUI's COOK: Chinese Dietary Therapy
By Bob Flaws & Honora Wolfe
ISBN 0-912111-05-4
ISBN 978-0-912111-05-6

THE PULSE CLASSIC:
A Translation of the Mai Jing
by Wang Shu-he, trans. by Yang Shou-zhong
ISBN 0-936185-75-9
ISBN 978-0-936185-75-0

THE SECRET OF CHINESE PULSE DIAGNOSIS
by Bob Flaws
ISBN 0-936185-67-8
ISBN 978-0-936185-67-5

SECRET SHAOLIN FORMULAS FOR THE TREATMENT OF EXTERNAL INJURY
by De Chan, trans. by Zhang Ting-liang & Bob Flaws
ISBN 0-936185-08-2
ISBN 978-0-936185-08-8

STATEMENTS OF FACT IN TRADITIONAL CHINESE MEDICINE   Revised & Expanded
by Bob Flaws
ISBN 0-936185-52-X
ISBN 978-0-936185-52-1

STICKING TO THE POINT: A Step-by-Step Approach to TCM Acupuncture Therapy
by Bob Flaws & Honora Wolfe   2 Condensed Books
ISBN 1-891845-47-0
ISBN 978-1-891845-47-5

A STUDY OF DAOIST ACUPUNCTURE
by Liu Zheng-cai
ISBN 1-891845-08-X
ISBN 978-1-891845-08-6

THE SUCCESSFUL CHINESE HERBALIST
by Bob Flaws and Honora Lee Wolfe
ISBN 1-891845-29-2
ISBN 978-1-891845-29-1

THE SYSTEMATIC CLASSIC OF ACUPUNCTURE & MOXIBUSTION
A translation of the Jia Yi Jing
by Huang-fu Mi, trans. by Yang Shou-zhong & Charles Chace
ISBN 0-936185-29-5
ISBN 978-0-936185-29-3

THE TAO OF HEALTHY EATING: DIETARY WISDOM ACCORDING TO CHINESE MEDICINE
by Bob Flaws   Second Edition
ISBN 0-936185-92-9
ISBN 978-0-936185-92-7

TEACH YOURSELF TO READ MODERN MEDICAL CHINESE
by Bob Flaws
ISBN 0-936185-99-6
ISBN 978-0-936185-99-6

TEST PREP WORKBOOK FOR BASIC TCM THEORY
by Zhong Bai-song
ISBN 1-891845-43-8
ISBN 978-1-891845-43-7

TEST PREP WORKBOOK FOR THE NCCAOM BIO-MEDICINE MODULE: Exam Preparation & Study Guide
by Zhong Bai-song
ISBN 1-891845-34-9
ISBN 978-1-891845-34-5

TREATING PEDIATRIC BED-WETTING WITH ACUPUNCTURE & CHINESE MEDICINE
by Robert Helmer
ISBN 1-891845-33-0
ISBN 978-1-891845-33-8

TREATISE on the SPLEEN & STOMACH: A Translation and annotation of Li Dong-yuan's *Pi Wei Lun*
by Bob Flaws
ISBN 0-936185-41-4
ISBN 978-0-936185-41-5

THE TREATMENT OF CARDIOVASCULAR DISEASES WITH CHINESE MEDICINE
by Simon Becker, Bob Flaws & Robert Casañas, MD
ISBN 1-891845-27-6
ISBN 978-1-891845-27-7

THE TREATMENT OF DIABETES MELLITUS WITH CHINESE MEDICINE
by Bob Flaws, Lynn Kuchinski & Robert Casañas, M.D.
ISBN 1-891845-21-7
ISBN 978-1-891845-21-5

THE TREATMENT OF DISEASE IN TCM, Vol. 1: Diseases of the Head & Face, Including Mental & Emotional Disorders   New Edition
by Philippe Sionneau & Lü Gang
ISBN 0-936185-69-4
ISBN 978-0-936185-69-9

THE TREATMENT OF DISEASE IN TCM, Vol. II: Diseases of the Eyes, Ears, Nose, & Throat
by Sionneau & Lü
ISBN 0-936185-73-2
ISBN 978-0-936185-73-6

THE TREATMENT OF DISEASE IN TCM, Vol. III: Diseases of the Mouth, Lips, Tongue, Teeth & Gums
by Sionneau & Lü
ISBN 0-936185-79-1
ISBN 978-0-936185-79-8

THE TREATMENT OF DISEASE IN TCM, Vol IV: Diseases of the Neck, Shoulders, Back, & Limbs
by Philippe Sionneau & Lü Gang
ISBN 0-936185-89-9
ISBN 978-0-936185-89-7

THE TREATMENT OF DISEASE IN TCM, Vol V: Diseases of the Chest & Abdomen
by Philippe Sionneau & Lü Gang
ISBN 1-891845-02-0
ISBN 978-1-891845-02-4

THE TREATMENT OF DISEASE IN TCM, Vol VI: Diseases of the Urogential System & Proctology
by Philippe Sionneau & Lü Gang
ISBN 1-891845-05-5
ISBN 978-1-891845-05-5

THE TREATMENT OF DISEASE IN TCM, Vol VII: General Symptoms
by Philippe Sionneau & Lü Gang
ISBN 1-891845-14-4
ISBN 978-1-891845-14-7

THE TREATMENT OF EXTERNAL DISEASES WITH ACUPUNCTURE & MOXIBUSTION
by Yan Cui-lan and Zhu Yun-long, trans. by Yang Shou-zhong
ISBN 0-936185-80-5
ISBN 978-0-936185-80-4

THE TREATMENT OF MODERN WESTERN MEDICAL DISEASES WITH CHINESE MEDICINE
by Bob Flaws & Philippe Sionneau
ISBN 1-891845-20-9
ISBN 978-1-891845-20-8

UNDERSTANDING THE DIFFICULT PATIENT: A Guide for Practitioners of Oriental Medicine
by Nancy Bilello, RN, L.ac.
ISBN 1-891845-32-2
ISBN 978-1-891845-32-1

WESTERN PHYSICAL EXAM SKILLS FOR PRACTITIONERS OF ASIAN MEDICINE
by Bruce H. Robinson & Honora Lee Wolfe
ISBN 1-891845-48-9
ISBN 978-1-891845-48-2

YI LIN GAI CUO (Correcting the Errors in the Forest of Medicine)
by Wang Qing-ren
ISBN 1-891845-39-X
ISBN 978-1-891845-39-0

70 ESSENTIAL CHINESE HERBAL FORMULAS
by Bob Flaws
ISBN 0-936185-59-7
ISBN 978-0-936185-59-0

160 ESSENTIAL CHINESE READY-MADE MEDICINES
by Bob Flaws
ISBN 1-891945-12-8
ISBN 978-1-891945-12-3

630 QUESTIONS & ANSWERS ABOUT CHINESE HERBAL MEDICINE: A Workbook & Study Guide
by Bob Flaws
ISBN 1-891845-04-7
ISBN 978-1-891845-04-8

260 ESSENTIAL CHINESE MEDICINALS
by Bob Flaws
ISBN 1-891845-03-9
ISBN 978-1-891845-03-1

750 QUESTIONS & ANSWERS ABOUT ACUPUNCTURE
Exam Preparation & Study Guide
by Fred Jennes
ISBN 1-891845-22-5
ISBN 978-1-891845-22-2